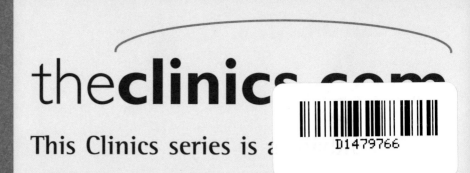

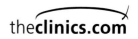

MAGNETIC RESONANCE IMAGING CLINICS

of North America

MR-Guided Interventions

Jonathan S. Lewin, MD
Guest Editor

August 2005 • Volume 13 • Number 3

SAUNDERS

An Imprint of Elsevier, Inc.
PHILADELPHIA   LONDON   TORONTO   MONTREAL   SYDNEY   TOKYO

W.B. SAUNDERS COMPANY
A Divison of Elsevier Inc.

Elsevier, Inc. • 1600 John F. Kennedy Boulevard • Suite 1800 • Philadelphia, Pennsylvania 19103-2899

http://www.theclinics.com

MRI CLINICS OF NORTH AMERICA	**Volume 13, Number 3**
August 2005	**ISSN 1064-9689**
Editor: Barton Dudlick	**ISBN 1-4160-2729-7**

Reprints: For copies of 100 or more, of articles in this publication, please contact the Commercial Re-prints Department, Elsevier Inc., 360 Park Avenue South, New York, New York 10010-1710. Tel. (212) 633-3813 Fax: (212) 462-1935 email: reprints@elsevier.com.

The ideas and opinions expressed in *Magnetic Resonance Imaging Clinics of North America* do not neces-sarily reflect those of the Publisher. The Publisher does not assume any responsibility for any injury and/or damage to persons or property arising out of or related to any use of the material contained in this periodical. The reader is advised to check the appropriate medical literature and the product in-formation currently provided by the manufacturer of each drug to be administered to verify the dosage, the method and duration of administration, or contraindications. It is the responsibility of the treating physician or other health care professional, relying on independent experience and knowledge of the patient, to determine drug dosages and the best treatment for the patient. Mention of any product in this issue should not be construed as endorsement by the contributors, editors, or the Publisher of the product or manufacturers' claims.

Magnetic Resonance Imaging Clinics of North America (ISSN 1064-9689) is published quarterly by the W.B. Saunders Company. Corporate and editorial offices: Elsevier, Inc., 1600 John F. Kennedy Boule-vard, Suite 1800, Philadelphia, PA 19103-2899. Accounting and circulation offices: 6277 Sea Harbor Drive, Orlando, FL 32887-4800. Periodicals postage paid at Orlando, FL 32862, and additional mailing offices. Subscription prices are $190.00 per year (US individuals), $290.00 per year (US institutions), $95.00 (US students and residents), $214.00 per year (Canadian individuals), $352.00 per year (Canadian institutions), $255.00 per year (foreign individuals), and $352.00 per year (foreign institutions). To re-ceive student and resident rate, orders must be accompanied by name of affiliated institution, date of term, and the *signature* of program/residency coordinator on institution letter-head. Orders will be billed at individual rate until proof of status is received. Foreign air speed delivery is included in all *Clinics* subscription prices. All prices are subject to change without notice. POSTMASTER: Send address changes to *Magnetic Resonance Imaging Clinics of North America*, W.B. Saunders Company, Periodicals Fulfillment, Orlando, FL 32887-4800. **Customer Service: 1-800-654-2452 (US). From outside of the US, call 1-407-345-4000. E-mail: hhspcs@harcourt.com.**

Magnetic Resonance Imaging Clinics of North America is covered in the *RSNA Index of Imaging Literature*, *Index Medicus*, *MEDLINE*, and *EMBASE/Excerpta Medica*.

Printed in the United States of America.

GUEST EDITOR

JONATHAN S. LEWIN, MD, Martin W. Donner Professor and Chairman, The Russell H. Morgan Department of Radiology and Radiological Science, The Johns Hopkins University School of Medicine; and Radiologist-in-Chief, Department of Radiology, The Johns Hopkins Hospital, Baltimore, Maryland

CONTRIBUTORS

ARAVIND AREPALLY, MD, Assistant Professor of Radiology and Surgery, The Russell H. Morgan Department of Radiology and Radiological Science, Division of Cardiovascular and Interventional Radiology, Johns Hopkins Medical Institutes, Baltimore, Maryland

ERGIN ATALAR, PhD, Professor, Departments of Radiology, BME, and ECE, The Johns Hopkins University, Baltimore, Maryland; and Electrical and Electronics Engineering Department, Bilkent University, Ankara, Turkey

DANIEL T. BOLL, MD, Department of Radiology, University Hospitals of Ulm, Ulm, Germany

JOHN A. CARRINO, MD, MPH, Department of Radiology, Brigham and Women's Hospital, Harvard Medical School, Boston, Massachusetts

BRUCE L. DANIEL, MD, Department of Radiology, Stanford University Medical Center, Stanford, California

JAMAL J. DERAKHSHAN, BS, Graduate Research Assistant and Graduate Student, Department of Biomedical Engineering; and School of Medicine, Case Western Reserve University, Cleveland, Ohio

JEFFREY L. DUERK, PhD, Professor of Radiology, Biomedical Engineering, and Oncology; and Director of Physics Research, Department of Radiology, Case Western Reserve University, University Hospitals of Cleveland, Cleveland, Ohio

KATRIN EICHLER, MD, Department of Diagnostic and Interventional Radiology, Universitätsklinikum Frankfurt/Main, Frankfurt, Germany

GUNTHER FISCHER, MD, Department of Pediatric Cardiology, University Hospital Schleswig-Holstein, Kiel, Germany

WALTER A. HALL, MD, Professor of Neurosurgery, Radiation Oncology, and Radiology, University of Minnesota School of Medicine, Minneapolis, Minnesota

CLAUDIA M. HILLENBRAND, PhD, Assistant Professor of Radiology, Department of Radiology, Case Western Reserve University, University Hospitals of Cleveland, Cleveland, Ohio

KULLERVO HYNYNEN, PhD, Professor of Radiology; and Director, Focused Ultrasound Laboratory, Department of Radiology, Brigham and Women's Hospital, Harvard Medical School, Boston, Massachusetts

MICHAEL JEROSCH-HEROLD, PhD, Advanced Imaging Research Center, Oregon Health and Science University, Portland, Oregon

FERENC A. JOLESZ, MD, B. Leonard Holman Professor of Radiology; Vice Chairman for Research; and Director, Division of MRI and Image-Guided Therapy Program, Department of Radiology, Brigham and Women's Hospital, Harvard Medical School, Boston, Massachusetts

DARA KRAITCHMAN, VMD, PhD, The Russell H. Morgan Department of Radiology and Radiological Science, The Johns Hopkins University, Baltimore, Maryland

HANS HEINER KRAMER, MD, Department of Pediatric Cardiology, University Hospital Schleswig-Holstein, Kiel, Germany

THOMAS LEHNERT, MD, Department of Diagnostic and Interventional Radiology, Universitätsklinikum Frankfurt/Main, Frankfurt, Germany

JONATHAN S. LEWIN, MD, Martin W. Donner Professor and Chairman, The Russell H. Morgan Department of Radiology and Radiological Science, The Johns Hopkins University School of Medicine; and Radiologist-in-Chief, Department of Radiology, The Johns Hopkins Hospital, Baltimore, Maryland

RAM LIEBENTHAL, MSc, Global Manager Interventional MR, General Electric Healthcare Technologies, Waukesha, Wisconsin

CHRISTINE H. LORENZ, PhD, Siemens Corporate Research, Imaging and Visualization, Princeton, New Jersey

MARTIN G. MACK, MD, PhD, Department of Diagnostic and Interventional Radiology, Universitätsklinikum Frankfurt/Main, Frankfurt, Germany

NATHAN McDANNOLD, PhD, Assistant Professor of Radiology, Focused Ultrasound Laboratory, Department of Radiology, Brigham and Women's Hospital, Harvard Medical School, Boston, Massachusetts

CYNTHIA MÉNARD, MD, Clinician Scientist and Assistant Professor, Princess Margaret Hospital, University Health Network, University of Toronto, Toronto, Ontario, Canada

ELMAR M. MERKLE, MD, Associate Professor of Radiology, Department of Radiology, Duke University Medical Center, Durham, North Carolina

SHERIF GAMAL NOUR, MD, Assistant Professor of Radiology and Biomedical Engineering, Departments of Radiology and Biomedical Engineering, Case Western Reserve University School of Medicine; Director, Interventional MRI Therapy Program, Department of Radiology, University Hospitals of Cleveland, Cleveland, Ohio; and Department of Diagnostic Radiology, Cairo University Hospitals, Cairo, Egypt

CARSTEN RICKERS, MD, Department of Pediatric Cardiology, University Hospital Schleswig-Holstein, Kiel, Germany

ROBERTO BLANCO SEQUEIROS, MD, PhD, Department of Radiology, Oulu University Hospital, Oulu, Finland; and Research Fellow, Department of Radiology, Brigham and Women's Hospital, Harvard Medical School, Boston, Massachusetts

CLARE TEMPANY, MD, Professor of Radiology; and Director of Clinical MRI, Division of MRI and Image-Guided Therapy Program, Department of Radiology, Brigham and Women's Hospital, Harvard Medical School, Boston, Massachusetts

CHARLES L. TRUWIT, MD, Professor of Radiology, Pediatrics, and Neurology, University of Minnesota School of Medicine, Minneapolis, Minnesota

MAURICE A.A.J. VAN DEN BOSCH, MD, PhD, Department of Radiology, University Medical Center Utrecht, Utrecht, The Netherlands

THOMAS J. VOGL, MD, PhD, Department of Diagnostic and Interventional Radiology, Universitätsklinikum Frankfurt/Main, Frankfurt, Germany

FRANK K. WACKER, MD, Professor of Radiology and Vice-Chairman, Department of Radiology, Klinik und Hochschulambulanz für Radiologie und Nuklearmedizin, Charité–Universitätsmedizin Berlin, Campus Benjamin Franklin, Berlin, Germany; and Adjunct Associate Professor of Radiology, Department of Radiology, Case Western Reserve University, University Hospitals of Cleveland, Cleveland, Ohio

CLIFFORD R. WEISS, MD, The Russell H. Morgan Department of Radiology and Radiological Science, Division of Cardiovascular and Interventional Radiology, Johns Hopkins Medical Institutes, Baltimore, Maryland

NORBERT WILKE, MD, Health Science Center, University of Florida, Jacksonville, Florida

CONTENTS

> Soon after the introduction of MR imaging as an imaging tool, researchers began to investigate its capabilities to guide interventional minimally invasive procedures, such as biopsies. These early efforts have encouraged vendors and numerous research groups worldwide to identify clinical problems in the field of image-guided intervention, for which MR imaging is beneficial as an imaging modality, and to develop and refine software and hardware components to meet the specific requirements of interventional MR imaging. Over nearly 20 years, continuous advances in magnet and system design have accelerated the progress of MR-guided intervention.

> This article reviews the latest developments in the field of interventional MR imaging, with special emphasis on the pulse sequences behind the advancements. Passive, semi-active, and active methods of device tracking along with ways to ensure the radiofrequency safety of interventional wires and a way to steer nonbraided catheters during interventional MR imaging are reviewed. This article addresses the use of catheter position and speed information to update pulse sequence parameters in real time for interactive and adaptive imaging. This article also reviews the extension of active tracking to high-resolution vessel wall imaging and the acquisition of images with a moving table and the application of active tracking to interventional MR imaging. Finally, the progress made on guiding and monitoring thermal therapy using the proton resonant frequency shift is examined.

> MR imaging has many potential advantages that make it an attractive tool to guide diagnostic and therapeutic procedures. To date, the use of endovascular MR

imaging–guidance techniques has been confined primarily to animal experiments, with only a few reports on MR-guided endovascular applications in patients. The most commonly used tracking methods are susceptibility artifact–based and microcoil- or antenna-based. Access to the patient within the scanner, dedicated devices, and safety issues remain major challenges. To face these challenges, attention from radiologists is required to make MR imaging-guided endovascular procedures a clinical reality.

The advent of interventional MR imaging techniques and the adoption of these techniques to guide percutaneous biopsies and aspirations have served as further steps along a series of technical refinements that commenced with the implementation of image-guided approaches for tissue sampling. Currently, the practice of and the expectations from these procedures are quite different from those of the blind percutaneous thrusts performed in the late nineteenth and early twentieth centuries. As the field of interventional MR imaging continues to flourish and to attract more radiologists who realize the many opportunities that this technology can offer to their patients, there is a need for a full comprehension of the concepts, techniques, limitations, and cost-effectiveness of MR imaging guidance to present this service to clinical partners in the appropriate setting. Radiologists also should recognize the need for their significant involvement in the technical aspects of MR-guided procedures, because several user-defined parameters and trajectory decisions can alter device visualization in the MR imaging environment and hence affect procedure safety.

In the last decade, cardiovascular MR imaging has made rapid progress. Developments in scanner technology and pulse sequence design have resulted in exquisite capabilities for imaging cardiac anatomy, function, and perfusion, including new capabilities for real-time imaging. MR imaging now is recognized as an excellent tool for the assessment of congenital cardiac malformations and for the accurate quantification of blood flow. This article provides an overview of the technical aspects of cardiovascular interventional MR imaging. The authors present important new applications, such as the repair of congenital defects and the injection of stem cells under MR imaging guidance, and review several pioneering studies that have proved the feasibility of these applications.

To improve the accuracy of biliary diagnosis and staging, the authors implemented intrabiliary MR imaging (IBMR), a new technique in the assessment of patients who have biliary obstruction. IBMR can create high-resolution cross-sectional images of the bile duct wall and adjacent tissues, which is vital in the assessment of these patients. Although this technique holds promise to provide an alternative means to image the biliary tree, it is still in infancy with methodology and applications. This article focuses on the rationale for IBMR, the current techniques for performing IBMR, and the results from a pilot clinical trial in patients who have biliary obstruction.

Prostate cancer is the most common noncutaneous cancer in men in the United States, with an estimated annual incidence of 230,000 cases in 2004. Despite an impressive scope of research efforts, difficult challenges persist in various aspects of prostate cancer care, including diagnosis, prognostication, and treatment. This article reviews recent developments in MR-guided needle interventions for prostate cancer, focusing primarily on interventional procedures conducted in the MR imaging scanner room. Researchers have shown that a number of minimally invasive procedures including biopsy, brachytherapy, and radiofrequency ablation can be conducted precisely under the imaging capabilities of MR imaging. The high soft tissue contrast provided by MR imaging has great potential to improve the effectiveness of these procedures.

Diagnostic MR imaging of the breast is used increasingly in clinical practice. Because of its high sensitivity, MR imaging of the breast can detect lesions that are clinically and mammographically occult. Techniques for MR-guided biopsy and ablation of breast cancer are reviewed. MR-guided preoperative needle localization and large-gauge core needle biopsy are discussed. Strategies for MR imaging guidance are compared, including stereotaxic and freehand methods. Methods for minimally invasive breast tumor ablation, including radiofrequency ablation, laser interstitial thermal ablation, cryosurgery, and focused ultrasound ablation are presented.

This article describes the procedural characteristics and techniques when performing musculoskeletal procedures under MR imaging guidance using a variety of platforms. MR-guided interventional procedures involving bone, soft tissue, intervertebral disks, and joints are safe and sufficiently effective for use in clinical practice. The main indications are biopsies, spinal interventions, and tumor ablation. MR-guided biopsy is advantageous if the lesion is not visible by other modalities, for regions adjacent to implants, or when subselective targeting is desired. MR-guided interventions also are used for periarticular cyst aspiration, needle localization, and intraoperative guidance. MR-guided musculoskeletal procedures should continue to be a growth area, particularly for the diagnosis and treatment of bone and soft tissue neoplasia and especially for providing the ability to monitor and control tumor ablation therapy. As image-guided therapy programs continue to proliferate, musculoskeletal applications are likely to become an essential aspect of interventional MR imaging deployments.

With the rapid evolution of technologic advances in neurosurgery, it is no surprise that the use of MR imaging to guide the performance of safe and effective surgical procedures is at the forefront of development. This article highlights the current capabilities of intraoperative MR-guided surgery for a variety of neurosurgical procedures and traces the evolution of the field to its present level of technical sophistication. The costs of intraoperative MR imaging and its future directions are discussed.

By integrating MR imaging and focused ultrasound, a real-time, image-controlled, non-invasive thermal ablation system has been developed and tested in multiple clinical applications in the breast and pelvis. MR imaging provides accurate localization and targeting of tumors. Temperature-sensitive imaging helps to identify the focal energy deposition and avoid thermal injury of normal tissues. Other advantages of MR imaging are the closed-loop feedback control of tissue heating and the direct measurement of the deposited thermal dose. Future applications include treatment of vascular malformations, targeted drug delivery, and gene therapy.

Radiofrequency Thermal Ablation: The Role of MR Imaging in Guiding and Monitoring Tumor Therapy

Sherif G. Nour and Jonathan S. Lewin

Performing radiofrequency ablation procedures under MR imaging involves two distinct processes: interactive guidance of the radiofrequency electrode into the targeted tumor and monitoring the effect of therapy. The justification for using MR imaging for electrode guidance is quite similar to its use to guide biopsy and aspiration procedures, where MR imaging offers advantages related to superior soft tissue contrast, multiplanar capabilities, and high vascular conspicuity that facilitate safe and accurate guidance in selected lesions. The major contribution of MR imaging to thermal ablation procedures is its ability to monitor tissue changes associated with the heating process instantaneously, an attribute that is not paralleled by any other currently available imaging modality. Such an ability facilitates a controlled approach to ablation by helping to detect inadequately treated tumor foci for subsequent interactive repositioning of the radiofrequency electrode during therapy. MR imaging guidance and monitoring enable treatment of the entire tumor on a single-visit basis while avoiding undue overtreatment and preserving often critically needed organ function.

MR-Guided Laser Ablation

Martin G. Mack, Thomas Lehnert, Katrin Eichler, and Thomas J. Vogl

Percutaneous MR-guided laser-induced interstitial thermotherapy (LITT) has received increasing attention as a promising technique for the treatment of a variety of primary and secondary malignant liver tumors. MR-guided LITT is a safe and effective treatment modality that improves survival in well-selected patients who have liver metastases. A major advantage of MR-guided LITT is that it can be easily performed under local anesthesia in an outpatient setting with a low complication rate. This article presents the results of local lesion control with MR-guided minimally invasive LITT and associated survival data.

MR-Guided Percutaneous Sclerotherapy of Low-Flow Vascular Malformations in the Head and Neck

Daniel T. Boll, Elmar M. Merkle, and Jonathan S. Lewin

MR-guided sclerotherapy is an excellent approach for the treatment of the predominant symptoms of congenital low-flow vascular malformations in the head and neck. This mode of treatment appears to be safe and efficient and allows the quantitative verification of therapeutic success during follow-up examinations. This article reviews the underlying pathophysiology of low-flow malformations and summarizes the MR imaging guidance and monitoring technique. Outcome data from the authors' experience at Case Western Reserve University/University Hospitals of Cleveland are summarized.

FORTHCOMING ISSUES

RECENT ISSUES

THE CLINICS ARE NOW AVAILABLE ONLINE!

Access your subscription at:
www.theclinics.com

GOAL STATEMENT

The goal of *Magnetic Resonance Imaging Clinics of North America* is to keep practicing radiologists and radiology residents up to date with current clinical practice in radiology by providing timely articles reviewing the state of the art in patient care.

ACCREDITATION

The *Magnetic Resonance Imaging Clinics of North America* is planned and implemented in accordance with the Essential Areas and Policies of the Accreditation Council for Continuing Medical Education (ACCME) through the joint sponsorship of the University of Virginia School of Medicine and Elsevier. The University of Virginia School of Medicine is accredited by the ACCME to provide continuing medical education for physicians.

The University of Virginia School of Medicine designates this educational activity for a maximum of 60 category 1 credits per year, 15 category 1 credits per issue, toward the AMA Physician's Recognition Award. Each physician should claim only those credits that he/she actually spent in the activity.

The American Medical Association has determined that physicians not licensed in the US who participate in this CME activity are eligible for AMA PRA category 1 credit.

Category 1 credit can be earned by reading the text material, taking the CME examination online at http://www.theclinics.com/home/cme, and completing the evaluation. After taking the test, you will be required to review any and all incorrect answers. Following completion of the test and evaluation, your credit will be awarded and you may print your certificate.

FACULTY DISCLOSURE

As a provider accredited by the Accreditation Council for Continuing Medical Education (ACCME), the Office of Continuing Medical Education of the University of Virginia School of Medicine must ensure balance, independence, objectivity, and scientific rigor in all its individually sponsored or jointly sponsored educational activities. All authors/editors participating in a sponsored activity are expected to disclose to the readers any significant financial interest or other relationship (1) with the manufacturer(s) of any commercial product(s) and/or provider(s) of commercial services discussed in an educational presentation and (2) with any commercial supporters of the activity (significant financial interest or other relationship can include such things as grants or research support, employee, consultant, stock holder, member of speakers bureau, etc). The intent of this disclosure is not to prevent authors/editors with a significant financial or other relationship from writing an article, but rather to provide readers with information on which they can make their own judgments. It remains for the readers to determine whether the author's/editor's interest or relationships may influence the article with regard to exposition or conclusion.

The authors/editors listed below have identified no professional or financial affiliations related to their presentation:
Aravind Arepally, MD; Ergin Atalar, PhD; Daniel T. Boll, MD; John A. Carrino, MD, MPH; Bruce L. Daniel, MD; Jamal J. Derakhshan, BS; Barton Dudlick, Acquisitions Editor; Katrin Eichler, MD; Gunther Fischer, MD; Claudia M. Hillenbrand, PhD; Kullervo Hynynen, PhD; Michael Jerosch-Herold, PhD; Dara Kraitchman, VMD, PhD; Hans Heiner Kramer, MD; Thomas Lehnert, MD; Martin G. Mack, MD, PhD; Nathan McDannold, PhD; Cynthia Ménard, MD; Elmar M. Merkle, MD; Sherif Gamal Nour, MD; Carsten Rickers, MD; Roberto Blanco Sequeiros, MD, PhD; Maurice A.A.J. van den Bosch, MD, PhD; Thomas J. Vogl, MD, PhD; Frank K. Wacker, MD; and Clifford R. Weiss, MD.

The authors listed below have identified the following professional or financial affiliation related to their presentation:
Jeffrey L. Duerk, PhD, is supported in part by a sponsored research agreement with Siemens Medical Solutions-MRI.
Walter A. Hall, MD, has a financial interest in Image-Guided Neurologics, Inc.
Ferenc A. Jolesz, MD, has research supported from Insightec, Inc.
Jonathan S. Lewin, MD, has research collaborations with Philips Medical, Siemens Medical Solutions, General Electric Healthcare, and Toshiba Medical Systems.
Ram Liebenthal, MSc, is Global Business Manager – Open and Interventional MR Programs, GE Healthcare Technologies.
Christine H. Lorenz, PhD, is a Siemens employee.
Clare Tempany, MD, is a consultant and received research support from Insightec, Inc.
Charles L. Truwit, MD, has a financial interest in Image-Guided Neurologics, Inc.
Norbert Wilke, MD, has received grant support for Siemens Medical Solutions and is a consultant to Barlex Laboratories.

Disclosure of discussion of non-FDA approved uses for pharmaceutical products and/or medical devices: The University of Virginia School of Medicine, as an ACCME provider, requires that all authors identify and disclose any "off label" uses for pharmaceutical and medical device products. The University of Virginia School of Medicine recommends that each physician fully review all the available data on new products or procedures prior to instituting them with patients.

All authors who provided disclosures will not be discussing off-label uses EXCEPT the following:
Aravind Arepally, MD, and **Clifford R. Weiss, MD,** will discuss the use of the Surgi-Vision intravascular wire in the biliary system; this has received FDA approval for intravascular use only.
Dara Kraitchman, VMD, PhD, will discuss the off label use of MR contrast agents, Feridex and Magnevist.

TO ENROLL

To enroll in the *Magnetic Resonance Imaging Clinics of North America* Continuing Medical Education program, call customer service at 1-800-654-2452 or visit us online at http://www.theclinics.com/home/cme. The CME program is available to subscribers for an additional fee of $165.00.

ELSEVIER
SAUNDERS

Magn Reson Imaging Clin N Am
13 (2005) xi–xii

MAGNETIC
RESONANCE
IMAGING CLINICS
of North America

Preface

MR-Guided Interventions

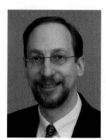

Jonathan S. Lewin, MD
Guest Editor

This issue of the *Magnetic Resonance Imaging Clinics of North America* is dedicated to the field of interventional MR. With the first insertion of a needle under MR image guidance in the 1980s, the future of MR imaging was irreversibly changed, creating a new frontier in diagnostic and therapeutic intervention. Minimally invasive therapy and image-guided biopsy, aspiration, and drainage had entered a new realm, taking advantage of the unequaled soft tissue contrast, multiplanar capabilities, and other attributes of MR that had previously been confined to noninvasive diagnostic examinations. In this issue, we have assembled a fine ensemble of physicians and scientists with experience in the theory, engineering, and wide range of clinical capabilities of interventional MR. With the accelerating interest in minimally invasive therapy under MR guidance over the last decade, it has become impossible to cover every clinical application in a single issue. However, this current compilation covers the basics of interventional MR hardware, software, interventional devices, and many clinical applications throughout the body.

Much of the debate during the 1990s centered on different concepts of interventional MR magnet and suite designs. In the last several years, it has been recognized that there are many different magnet designs that are suitable for MR image–guided intervention. In the first article in this issue, Dr. Elmar Merkle and colleagues cover these basic concepts in suite design and describe the most frequently applied equipment configurations. In their overview on pulse sequences for interventional MR imaging, Jamal Derakshan and Dr. Jeffrey Duerk highlight recent advances in pulse sequence design, taking advantage of the newest capabilities of MR imaging systems for interventional applications. Next appears a series of articles that describe the most common or most promising interventional applications throughout the body, written by experts in the development and performance of clinical applications. Lastly, Drs. Walter Hall and Chip Truwit provide a summary of intraoperative MR applications in neurosurgery. As with any developing technology, some of these applications are more mature than others: a few are primarily restricted to animal models, while most are applied routinely in clinical settings.

As you read this issue, it is my hope that you see the many ways in which the unique imaging capabilities of MR can be exploited for unsurpassed guidance and monitoring of interventional procedures. In addition to those benefits of MRI for device placement, several of the articles describe therapeutic applications in which the unique ability of MRI to accurately image tissue changes during thermal or chemical therapies can be used to great advantage. In particular, the ability to image thermal changes is a fundamental aspect of the use of MR for high intensity focused ultrasound therapy, as described in the article by Ferenc Jolesz, MD, one of the true pioneers of MR image–guided therapy, and colleagues. This capability is also evident in the articles on MR-guided radiofrequency ablation by Dr. Sherif Nour and coauthors, on MR-guided laser ablation by Dr. Martin Mack and colleagues, and on sclerotherapy by Dr. Daniel Boll and coauthors. It is the combination of accurate guidance capabilities and sensitive tissue monitoring that combine to make interventional MR a tremendously potent interventional modality.

By the end of the issue, it is my hope that readers will have gained a deepened understanding of the underlying concepts in interventional MRI, and will also have an appreciation of the wide range of applications in current clinical practice, as well as some of those that are just over the horizon. Yogi Berra once said, "The future ain't what it used to be." In fact, with respect to interventional MR, it is brighter than ever.

Jonathan S. Lewin, MD
*The Russell H. Morgan Department of Radiology
and Radiological Science
The Johns Hopkins University
600 North Wolfe Street
Baltimore, MD 21287, USA*

E-mail address: jlewin2@jhmi.edu

ELSEVIER
SAUNDERS

Magn Reson Imaging Clin N Am
13 (2005) 401–413

MAGNETIC
RESONANCE
IMAGING CLINICS
of North America

The Interventional MR Imaging Suite: Magnet Designs and Equipment Requirements

Elmar M. Merkle, MD[a],*, Jonathan S. Lewin, MD[b],
Ram Liebenthal, MSc[c], Christine H. Lorenz, PhD[d]

[a]Department of Radiology, Duke University Medical Center, Erwin Road,
Duke North–Room 1417, Durham, NC 27710, USA
[b]The Russell H. Morgan Department of Radiology and Radiological Science, The Johns Hopkins University,
601 North Caroline Street, Room 4210, Baltimore, MD 21287–0842, USA
[c]General Electric Healthcare Technologies, 3200 Grandview Boulevard, Waukesha, WI 53188, USA
[d]Siemens Corporate Research, Imaging and Visualization, 755 College Road East, Princeton, NJ 08540, USA

Soon after the introduction of MR imaging as an imaging tool, researchers also began to investigate its capabilities to guide interventional minimally invasive procedures, such as biopsies [1–7]. These early efforts have encouraged vendors as well as numerous research groups all over the world to identify clinical problems in the field of image-guided intervention for which MR imaging is beneficial as an imaging modality and to develop and refine software and hardware components to meet the specific requirements of interventional MR (IMR) imaging. Over nearly 20 years, continuous advances in magnet and system design have accelerated the progress of MR-guided intervention.

Image quality versus "openness"

Many different MR imaging system configurations have been used to guide percutaneous and surgical procedures. Each of these systems has advantages and disadvantages for interventional and intraoperative imaging, with a constant trade-off between signal-to-noise ratio, patient access, usable field of view, and expense. Understanding the role of different MR imaging system designs in intervention requires a distinction between image guidance and procedural monitoring.

There are many procedures in which the information provided by MR imaging can be used to monitor therapeutic intervention. Examples include thermal ablation, in which thermal energy is deposited and the resulting tissue changes are continuously or intermittently observed, and surgical intervention, in which the status of tumor resection or cyst aspiration may be intermittently examined. These forms of interventional MR imaging require much less modification to standard imaging systems, because patient access is not necessarily required during the monitoring process. Both types of procedures have already been performed on conventional cylindrical superconducting systems [8–11].

The use of MR imaging for interventional guidance includes its use by radiologists during the manipulation of needles, electrodes, catheters, or thermal devices as well as its application by surgeons for guiding endoscopes, scalpels, or curettes. This form of more active intervention requires a significant departure from conventional diagnostic concepts and traditional imaging systems. The most basic form of this type of guidance can be provided from a retrospective data set through the use of frameless or frame-based stereotactic systems, but there has been increasing emphasis on the use of real-time or near–real-time guidance for interventional MR imaging procedures. The factors contributing to high image quality in diagnostic MR imaging include system field strength and the homogeneity and stability of

---

* Corresponding author.
E-mail address: elmar.merkle@duke.edu
(E.M. Merkle).

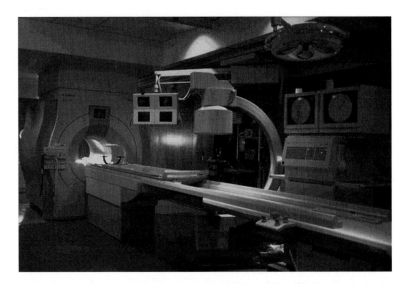

Fig. 1. Superconducting short-bore system. The solution proposed by Phillips Medical Systems, cited in this example at the University of Minnesota, includes a standard short-bore superconducting 1.5-T MR imager adjacent to a surgical workspace that includes C-arm fluoroscopy. A custom table can slide from the surgical workspace into the magnet for intermittent imaging at appropriate times during the surgical intervention. The C-arm fluoroscopic unit can also assist with angiographic procedures. The most recent generation includes a 3-T imaging system, installed at Hennepin County Medical Center. (Courtesy of C.L. Truwit, MD, University of Minnesota, Minneapolis, Minnesota.)

the static and gradient magnetic fields. These factors are most easily obtained by decreasing the "openness" of an imaging system. The optimal design of a magnet with regard to field homogeneity would be a complete sphere without any opening [12]. In contrast, the environment best suited to radiologic or surgical intervention is one with maximum patient access, thus allowing complete freedom for the interventional approach and maintaining close proximity to the monitoring and therapeutic devices. These attributes are in direct opposition to those facilitating image quality [12]. The use of MR imaging for guidance of interventional procedures has required compromise between these opposing forces; this balance has been achieved through a number of different concepts and solutions. Some of the first interventional procedures under MR imaging guidance were performed on conventional cylindrical systems, thereby simplifying the imaging but significantly compromising the patient access that is necessary for performance of the procedure and for monitoring patient discomfort and safety. Biopsy and aspiration procedures have been and can be performed using these cylindrical superconducting systems, but the patient must be withdrawn from the magnet between scans to reposition the needle [11]. In the late 1980s, this requirement resulted in

relatively long procedure times and contributed to the lack of the widespread use of MR imaging for biopsy and aspiration. In particular, when the lesion in question was visible and accessible for biopsy under CT or sonography, these more conventional methods for procedural guidance were clearly preferable techniques. These disadvantages were overcome in part by the patient access provided by permanent or resistive "open"-magnet imaging systems [2–5]. Unfortunately, the open low-field imaging systems available in the late 1980s often required significant imaging time to obtain a sufficient signal-to-noise ratio to allow needle insertion under MR imaging guidance. Nonetheless, the patient access provided by these systems led to an increased number of reports of its use, primarily for biopsies in the head and neck region [6,7,13]. Since then, many magnet, gradient, and receiver chain design improvements have led to a number of approaches for interventional imaging. The following is a brief description of the most commonly used current designs for intervention. Each system has benefits and limitations for interventional procedure guidance, because each has chosen a different balance between the spatial constraints necessary for high-quality imaging and the freedom necessary for surgical or radiologic intervention.

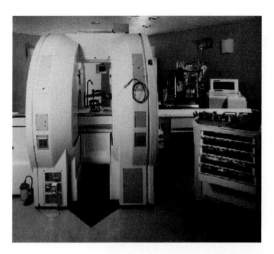

Fig. 2. The double-donut design is shown. The General Electric Health Care Signa SP scanner consists of two short superconducting cylindrical magnets separated by a 54-cm space to allow physician or nurse access. The space between the two magnet halves allows patient access from the top or sides, typically used with the surgeon and assistant on opposite sides of the patient's head. An optically linked frameless stereotactic tracking system is integrated into the top support piece. The scanner is designed for an operating room environment with electrical outlets and anesthesia gases integrated into the magnet covers. This system has a large fringe field, and all surgical instruments and accessory equipment in proximity to the system must be safe and compatible for MR imaging. (Courtesy of General Electric Health Care, Milwaukee, Wisconsin; with permission.)

1990s: when interventional MR imaging came into vogue

During the past 15 years, IMR imaging has become popular and multiple high-profile research groups have focused a substantial part of their resources and efforts on establishing IMR imaging programs. During that time, three different magnet concepts have been used primarily:

1. Cylindrical superconducting high-field MR imaging systems (1.0–1.5 T) that can be combined with an in-room fluoroscopy radiographic unit
2. The midfield "double-donut" configuration (0.5 T)
3. Biplanar low-field MR imaging systems (0.064–0.3 T)

These systems are described in more detail in the following sections.

Cylindrical superconducting systems

From an image quality point of view, cylindrical superconducting systems enjoy many significant advantages relative to static magnetic field strength and homogeneity, and the adoption of this system design as the standard for image quality in the diagnostic arena is not a chance occurrence. The limited patient access for procedural performance and direct visual observation of the patient is a compromise that still allows the successful performance of certain procedures. The excellent signal-to-noise ratio achieved with these systems is well suited to thermal monitoring during ablation and has been used during laser and radiofrequency (RF) ablation procedures in the brain, liver, and head and neck [1,9,14–17]. The investigators in these studies limited the use of MR imaging to the thermal monitoring of the tumor destruction process; they typically inserted the laser fiber or RF electrode under CT guidance or used a neurosurgical stereotactic approach based on retrospective MR imaging data. Nonetheless, the insertion of a thermal device, such as an RF electrode, is feasible using a cylindrical superconducting MR imaging system if the tumor location is unfavorable for CT-guided or ultrasound-guided puncture (eg, subphrenic metastases or if a double-oblique puncture tract is required) [18]. The RF electrode must be bent manually before the puncture, however, because there is only limited space in the gantry of a closed-bore MR imaging scanner [18].

Another approach to the use of cylindrical superconducting systems for interventional monitoring has been the siting of a superconducting system in a surgical environment. With the rapid falloff of the static magnetic field achieved by actively shielded magnet designs, it is possible to site a superconducting system in near proximity to a surgical workspace. This design was first adopted for a system constructed by Philips Medical Systems (Eindhoven, The Netherlands) (Fig. 1), in which a procedure suite with most of the amenities of a conventional surgical theater was constructed just outside the fringe field of a superconducting, short-bore, 1.5-T imaging system. Surgery can be performed in the surgical portion of the suite much as in a conventional operating room. When desired, however, intermittent images can be obtained by sliding the patient into the cylindrical imaging system. The imaging system offers all the standard capabilities of a high-field system, including functional imaging

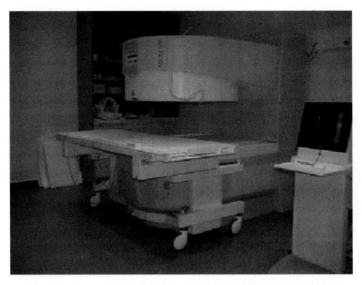

Fig. 3. Siemens Magnetom Concerto system. In this design, a single column on one side of the patient supports the upper magnet pole, thereby allowing access from the contralateral side as well as from the head and foot ends of the magnet. (Courtesy of Siemens Medical Solutions, Erlangen, Germany; with permission.)

with high image quality. Although there are few compromises to the surgical or imaging portion of this environment, this configuration does not allow interactive guidance of the intervention, because access to the patient is markedly limited. Direct patient observation by the anesthesiologist is also not possible during scanning, and antisepsis is a challenge because the inside of the cylindrical magnet cannot be draped easily. This intraoperative concept has been adopted by General Electric Health Care (Milwaukee, Wisconsin) and Siemens Medical Solutions (Erlangen, Germany), and large neurosurgical series with up to 200 patients have recently been reported [19]. Currently, these 1.5-T intraoperative MR imaging systems are capable of intraoperative diffusion tensor imaging that can depict shifting of major white matter tracts caused by the surgical intervention itself [20].

Another recent area of research interest has been the development of MR imaging methods for the guidance of angiographic procedures. Although access to the patient's anatomy in the magnet isocenter of a cylindrical magnet is limited, short-bore superconducting cylindrical systems do allow a degree of access to the patient's groin. Several groups are investigating the use of this type of system for catheter-based intervention with the radiologist or interventional cardiologist controlling the procedure from the groin near the magnet aperture [21–26]. The Philips system shown in

Fig. 1 includes a "C-arm" fluoroscope to facilitate this type of procedure. To date, MR imaging methods for catheter guidance remain rather elementary; however, Razavi et al [27] from King's College in London have recently shown in a series of 16 patients that cardiac catheterization guided by MR imaging is safe and practical. According to their study, MR-guided cardiac catheterization allows better soft tissue visualization, provides more pertinent physiologic information, and results in lower radiation exposure than do fluoroscopically guided procedures. MR imaging guidance could therefore become the method of choice for diagnostic cardiac catheterization in patients with congenital heart disease as well as an important tool for interventional cardiac catheterization and RF ablation. Another recent article by Paetzel et al [28] reports the successful MR-guided balloon dilatation of femoral and popliteal artery stenoses supported by real-time imaging and intra-arterial MR angiography in 3 patients.

Finally, the use of cylindrical magnets has also been applied for guidance of stereotactic biopsy for breast lesions and for monitoring thermal ablation procedures for these lesions [29–32].

Double-donut configuration

A novel approach to obtaining access to a patient in a cylindrical system is exemplified in

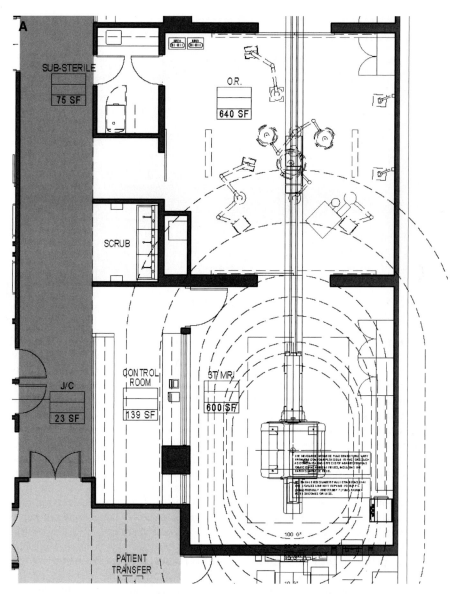

Fig. 4. MR-guided surgical suite concept from General Electric Health Care, which is planned to include the latest version of the Signa 1.5- or 3.0-T Excite High Definition magnet; it is planned to be integrated into the operating room area in a two-room layout connected through RF-shielded sliding doors, where the magnet and surgical bed are to be installed in a line. (A) The floor plan of a two-room layout illustrates the setup of the operating room and the MR imaging room, which are connected through RF-shielded doors. (B) Graphic illustration of the intraoperative MR imaging suite concept. Please note the RF-shielded doors at each side of the illustration. (Courtesy of General Electric Health Care, Milwaukee, Wisconsin; with permission.)

the double-donut configuration of the Signa SP system (General Electric Health Care) designed specifically for interventional applications (Fig. 2) [33–35]. This design has taken the central segment out of a cylindrical system, thereby allowing patient access from the sides and top at the isocenter of the imaging system. This product design has been directed toward use in a surgical environment and allows enough room in the gaps between the halves (54 cm) for two small- to medium-sized physicians or nurses, one on either side of the patient [12]. This system provides

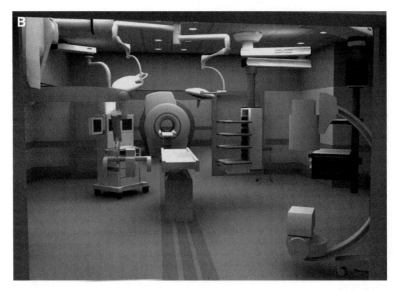

Fig. 4 (*continued*)

a marked improvement in patient access compared with a closed-bore cylindrical system. This concept represented the first system designed and constructed specifically for interventional guidance, and it is the only system that currently allows complete vertical and side patient access at the imaging isocenter. This magnet design has been used to guide and to monitor a large number of surgical procedures in addition to being the design used in several published series of biopsies and aspirations [34,36–39]. Nonetheless, the marked improvement in patient access is achieved at the expense of decreased field strength at the imaging isocenter (0.5 T) compared with the field strength generated by each superconducting half and therefore compromises magnetic field homogeneity [12]. The unobstructed side and vertical access to the patient also complicates engineering of the RF coil, thus requiring a local transmit-receive coil with a somewhat limited field of view.

At Stanford University, a digital flat-panel radiographic system with a spatial resolution of 1024^2 and a temporal resolution of 30 frames per second was integrated into the double-donut setup. This hybrid system is capable of MR imaging and radiographic imaging of the same field of view without patient movement [40,41].

Biplanar magnet designs

Another approach that has found widespread application for diagnostic MR imaging in the burgeoning open MR imaging market has been the use of a biplanar magnet design. With these magnets, the patient is positioned between flat magnetic poles, thereby permitting patient access from a range of side approaches. These systems typically use lower field permanent or resistive magnets with field strengths ranging from 0.064 to 0.3 T, although superconducting midfield models of this design have also been introduced. The degree of access around the circumference of the biplanar magnet depends on the number and position of the supports separating the two magnetic poles. A large degree of access around the circumference is afforded by the C-arm designs produced by Siemens Medical Solutions and Philips Medical Systems. In this design, a single column on one side of the patient supports the upper pole, thus allowing access from the contralateral side of the supporting post as well as at the head and foot ends of the magnet (Fig. 3). Several manufacturers produce biplanar systems with two supporting posts, thus resulting in slightly more restricted patient access. These include systems produced by Fonar Corporation (Melville, New York), Hitachi Medical Corporation of America (Twinsburg, Ohio), and General Electric Health Care. There are also designs with four support posts from Toshiba America Medical Systems (San Francisco, California) and Fonar Corporation. The biplanar concept has the advantage of a fairly homogeneous static magnetic field, but it is limited to

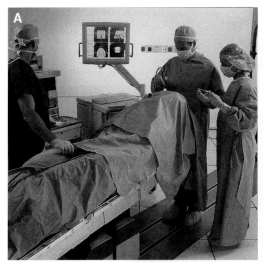
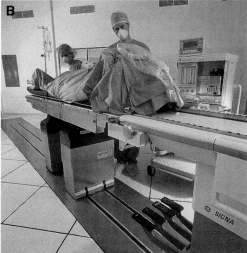
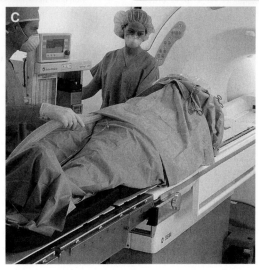

Fig. 5. Potential work flow in a single operating room layout illustrating the various patient locations during surgery, transportation, and imaging using a newly designed surgical bed with implemented vascular interventional workplace for advanced surgery (VIWAS) technology. (*A*) In the operating room, the new table is supposed to allow all patient positions offered by a standard surgical bed. (*B*) This image illustrates the transfer from the operating room to the magnet room. (*C*) This image illustrates the patient transfer onto the imaging table. (Courtesy of General Electric Health Care, Milwaukee, Wisconsin; with permission.)

lower field strength than cylindrical superconducting designs. The side access provided by these systems is analogous to that of C-arm fluoroscopy and is amenable to needle- or catheter-directed procedures [42–45]. Anterior or posterior interventional approaches require decubitus or oblique patient positioning, however, which may not be possible with large patients because of the relatively limited space between the poles of the biplane magnet. A true direct vertical approach to the patient is only possible for small body parts, such as the extremities, or when the patient table is brought outside the magnet.

New magnet designs

The experience gained during the past decade has led to new and more sophisticated magnet concepts. Overall, a trend toward high-field imaging is obvious. IMR imaging systems, which are primarily used to guide intraoperative procedures, are now combined on a more frequent basis

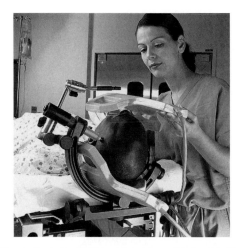

Fig. 6. Optimized MR imaging–compatible head holder and dedicated six-element phased-array RF coil. (Courtesy of General Electric Health Care, Milwaukee, Wisconsin; with permission.)

with high-end radiographic angiography units. Conversely, IMR imaging systems, which are primarily used for biopsies, thermal ablation procedures, and placement of drainage catheters, now allow more patient access while maintaining high-field image quality. Economic issues have also been taken into account during the development of these new IMR imaging systems. Over the last 15 years, it has become obvious that even major academic institutions only rarely have the workload to occupy a dedicated interventional MR imaging system with interventional and/or intraoperative cases alone. Thus, IMR imaging systems must also be capable of performing diagnostic MR imaging scans with excellent image quality during "dead time" to justify their purchase. In this section, various new IMR imaging systems are discussed.

High-end intraoperative MR imaging

Based on feedback from prestigious research sites, such as the group established by Dr. F. Jolesz at the Brigham and Women's Hospital in Boston and other institutions that have been using the General Electric 0.5-T Signa SP (double donut) during the past 10 years, General Electric Health Care has identified several design parameters that seem to be critical to the success and acceptance of high-end intraoperative MR imaging so as to meet today's application's needs and expectations. These expectations are outlined as follows:

It is important to maintain standard surgical procedures inside the operating room. The

key parameter is to maintain the best possible patient positioning with an uncompromised surgical bed. In addition, this would include the use of standard ferrous surgical tools as well as standard ancillary equipment.

It is critical to use higher field magnets to benefit from advanced imaging techniques, such as diffusion tensor echo planar imaging, spectroscopy, and functional MR imaging studies.

Patient positioning and patient safety are critical to the success and quality of the procedure.

An investment return is important for the hospital to justify the relatively substantial investment; therefore, the design should have a multimodality and multiapplication nature. For example, the design should be MR imaging and radiographically compatible for integrated vascular procedures.

A modular approach to the system design seems to be necessary to enable the integration of emerging technologies (eg, focused ultrasound).

A newly designed MR-guided surgical suite from General Electric Health Care is supposed to be installed at the Brigham and Women's Hospital in Boston during 2005. The latest version of the Signa Excite High Definition magnet is planned to be integrated into the operating room in a two-room layout connected through RF-shielded sliding doors (Fig. 4). This magnet is currently available at 1.5-T and 3.0-T field strengths. A newly designed surgical bed is also considered (Maquet, Rastatt, Germany) with the features of a standard surgical bed as well as the ability to transfer a patient into the magnet (Fig. 5). This system concept is supposed to offer MR imaging and radiographic compatibility for integrated vascular procedures as well.

Further optimization for neurosurgery is supposed to be provided by a newly developed MR imaging–compatible head holder (Mayfield, Integra NeuroSciences, Plainsboro, New Jersey) and a dedicated six-element phased-array RF coil (Fig. 6).

Finally, focused ultrasound surgical technology (ExAblate 2000; InSightec, Dallas, Texas) for minimally invasive treatment of uterine fibroids is planned to be integrated as part of the MR-guided surgical suite.

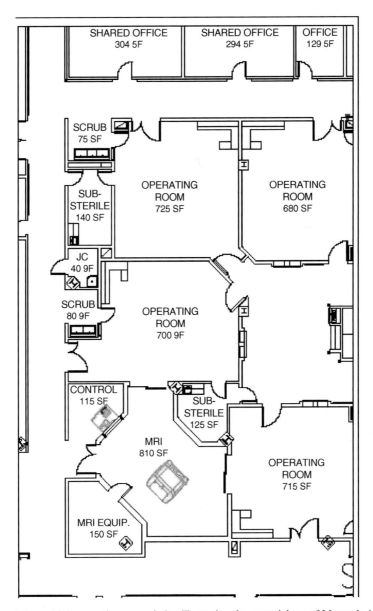

Fig. 7. Floor plan of the multiple operating room design illustrating the potential use of Maquet's AlphaMaquet 1150 surgical bed combined with the General Electric Signa patient bed for patient transfer. This setup may be more cost-effective, because this intraoperative MR imaging system may be able to serve more than one operating room, thus improving the return on the investment and facilitating the scheduling of intraoperative imaging cases. (Courtesy of General Electric Health Care, Milwaukee, Wisconsin; with permission.)

Economic issues have also been considered, because this intraoperative MR imaging concept should be able to serve more than one operating room simultaneously, thus improving the return of the investment and facilitating scheduling of intraoperative imaging cases (Fig. 7).

Other vendors, such as Siemens Medical Solutions and Philips Medical Systems, offer similar hybrid MR imaging and radiographic systems. When placed within the radiology department outside the operating room area, these systems are used together primarily for optimization of regional tumor therapy; however, they can also be used separately as an MR imaging unit and a radiographic angiography unit to increase cost-effectiveness [46,47].

A

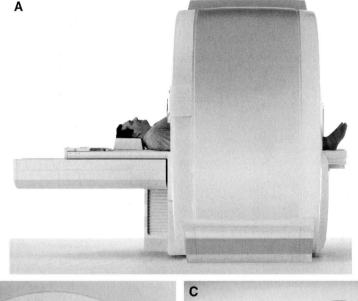

B

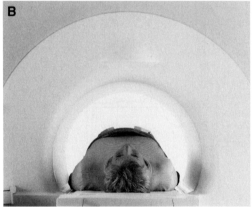

C

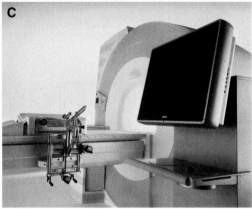

Fig. 8. Magnetom Espree, a new 1.5-T open-bore MR imaging system. With a total bore length of only 125 cm (A), a bore width of 70 cm (B), and an 18-inch in-room monitor (C), this MR imaging system allows interventions in a manner similar to procedures performed under CT guidance. (Courtesy of Siemens Medical Solutions, Erlangen, Germany; with permission.)

A different approach has been taken by Interventional MRI System (IMRIS; Winnipeg, Alberta, Canada), which uses a short, large-diameter, 1.5-T scanner mounted onto ceiling rails. This magnet can be moved while the patient remains still [48,49].

Open-bore high-field MR imaging systems

Siemens Medical Solutions recently introduced the Magnetom Espree, a so-called "open-bore" 1.5-T MR imaging system, with the first one installed at the Mayo Clinic in Jacksonville, Florida in September 2004. This magnet design features the total imaging matrix (Tim) system, which allows simultaneous acquisition with as many as 32 coil elements and also offers wireless vectorcardiographic triggering. This MR imaging system is compatible with the Angio CT Miyabi (Siemens Medical Solutions) patient transport system, which allows patient transport from the angiography or operating suite to the MR imaging scanner. The MR imaging table itself has a 205-cm extension and can be cantilevered out the rear of the scanner for access from both ends of the scanner. This MR imaging system seems to be well suited to perform MR-guided neurosurgery and percutaneous interventions, because the bore is only 1.25 m long but 70 cm wide,

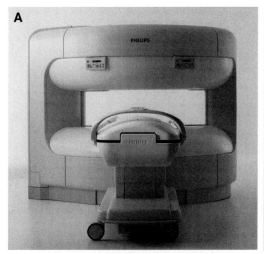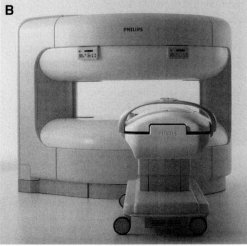

Fig. 9. Philips 1.0-T open Panorama MR imaging system. This system allows table movement not only in a longitudinal direction (*A*) but in a lateral direction (*B*). This increases the range of freedom for patient positioning during interventional procedures. (Courtesy of Philips Medical Systems, Eindhoven, The Netherlands; with permission.)

making any intervention similar to procedures performed under CT guidance (Fig. 8). This advantage has the potential to increase its acceptance as an interventional MR imaging system primarily in imaging centers where there is no dedicated interventional MR imaging research group. To the best of the authors' knowledge, however, no interventional procedures have been performed yet with the Magnetom Espree MR imaging system used for guidance purposes.

In-room scan control is possible with the Magnetom Espree using the in-room monitor (see Fig. 8). A prototype software application has also been developed to control the scanner using four-dimensional visualization.

In addition to being well suited for interventional procedures, the open-bore Magnetom Espree offers two other advantages that may justify its purchase. With a bore opening of 70 cm in diameter, the average distance between a patient's head and the magnet is 30 cm, thus easing claustrophobia issues for diagnostic examinations. Secondly, the Magnetom Espree is the only 1.5-T scanner that can provide enough room for severely obese patients (see Fig. 8).

Open high-field MR imaging systems

Another new development in the field of interventional MR imaging is the recent introduction of open high-field MR imaging systems as realized by Philips Medical Systems with the introduction of the open 1.0-T Philips Panorama

MR imaging system (Fig. 9). This magnet design allows maximized patient access while maintaining high-field image quality. In addition, the table can be moved in two directions: longitudinal and lateral (see Fig. 9). This offers increased freedom in patient positioning during interventional procedures as well as optimized off-center patient positioning with the region of interest (eg, shoulder, elbow) being in the isocenter of the magnet during regular MR imaging. Finally, the new receiver coil design offers access for biopsy needles

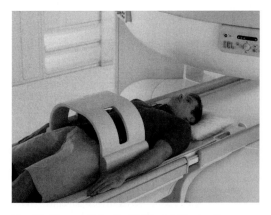

Fig. 10. Torso coil for the Philips 1.0-T open-Panorama MR imaging system. The opening within the coil may provide enough space to allow insertion of a biopsy needle or a thermal device, such as a laser fiber. (Courtesy of Philips Medical Systems, Eindhoven, The Netherlands; with permission.)

or thermal ablation devices while maintaining high-field image quality (Fig. 10). As mentioned previously for the open-bore high-field MR imaging systems, this magnet design also offers two additional advantages to justify its purchase: first, it is likely to be preferred by claustrophobic patients, thus markedly reducing the required rate of sedation, and, second, severely obese patients are also likely to prefer being examined in a more spacious MR imaging system.

References

[1] Mueller PR, Stark DD, Simeone JF, et al. MR-guided aspiration biopsy: needle design and clinical trials. Radiology 1986;161(3):605–9.

[2] Lufkin R, Teresi L, Hanafee W. New needle for MR-guided aspiration cytology of the head and neck. AJR Am J Roentgenol 1987;149(2):380–2.

[3] Lufkin R, Duckwiler G, Spickler E, et al. MR body stereotaxis: an aid for MR-guided biopsies. J Comput Assist Tomogr 1988;12(6):1088–9.

[4] Kaufman L, Arakawa M, Hale J, et al. Accessible magnetic resonance imaging. Magn Reson Q 1989; 5(4):283–97.

[5] Gronemeyer DH, Kaufman L, Rothschild P, et al. New possibilities and aspects of low-field magnetic resonance tomography. Radiol Diagn (Berl) 1989; 30(4):519–27 [in German].

[6] Lufkin R, Teresi L, Chiu L, et al. A technique for MR-guided needle placement. AJR Am J Roentgenol 1988;151(1):193–6.

[7] Duckwiler G, Lufkin RB, Teresi L, et al. Head and neck lesions: MR-guided aspiration biopsy. Radiology 1989;170(2):519–22.

[8] Kahn T, Harth T, Bettag M, et al. Preliminary experience with the application of gadolinium-DTPA before MR imaging-guided laser-induced interstitial thermotherapy of brain tumors. J Magn Reson Imaging 1997;7(1):226–9.

[9] Vogl TJ, Mack MG, Muller P, et al. Recurrent nasopharyngeal tumors: preliminary clinical results with interventional MR imaging—controlled laser-induced thermotherapy. Radiology 1995;196(3): 725–33.

[10] Liu H, Martin AJ, Truwit CL. Interventional MRI at high-field (1.5 T): needle artifacts. J Magn Reson Imaging 1998;8(1):214–9.

[11] Salomonowitz E. MR imaging-guided biopsy and therapeutic intervention in a closed-configuration magnet: single-center series of 361 punctures. AJR Am J Roentgenol 2001;177(1):159–63.

[12] Hinks RS, Bronskill MJ, Kucharczyk W, et al. MR systems for image-guided therapy. J Magn Reson Imaging 1998;8(1):19–25.

[13] Wenokur R, Andrews JC, Abemayor E, et al. Magnetic resonance imaging-guided fine needle aspiration for the diagnosis of skull base lesions. Skull Base Surg 1992;2:167–70.

[14] Castro DJ, Lufkin RB, Saxton RE, et al. Metastatic head and neck malignancy treated using MRI guided interstitial laser phototherapy: an initial case report. Laryngoscope 1992;102(1):26–32.

[15] Kahn T, Bettag M, Ulrich F, et al. MRI-guided laser-induced interstitial thermotherapy of cerebral neoplasms. J Comput Assist Tomogr 1994;18(4): 519–32.

[16] Anzai Y, Lufkin R, DeSalles A, et al. Preliminary experience with MR-guided thermal ablation of brain tumors. AJNR Am J Neuroradiol 1995;16(1):39–48.

[17] Jager L, Muller-Lisse GU, Gutmann R, et al. Initial results with MRI-controlled laser-induced interstitial thermotherapy of head and neck tumors. Radiologe 1996;36(3):236–44 [in German].

[18] Mahnken AH, Buecker A, Spuentrup E, et al. MR-guided radiofrequency ablation of hepatic malignancies at 1.5 T: initial results. J Magn Reson Imaging 2004;19(3):342–8.

[19] Nimsky C, Ganslandt O, Von Keller B, et al. Intraoperative high-field-strength MR imaging: implementation and experience in 200 patients. Radiology 2004;233(1):67–78.

[20] Nimsky C, Ganslandt O, Hastreiter P, et al. Intraoperative diffusion-tensor MR imaging: shifting of white matter tracts during neurosurgical procedures—initial experience. Radiology 2005;234(1): 218–25.

[21] Strother CM, Unal O, Frayne R, et al. Endovascular treatment of experimental canine aneurysms: feasibility with MR imaging guidance. Radiology 2000; 215(2):516–9.

[22] Hillenbrand CM, Elgort DR, Wong EY, et al. Active device tracking and high-resolution intravascular MRI using a novel catheter-based, opposed-solenoid phased array coil. Magn Reson Med 2004;51(4):668–75.

[23] Wacker FK, Elgort D, Hillenbrand CM, et al. The catheter-driven MRI scanner: a new approach to intravascular catheter tracking and imaging-parameter adjustment for interventional MRI. AJR Am J Roentgenol 2004;183(2):391–5.

[24] Quick HH, Kuehl H, Kaiser G, et al. Interventional MR angiography with a floating table. Radiology 2003;229(2):598–602.

[25] Bock M, Volz S, Zuhlsdorff S, et al. MR-guided intravascular procedures: real-time parameter control and automated slice positioning with active tracking coils. J Magn Reson Imaging 2004;19(5):580–9.

[26] Wilson MW, Fidelman N, Weber OM, et al. Experimental renal artery embolization in a combined MR imaging/angiographic unit. J Vasc Interv Radiol 2003;14(9 Pt 1):1169–75.

[27] Razavi R, Hill DL, Keevil SF, et al. Cardiac catheterisation guided by MRI in children and adults with congenital heart disease. Lancet 2003; 362(9399):1877–82.

[28] Paetzel C, Zorger N, Bachthaler M, et al. Feasibility of MR-guided angioplasty of femoral artery stenoses using real-time imaging and intraarterial contrast-enhanced MR angiography. Rofo Fortschr Geb Rontgenstr Neuen Bildgeb Verfahr 2004; 176(9):1232–6.

[29] Orel SG, Schnall MD, Newman RW, et al. MR imaging-guided localization and biopsy of breast lesions: initial experience. Radiology 1994;193(1): 97–102.

[30] Heywang-Kobrunner SH, Heinig A, Pickuth D, et al. Interventional MRI of the breast: lesion localisation and biopsy. Eur Radiol 2000;10(1):36–45.

[31] Hall-Craggs MA. Interventional MRI of the breast: minimally invasive therapy. Eur Radiol 2000;10(1): 59–62.

[32] Pfleiderer SO, Reichenbach JR, Azhari T, et al. A manipulator system for 14-gauge large core breast biopsies inside a high-field whole-body MR scanner. J Magn Reson Imaging 2003;17(4):493–8.

[33] Schenck JF, Jolesz FA, Roemer PB, et al. Superconducting open configuration MR imaging system for image-guided therapy. Radiology 1995;195(3): 805–14.

[34] Silverman SG, Collick BD, Figueira MR, et al. Interactive MR-guided biopsy in an open-configuration MR imaging system. Radiology 1995;197(1): 175–81.

[35] Silverman SG, Jolesz FA, Newman RW, et al. Design and implementation of an interventional MR imaging suite. AJR Am J Roentgenol 1997;168(6): 1465–71.

[36] Black PM, Moriarty T, Alexander E III, et al. Development and implementation of intraoperative magnetic resonance imaging and its neurosurgical applications. Neurosurgery 1997;41(4):831–42.

[37] Schwartz RB, Hsu L, Wong TZ, et al. Intraoperative MR imaging guidance for intracranial neurosurgery: experience with the first 200 cases. Radiology 1999; 211(2):477–88.

[38] Gould SW, Martin S, Agarwal T, et al. Image-guided surgery for anal fistula in a 0.5T interventional MRI unit. J Magn Reson Imaging 2002; 16(3):267–76.

[39] Genant JW, Vandevenne JE, Bergman AG, et al. Interventional musculoskeletal procedures performed by using MR imaging guidance with a vertically open MR unit: assessment of techniques and applicability. Radiology 2002;223(1): 127–36.

[40] Fahrig R, Butts K, Wen Z, et al. Truly hybrid interventional MR/X-ray system: investigation of in vivo applications. Acad Radiol 2001;8(12): 1200–7.

[41] Fahrig R, Heit G, Wen Z, et al. First use of a truly-hybrid X-ray/MR imaging system for guidance of brain biopsy. Acta Neurochir (Wien) 2003;145(11): 995–7.

[42] Lewin JS, Petersilge CA, Hatem SF, et al. Interactive MR imaging-guided biopsy and aspiration with a modified clinical C-arm system. AJR Am J Roentgenol 1998;170(6):1593–601.

[43] Gehl HB, Frahm C, Schimmelpenning H, et al. A technique of MRT-guided abdominal drainage with an open low-field magnet. Its feasibility and the initial results. Rofo Fortschr Geb Rontgenstr Neuen Bildgeb Verfahr 1996;165(1):70–3 [in German].

[44] Lewin JS, Nour SG, Connell CF, et al. Phase II clinical trial of interactive MR imaging-guided interstitial radiofrequency thermal ablation of primary kidney tumors: initial experience. Radiology 2004; 232(3):835–45.

[45] Kettenbach J, Kostler W, Rucklinger E, et al. Percutaneous saline-enhanced radiofrequency ablation of unresectable hepatic tumors: initial experience in 26 patients. AJR Am J Roentgenol 2003;180(6): 1537–45.

[46] Vogl TJ, Balzer JO, Mack MG, et al. Hybrid MR interventional imaging system: combined MR and angiography suites with single interactive table. Feasibility study in vascular liver tumor procedures. Eur Radiol 2002;12(6):1394–400.

[47] Wilson MW, Kerlan RK Jr, Fidelman NA, et al. Hepatocellular carcinoma: regional therapy with a magnetic targeted carrier bound to doxorubicin in a dual MR imaging/conventional angiography suite—initial experience with four patients. Radiology 2004;230(1):287–93.

[48] Hoult DI, Saunders JK, Sutherland GR, et al. The engineering of an interventional MRI with a movable 1.5 Tesla magnet. J Magn Reson Imaging 2001; 13(1):78–86.

[49] Fenchel S, Boll DT, Lewin JS. Intraoperative MR imaging. Magn Reson Imaging Clin N Am 2003; 11(3):431–47.

ELSEVIER
SAUNDERS

Magn Reson Imaging Clin N Am
13 (2005) 415–429

MAGNETIC
RESONANCE
IMAGING CLINICS
of North America

Update to Pulse Sequences for Interventional MR Imaging

Jamal J. Derakhshan, BS[a,b], Jeffrey L. Duerk, PhD[a,c,*]

[a]Department of Biomedical Engineering, Case Western Reserve University, Cleveland, OH 44106, USA
[b]School of Medicine, Case Western Reserve University, Cleveland, OH 44106, USA
[c]Department of Radiology, Case Western Reserve University, University Hospitals of Cleveland,
11100 Euclid Avenue, Cleveland, OH 44106, USA

Interventional MR imaging has been defined as the use of MR images for the rapid guidance or monitoring of diagnostic or therapeutic procedures including surgery, percutaneous procedures, vascular interventions, and cancer therapy monitoring [1]. The field of interventional MR imaging has continued to develop over the past decade. This article presents some of the advancements in the field of interventional MR imaging since the last review almost 5 years ago and highlights some of the new and emerging imaging techniques. In particular, the authors have identified specific advancements in pulse sequences and reconstruction algorithms; interventional device visualization, tracking, manipulation, and safety; real-time pulse sequence parameter control and adaptive imaging; high-resolution vessel wall imaging; moving table acquisitions; and guiding and monitoring thermal therapy.

Pulse sequences and reconstruction algorithms

The basic interventional MR imaging pulse sequences

Interventional procedures on humans at fields from 0.2 T to 0.5 T have demonstrated that there is no ideal MR imaging pulse sequence for all interventional procedures. Aside from the requirement that the pulse sequence used for the guidance phase of the procedure must be fast (ie, short repetition time [TR]) to deliver high temporal resolution, the best pulse sequence is dependent on the interventional task, anatomic location, and preferred contrast for the procedure being performed. Interventional biopsies of the head and neck are best accomplished with fast imaging with steady precession (FISP) or FISP with balanced gradients in all directions (True-FISP) sequences in which blood appears bright and thus produce excellent vessel conspicuity. Interventional liver procedures are best performed using T2-weighted turbo spin-echo or a time-reversed version of FISP sequences due to better lesion depiction, although blood appears dark in these sequences [2]. In certain interventional body imaging applications such as MR–guided transgluteal biopsy of the prostate gland, some prefer the use of spoiled steady-state acquisitions (fast low-angle shot [FLASH]) with T1 weighting to increase the visibility of the needle at the expense of losing lesion depiction (which must be inferred from previously acquired T2-weighted turbo spin-echo images) [3].

Measuring velocity with steady-state free precession

Although two-dimensional CINE phase-contrast flow velocity quantification has been well described since the mid-1980s, its use in rapid/steady-state imaging has been limited. A new method for measuring blood flow velocity based

J.J. Derakhshan is supported in part by NIH grant T32 GM07250 and the Case Medical Scientist Training Program. The Case Western Reserve University MR program gratefully acknowledges research support from Siemens Medical Solutions-MRI (Erlangen, Germany).

* Corresponding author. Department of Radiology-MRI, University Hospitals of Cleveland, 11100 Euclid Avenue, Cleveland, OH 44106.
E-mail address: Duerk@uhrad.com (J.L. Duerk).

on phase-contrast and balanced steady-state free precession (SSFP) called phase-contrast SSFP has been developed that works by inverting all gradients in the slice-select direction (Fig. 1A). There is no need for additional flow-encoding gradient lobes that would lengthen TR. This method has a higher intrinsic signal-to-noise ratio (SNR) and lower phase noise compared with previous phase-contrast methods and is less dependent on in-flow enhancement (see Fig. 1B). These benefits make this sequence better for measuring slow flow and pulsatile flow [4], yet it is limited to quantitative assessment of through-plane flow.

Magnetization preparation to induce the steady state

Steady-state pulse sequences are important for interventional imaging due to the high temporal and spatial resolution and high SNR. Magnetization preparation is necessary to speed up the approach to the steady state and reduce signal oscillations during data collection. For many applications, a single $\alpha/2$ flip angle pulse is sufficient magnetization preparation. In applications that are sensitive to magnetization oscillations, a sequence of $\alpha/2$ flip angle pulses can be used to reduce

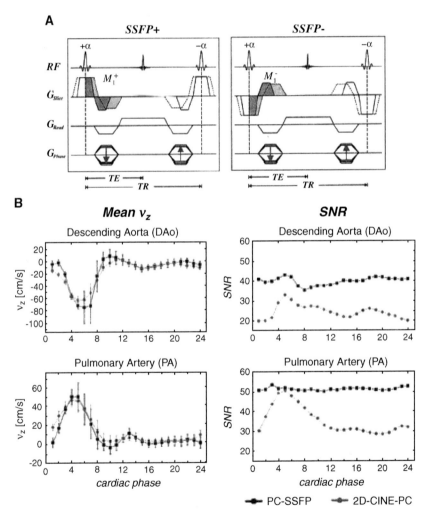

Fig. 1. (*A*) The pulse sequence for phase-contrast (PC) SSFP showing alternating slice-select gradient polarity that gives rise to velocity encoding. G, gradient; M_1^+ and M_1^-, moments. (*B*) Plots of mean velocity and the signal-to-noise ratio (SNR) of blood in the descending aorta and pulmonary artery for phase-contrast SSFP and traditional two-dimensional CINE phase-contrast. TE, echo time. (*From* Markl M, Alley MT, Pelc NJ. Balanced phase-contrast steady-state free precession [PC-SSFP]: a novel technique for velocity encoding by gradient inversion. Magn Reson Med 2003;49(5):945–52. © 2003 Wiley-Liss, Inc. Reprinted with permission from Wiley-Liss, Inc., a subsidiary of John Wiley & Sons, Inc.)

oscillations in the steady state magnetization at the expense of spending more time on magnetization preparation. In these cases, using a linearly increasing series of radiofrequency (RF) pulses for magnetization preparation (instead of a set of constant $\alpha/2$ flip angle pulses) increases image SNR and image quality and decreases artifacts due to signal oscillations caused by off-resonant spins. This method may allow fewer preparatory RF pulses to be used to establish the steady state, hence reducing the acquisition time and increasing temporal resolution [5].

Real-time steady-state free precession with intermittent inversion pulses for myocardial infarct enhancement

It is possible to acquire a myocardium-nulled image between every few temporal frames during interactive SSFP imaging by periodically adding a nonselective 180° inversion pulse during SSFP imaging (Fig. 2A). This method does not use ECG gating or breath-holding and is the first demonstration of visualization of infarcted myocardium during interactive imaging. The images are collected fast enough to allow monitoring of cardiac function including segmental akinesia. The inversion pulse can be disabled interactively if nulled images are not needed during navigation to the heart; further, the delay time following the inversion pulse can be changed interactively to achieve optimal myocardium nulling during the procedure. The infarcted myocardium is selectively enhanced by the delayed hyperenhancement effect following injection of contrast agent. It is possible to null normal myocardium and blood and produce a high contrast-to-noise ratio between the infarcted tissue border, normal tissue, and blood to facilitate infarct identification (see Fig. 2B, C). The pulse sequence has been used in conjunction with an active catheter to achieve good discrimination between healthy and infarcted myocardium, cavitary blood, and the interventional catheter. Frame rates as high as seven frames per second have been acquired with $2 \times 1.8 \times 6$ mm^3 resolution. Hence, the technique allows diagnosis of infarcted tissue and interventional positioning of a catheter in the infarcted region of the beating heart [6].

Parallel imaging to increase frame rate

Parallel imaging techniques such as sensitivity encoding (SENSE) and simultaneous acquisition of spatial hormones (SMASH) can decrease the amount of time it takes to acquire an image of a given resolution or increase the image resolution at a given frame rate; the techniques employ multiple receive coils with different spatial sensitivities to correct for aliasing artifacts that occur due to undersampling k-space. The acceleration gain comes at the cost of decreased SNR and some incomplete aliasing artifact suppression. To employ parallel imaging, the sensitivity profile of the coils must be determined in vivo. Changes in scan plane orientation, magnetization preparation, and device location during interventional procedures make it difficult to use previously acquired sensitivity profiles; however, the sensitivity maps may be estimated adaptively using the time-adaptive SENSE (TSENSE) method. Using the TSENSE method to estimate the time-varying coil sensitivities during interventional MR imaging, parallel imaging with an acceleration factor of two has been accomplished, resulting in seven frames per second with a resolution of $1.8 \times 3.5 \times 8$ mm^3. This high frame rate has made it possible to depict in real-time the three-dimensional motion of the cardiac wall. By disabling TSENSE reconstruction for a few frames after a change in scan plane orientation, artifacts caused by errors in sensitivity map estimation can be reduced. TSENSE reconstruction tolerates changes in magnetization preparation, indicating that the sensitivity maps remain valid despite saturation preparation and injection of contrast agents. Using TSENSE to accelerate imaging has been shown to cause less temporal blurring of wall motion than view sharing [7].

Temporal filtering to increase frame rate

It is possible to increase the frame rate in interventional MR imaging without changing the spatial resolution by using radial imaging and reducing the number of projections acquired; however, the increase in frame rate is limited by increasing aliasing artifacts as the number of projections is reduced (Fig. 3A). Image reconstruction techniques such as view sharing, in which k-space data from the previous acquisition are combined with the newly acquired k-space data, can reduce the aliasing artifacts but blur objects that have moved between acquisitions. By using reduced field-of-view (FOV) processing in conjunction with undersampled radial k-space acquisitions (number of projections ≥ 32), interventional images have been acquired and reconstructed on-line at eight true frames per second with $2 \times 2 \times 8$ mm^3 resolution (see Fig. 3B). The

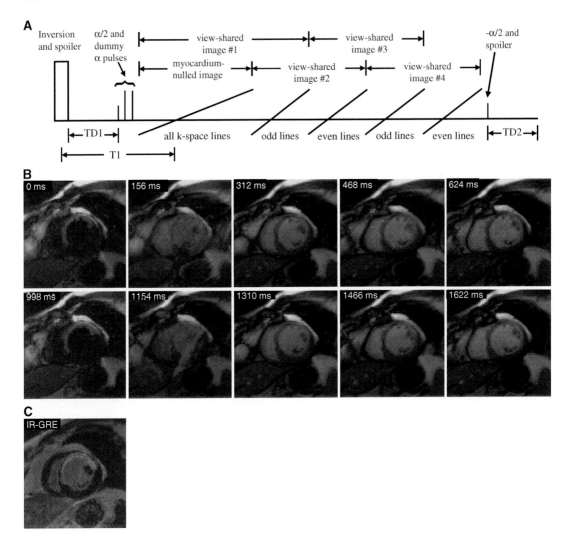

Fig. 2. (*A*) The pulse sequence for acquiring inversion recovery real-time SSFP images. (*B*) Consecutive short-axis images over two inversion cycles from a human patient with a previous myocardial infarction 12 minutes after contrast agent injection. Infarcted tissue is seen at 0 and 998 milliseconds from the 8 to 2 o'clock position in the images. (*C*) Conventional inversion recovery gradient recalled echo delayed hyperenhancement effect image acquired 22 minutes post contrast injection for comparison. The location of infarction is the same as that shown using the inversion recovery real-time SSFP method. (*From* Guttman MA, Dick AJ, Raman VK, et al. Imaging of myocardial infarction for diagnosis and intervention using real-time interactive MRI without ECG-gating or breath-holding. Magn Reson Med 2004;52(2): 354–61. © 2004 Wiley-Liss, Inc. Reprinted with permission from Wiley-Liss, Inc., a subsidiary of John Wiley & Sons, Inc.)

reduced FOV reconstructed images have the same image quality (artifact degradation) as unfiltered images with twice as many projections, thus enabling a twofold increase in frame rate. A comparison of Cartesian reduced FOV processing with radial reduced FOV demonstrated that radial reduced FOV images had better artifact suppression: in radial imaging, aliasing artifacts are manifested as incoherent streaks of low signal intensity throughout the image as opposed to

forming discrete ghosts in Cartesian acquisitions; therefore, any remaining aliasing artifacts are less obtrusive [8].

Device visualization, tracking, manipulation, and safety

There is a growing interest in using interventional MR imaging to perform catheterizations that are currently performed under fluoroscopy

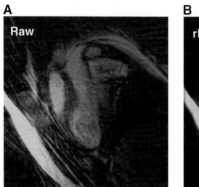
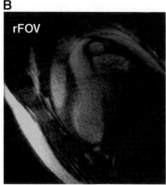

Fig. 3. (*A*) Raw (unfiltered) image acquired with 32 radial projections demonstrating significant undersampling artifacts. (*B*) The same image processed with the reduced FOV (rFOV) method demonstrating significant reduction of the undersampling artifacts. (*From* Peters DC, Guttman MA, Dick AJ, et al. Reduced field of view and undersampled PR combined for interventional imaging of a fully dynamic field of view. Magn Reson Med 2004;51(4):765. © 2004 Wiley-Liss, Inc. Reprinted with permission from Wiley-Liss, Inc., a subsidiary of John Wiley & Sons, Inc.)

because MR imaging provides better soft tissue contrast, can generate tomographic views in arbitrary orientations, and can calculate intravascular flow velocity without the use of ionizing radiation [9]. To perform these endovascular interventions, the catheter must be adequately visualized spatially and temporally. Methods for visualization can be grouped into the broad categories of passive, semiactive, and active [10].

Passive visualization

Passively visualized objects rely on the difference in magnetic susceptibility between an exogenous marker and the surrounding tissue to create a signal void (or enhancement) at the location of the device in the image. SSFP sequences such as balanced fast field echo (FFE) or TrueFISP are ideally suited for imaging passive devices due to their high SNR and high spatial and temporal resolution [11]. The major benefit of passively visualized devices is that there are relatively few concerns regarding RF heating [10]. One of the

first studies to demonstrate completely MR–guided cardiac catheterizations in humans was performed in children to repair congenital heart defects; the study used passively visualized carbon dioxide–filled catheters with SSFP imaging to eliminate the danger of RF heating (Fig. 4) [12].

Devices that contain susceptibility markers can disrupt the steady state signal from blood that passes near the magnetic field inhomogeneity. The disturbance manifests as a signal void that extends beyond the localized region of susceptibility-induced magnetic field inhomogeneity in regions of blood flow. The effect is typically worse at higher blood velocities. T1-shortening contrast agents such as gadolinium have been shown to dramatically reduce these effects by reducing the time taken to re-achieve the steady state [11].

Magnetic susceptibility markers can be difficult to see in an image due to the relatively low contrast between the marker and the surrounding anatomy [13]. One way to increase the visibility of passively visualized objects such as catheters filled

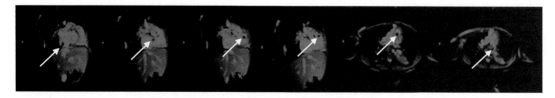

Fig. 4. MR images of a passively visualized catheter (*arrows*) being guided from the inferior vena cava to the right pulmonary artery in a human. (*From* Razavi R, Hill DL, Keevil SF, et al. Cardiac catheterisation guided by MRI in children and adults with congenital heart disease. Lancet 2003;362(9399):1879.)

with T1-reducing contrast agent is to add an inversion or pi (180°) pulse in the pulse sequence and collect image data at the inversion time of the surrounding tissue. This magnetization-prepared or inversion-recovery FLASH sequence decreases the background signal amplitude and increases the catheter-to-background ratio by up to 200% [14].

Active visualization

Active visualization of a device is accomplished by capacitively coupling a resonant coil (microcoil) on the device to a receive channel on the MR scanner. The signal from the microcoil is used to calculate the device position, which is then combined with the image from a surface coil to depict the location of the device with regard to the surrounding anatomy. The position of the microcoil can be calculated using the same fast gradient-echo sequence used for imaging without any additional RF pulses; therefore, no additional time is needed for active tracking. The current method of acquiring image data and tracking information simultaneously eliminates distortions caused by motion that used to be present when real-time tracking information was superimposed on a previously acquired vascular "roadmap."

Radiofrequency safety of wires in interventional MR imaging

Empiric studies of RF heating of wires and anecdotal reports of wire heating during interventional procedures have raised concerns regarding the safety of wires and conductive structures used during interventional MR imaging. A theoretic model of wire tip heating has been developed that is able to determine the absolute amount of heating of a straight wire that is completely embedded in tissue and exposed to a uniform RF field. By using this method, it is possible to ascribe such an interventional wire a safety index (degrees Celsius divided by watts per kilogram). When this index is multiplied by the specific absorption rate (SAR), it gives the temperature increase that an RF pulse is expected to produce. After choosing which wires are needed during an interventional procedure and determining the safety index of those wires, this model can be used to determine the peak SAR that will keep the temperature increase below a certain safe level. By limiting the peak SAR of the pulse sequence to this value during the procedure, the RF heating will not exceed the predetermined value and unexpected heating can be avoided. Further refinement of the model for curved wires, wires that extend out of tissue, and inhomogeneous RF pulses is needed to apply this model for the safe use of wires in clinical interventional MR imaging [15].

Semiactive visualization

Semiactive devices (also known as wireless active devices) contain tuned resonant circuits that are inductively coupled to surface coils (Fig. 5A) instead of being capacitively connected to the MR scanner. The resonant circuits provide local gain to an RF pulse to enhance the signal around a resonant loop. Due to the local increase in tip angle near the resonant loop, the spins around the loop and the spins far from the loop will experience different tip angles and thus the detected signal from the surface coil is different (see Fig. 5B). The contrast between the catheter and background tissue varies as a function of flip angle (see Fig. 5C). By varying the flip angle of the steady-state pulse sequence, the catheter conspicuity and tissue contrast can be manipulated (see Fig. 5D). At low tip angles, instrument-only images are produced. At intermediate tip angles, the instrument and the surrounding tissue are seen. At high tip angles, the catheter is no longer seen and tissue-only images are produced. The optimal flip angle for maximal catheter signal and catheter-to-background contrast-to-noise ratio was found to be 10° to 20°. The method was able to produce and display six to nine frames per second. This method eliminates the need for long conductive wires that cause the majority of the RF heating safety concerns in active visualization, allows visualization along the distal 12 cm of the catheter including the catheter tip, and makes catheter handling much easier because there is no physical connection to the scanner. The precise location of the catheter, however, cannot be fed back to the scanner for parameter adjustment, as can be done with active devices, unless image-based segmentation is performed [16].

A different way to localize resonant circuits, which also reduces RF heating of the loop itself, is to perform optical decoupling of the resonant circuits [17]. In this method, optical signals are sent to the resonant circuit to detune and retune the circuit during RF pulse transmission. By using this method, it is possible to localize optically detunable resonant circuits in real time with no capacitive connection to the scanner [13]; however, this method requires a fiber-optic cable to be

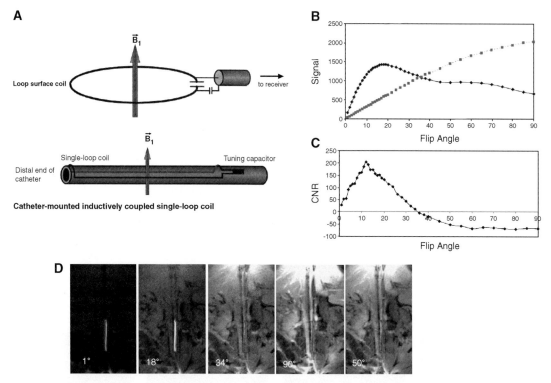

Fig. 5. (*A*) Schematic diagram depicting inductive coupling between a tuned resonant loop on a catheter and a loop surface coil capacitively coupled to the MR scanner. (*B*) Catheter signal (*black line*) and background signal (*gray line*) as a function of flip angle. (*C*) Catheter contrast-to-noise ratio (CNR) as a function of the flip angle. (*D*) Images of a catheter with a tuned resonant loop located in the aorta of a pig and being visualized inductively using 1°, 18°, 34°, 50°, and 99° flip angles. (*From* Quick HH, Zenge MO, Kuehl H, et al. Interventional magnetic resonance angiography with no strings attached: wireless active catheter visualization. Magn Reson Med 2005;53(2):446–55. © 2005 Wiley-Liss, Inc. Reprinted with permission from Wiley-Liss, Inc., a subsidiary of John Wiley & Sons, Inc.)

attached to the device, which can hamper instrument handling.

Steering interventional catheters

Potential heating of braiding material in conventional semirigid steerable catheters is one major drawback to MR–guided catheterizations [10]. To date, MR–guided catheter interventions have had to rely on nonbraided, low-torquing, low-steerable catheters [12]. One proposed solution to circumvent this problem uses the high magnetic field environment of the scanner to help guide the catheter (a 1.5-F catheter was modified with a three-axis coil on its tip; electrical current of varying strength was applied to specific coils when turns were to be made). Specifically, the current causes magnetic moments that interact with the main magnetic field to produce a torque to deflect the tip of the catheter. The catheter is

visualized by the local magnetic field inhomogeneity artifact that the coil at the tip produces; if this artifact is not large enough for easy localization, then a "visualization current" can be applied to the catheter tip to increase the size of the tip artifact [9]. This method has been used to successfully guide a catheter through a three-dimensional maze.

Real-time pulse sequence parameter control and adaptive imaging

Because MR produces thin tomographic views, it is possible for an interventional device to move out of a predefined slice during a procedure, resulting in partial or complete loss of visualization of the device. This problem is not encountered in fluoroscopy due to the projection images acquired. To solve this problem, it is possible to perform automated slice tracking during which the calculated position of an active microcoil is continuously used by the pulse sequence to adjust the imaging plane so that it remains centered on the location of the microcoil as the device is manipulated [18]. Because the device always remains in the imaging plane, time is not wasted by manually repositioning the slice during the intervention. The interventionalist can continuously see the device and its surroundings and continue working without having to stop and change the slice position when the device would otherwise go out of the imaging plane (Fig. 6A–C). Automated slice tracking decreases the overall procedure time and increases interventionalist satisfaction.

User interfaces have been developed that allow changing other pulse sequence parameters interactively from within the scanner room and allow a greater variety of images to be acquired. The slice orientation (transverse, coronal, or sagittal) (see Fig. 6D, E) and contrast mechanism

(FLASH, TrueFISP, or projection MR digital subtraction angiography) (see Fig. 6F, G) can be changed "on the fly" during the procedure [19].

In adaptive imaging, other parameters such as spatial resolution, FOV, echo time, TR, bandwidth, temporal resolution, flip angle, and slice thickness are continuously updated according to a predefined algorithm related to the calculated speed of catheter movement. Adaptive imaging eliminates the need for manual adjustment of these parameters during the procedure and optimizes the values of these parameters based the speed at which the catheter is moved [20].

High-resolution vessel wall imaging

The idea of using resonant loops to localize a catheter tip (active tracking) has been expanded to create sensitive coils that are able to directly

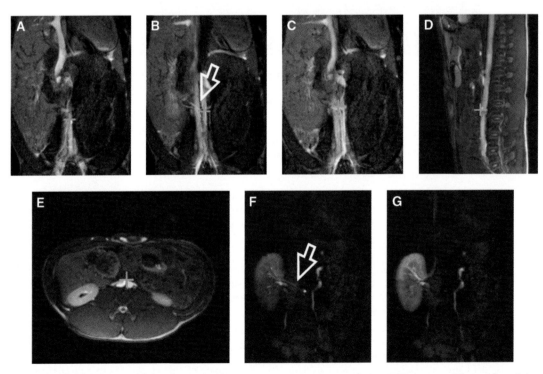

Fig. 6. (*A–C*) Example of automated slice tracking using an active catheter and TrueFISP contrast. The position of the active coil is demonstrated by the "+" symbol in the images (*A–E*). The coronal imaging plane has changed to keep the coil in the imaging plane. (*D*) The slice orientation has been interactively changed to the sagittal plane and (*E*) the transverse plane. (*F, G*) Example of changing the contrast interactively to MR-digital subtraction angiography projection technique, showing enhancement of the upper pole of the right kidney after contrast agent injection. (*From* Bock M, Volz S, Zuhlsdorff S, et al. MR-guided intravascular procedures: real-time parameter control and automated slice positioning with active tracking coils. J Magn Reson Imaging 2004;19(5):586. © 2004 Wiley-Liss, Inc. Reprinted with permission from Wiley-Liss, Inc., a subsidiary of John Wiley & Sons, Inc.)

image blood vessels and their surroundings (like a miniature surface coil). One recent design is the intravascular extended sensitivity loopless antenna, which is a long coaxial cable with an extended inner conductor (whip). The antenna is insulated to increase the longitudinal distance over which imaging can be performed, and the whip is wound helically to allow imaging at the antenna tip. This antenna has a high and homogeneous sensitivity along its length that allows imaging along its length (20 cm) without repositioning the catheter; it also allows imaging at the tip of the device [21].

Active device localization with automated scan plane adjustment has been combined with high-resolution vessel wall imaging. In one study in porcine using a True FISP pulse sequence [22], two solenoids wound in opposite directions concentric to the catheter and separated by 1cm were independently connected to two receive channels on the MR scanner. The signal from each channel was analyzed independently to localize each solenoid and adjust the scan plane position and orientation such that both solenoids remained in the scan plane throughout the procedure. The signals from the solenoids were combined using the sum-of-squares method to perform high-resolution vessel wall imaging in a manner similar to intravascular imaging done previously with a single-channel opposed solenoid design. Using this method, the investigators reported tracking and updating the scan plane at 1.5 frames per second and acquiring high-resolution vessel wall images in 15 seconds with an in-plane resolution of 240 μm. Using the opposed solenoid method, it was possible to acquire high-resolution vessel wall images along roughly 2 cm without repositioning the catheter.

Continuously moving table imaging (extended field-of-view imaging, incremental field-of-view imaging, whole-body imaging)

Interventional MR imaging suffers from two competing requirements. The physician must not only have access to the patient and perform the procedure in a manner as comfortable as possible but the images must also be acquired with as high an SNR, resolution, and frame rate as possible (which requires long, small-diameter bore magnets with high magnetic fields) [23]. One possible way to satisfy both requirements is to use extended FOV imaging. To acquire such images, the patient bed is moved through the active area of the magnet, allowing a region larger than the active area to

be imaged. Alternatively, this technique allows the same FOV to be acquired with a shorter magnet, thus improving access to the patient while maintaining the benefits of the longer-bore magnets [24].

Initially, a multistation approach was used to increase the FOV. Several standard FOVs were acquired and then stitched together in the spatial domain to form the extended FOV image [25]. These methods suffered from discontinuity artifacts at the border between joined regions of interest (ROIs) and longer scan times due to multiple table repositionings and waiting at each location for the re-establishment of the steady state [24]. Newer extended FOV methods acquire data in a more continuous manner to avoid these shortcomings.

There are several methods to perform continuously moving table acquisitions. K-space traversal can be done in a rectilinear or nonrectilinear manner. For rectilinear encoding, slice selection, phase encoding, or frequency encoding can be done along the direction of motion. When frequency encoding is done along the direction of motion, the data at each phase-encoding step belong to a different location along the z-axis in addition to the expected different position along the phase-encoding (x or y) dimension. To move the frequency-encoded data to the correct z locations, the frequency-encoded data are Fourier-transformed and then shifted along the frequency-encoding (z) direction by an amount equal to the distance the table has moved since the previous phase-encoding step. Finally, the data are Fourier transformed in the other dimensions to get a regional FOV [26].

A different method of doing frequency encoding along the direction of motion in which coherent data sets are directly acquired is called frequency-adapted sliding-table acquisition [24]. Data from the same region along the cranial caudal axis are directly obtained by adjusting the center frequency of the receiver from view to view (Fig. 7A). The center frequency change (Δf) between two consecutive phase-encoding views (equation 1) is

$$\Delta f = \gamma G_z V T_R \qquad (1)$$

where γ is the gyromagnetic ratio, G_z is the slice select gradient, V is the speed of table motion, and T_R is the sequence repetition time. The multiple resulting FOVs (called regional FOVs) are cropped and concatenated in the spatial domain to obtain the extended FOV image. This method

A

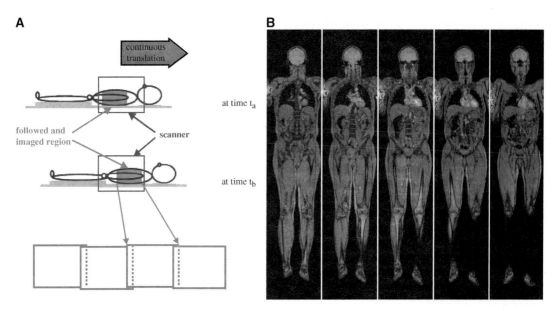

B

Fig. 7. (*A*) A schematic representation of following the same region of the object during continuously moving table translation by adjusting the center frequency of the receiver. (*B*) Five coronal head to toe images acquired using the frequency-adapted sliding table acquisition technique in 2.5 minutes. (*From* Zhu Y, Dumoulin CL. Extended field-of-view imaging with table translation and frequency sweeping. Magn Reson Med 2003;49(6):1106–12. © 2003 Wiley-Liss, Inc. Reprinted with permission from Wiley-Liss, Inc., a subsidiary of John Wiley & Sons, Inc.)

allows 5 to 10 body-length tomographic slices to be acquired in 2.5 minutes (see Fig. 7B).

In "helical MR" [27], radial projections are acquired equidistantly along the z-direction as the patient passes through the magnet. Consecutive radial projections circulate about the z-axis (Fig. 8A). Axial slices are reconstructed by interpolating k-space data acquired superior and inferior to the physical location of the slice. The data are then gridded and Fourier transformed to form two-dimensional axial slices (see Fig. 8B–G). Collecting data in the axial plane exploits the region of highest main magnet homogeneity and gradient linearity. It was found that using only the center lobe of a sinc RF pulse reduced oscillations in the magnetization compared with a fully rectangular slice profile due to what has been termed the "catalyzing effect" of the imperfect slice profile (the magnetization achieves steady state more rapidly). This method predicts good image quality for table speeds up to 1.69 cm/s and allows reconstruction and viewing of axial slices in real time (up to five frames per second), with a total body scan time of approximately 2 minutes and in-plane resolution of 1.56×1.56 mm^2. It is unfortunate that the SNR achieved in this experiment is equivalent to that of a two-dimensional acquisition rather than a three-dimensional scan.

Gradient nonlinearity is more detrimental to moving table imaging than traditional stationary acquisition [24] because during moving table acquisition, gradient nonlinearity produces blurring in addition to spatial distortion [26]. Correction for gradient nonlinearity by spatially remapping data along with intensity correction has been extended to moving table acquisition with rectilinear frequency encoding along the direction of motion (Fig. 9) [26]. This method reduces gradient nonlinearity artifacts at the expense of increased reconstruction time because the correction is applied at each phase-encoding step (to save additional time, up to 128 steps can be grouped together). The correction technique allows acquisition to be done more quickly because the patient table can be moved at higher speeds (2.66 cm/s in this study). One benefit of helical MR is that the gradient nonlinearity correction is not necessary near the magnet isocenter [28].

Some future enhancements that need to be made to improve moving table image quality include developing ways to perform position-dependent frequency, shim, and transmit-power calibrations [24]. In addition, most studies to date have used the body coil for RF transmission and reception. By using phased-array coils, it is hoped that SNR will be increased [27].

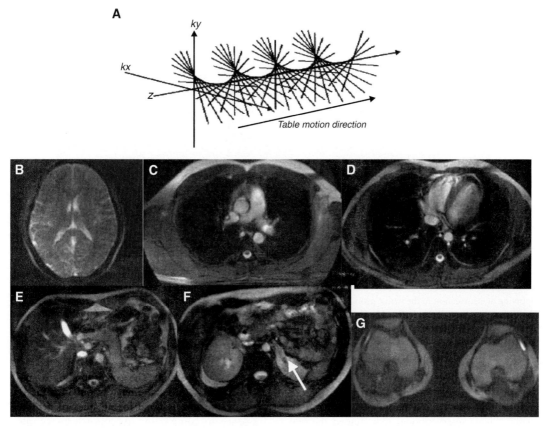

Fig. 8. (A) Helical trajectory in kx-ky-z space. (B–G) Images from the helical data set acquired in approximately 2 minutes. (*From* Shankaranarayanan A, Herfkens R, Hargreaves BM, et al. Helical MR: continuously moving table axial imaging with radial acquisitions. Magn Reson Med 2003;50(5):1053–60. © 2003 Wiley-Liss, Inc. Reprinted with permission from Wiley-Liss, Inc., a subsidiary of John Wiley & Sons, Inc.)

Helical MR has already shown that it is possible to acquire and display two to five axial frames per second. By modifying the technique to move the table at varying rates depending on the speed of catheter insertion, it may be possible to use moving table acquisition to track an interventional device. This methodology might allow interventional MR imaging to be done on even shorter-bore magnets, which would further enhance patient access during interventional procedures on cylindric-bore magnets.

Guiding and monitoring thermal therapy

Thermal therapy has been performed most commonly on brain, liver, and uterine tumors by decreasing the temperature of the targeted tissue by cryotherapy or by increasing the temperature by laser, RF, microwave, or focused ultrasound [23]. Currently, proton resonance frequency (PRF) shift is the method of choice for monitoring thermal therapy at mid to high magnetic fields (≥ 1 T) [29]. In the PRF method, the change in phase during a gradient recalled echo pulse sequence is used to calculate the temperature change (ΔT) [30]:

$$\Delta T = \frac{\Phi - \Phi_{baseline}}{\alpha \gamma \beta_0 TE} \tag{2}$$

where $\alpha = -0.01$ ppm/°C is the PRF change coefficient for aqueous tissue, γ is the gyromagnetic ratio, B_0 is the main magnetic field strength, TE is the echo time, and Φ_0 is the initial phase before heating. To generate accurate temperature maps, the image of interest must be completely registered with the baseline image. Any misregistration of the treatment and baseline images will be incorrectly interpreted as temperature variations, which can be detrimental to effective

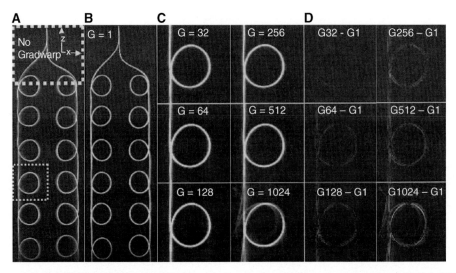

Fig. 9. (*A*) Uncorrected data that are blurred due to the moving acquisition and gradient nonuniformity. (*B*) Result when the correction is applied at each phase encoding step. (*C*) Result of grouping G phase encoding steps together and applying one correction to the whole group. (*D*) Subtraction images that show the worsening effect of grouping more and more steps together. (*From* Polzin JA, Kruger DG, Gurr DH, et al. Correction for gradient nonlinearity in continuously moving table MR imaging. Magn Reson Med 2004;52(1):185. © 2004 Wiley-Liss, Inc. Reprinted with permission from Wiley-Liss, Inc., a subsidiary of John Wiley & Sons, Inc.)

performance of thermal therapy. Breathing during hepatic tumor ablations is a good example of motion that has caused temperature estimation errors during interventional MR–guided thermal therapy.

To generate more accurate temperature maps during long, free-breathing interventional liver procedures, a method employing multiple background images and navigated images has been employed. The pulse sequence for the process is shown in Fig. 10A. In the pretreatment phase, a series of 8 to 12 baseline data sets are acquired. For each data set, the respiratory trigger point is incremented by 3% of the respiratory period to have baseline images over a wide range of diaphragm positions. The position of the diaphragm for each data set is calculated from the navigator data and is plotted for the user to see. Because the respiration is variable, there may be diaphragm positions that have been missed; therefore, the user can specify more trigger locations to have baseline images evenly distributed over all possible diaphragm locations. During the intervention, the following procedure is used to calculate the temperature map for each image (see Fig. 10C). For each line of k-space that is acquired, the position of the diaphragm from the corresponding navigator is calculated. The baseline navigators are searched for the navigator that has the closest

diaphragm position. The corresponding k-space line from the baseline image is put in a matrix. This procedure is done for all lines of acquired k-space to compile the appropriate background k-space image. The acquired k-space data are corrected for any linear phase distortions caused by small differences in diaphragm position between the acquired data and the compiled background k-space data, and then both data sets are inverse Fourier transformed. Calculation of the temperature change is done according to equation 2. This method of applying respiratory triggering with navigator diaphragm localization and multiple baseline image correction produces temperature maps with less distortions than simpler methods that use respiratory triggering only or respiratory triggering with navigator correction using a single baseline image (see Fig. 10D) [31].

Another approach using PRF involves eliminating the need for baseline images altogether by deriving the baseline phase in the treatment (heated) area from regions outside the thermal lesion in the same image [30]. In this method, a polynomial is fit to the phase outside of the heated region. The baseline phase in the heated region is extrapolated using the polynomial. This method produces images with less erroneous temperature variations than those obtained using a separate image for the background-phase estimation.

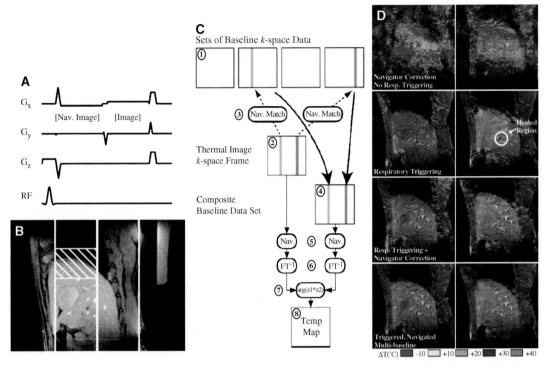

Fig. 10. (*A*) The pulse sequence used to acquire navigator (Nav.) and full-sized images. (*B*) Sagittal image of pig showing the location of the navigator over the diaphragm. (*C*) Schematic of the process used to determine the baseline image, correct for linear phase distortion, and generate the temperature map. (*D*) Temperature maps during laser heating of a porcine liver demonstrating the benefit of using the triggered, navigated, multibaseline method compared with using only navigator correction, doing only respiratory triggering, or using triggering and navigator correction without multiple baseline images. FT^{-1}, inverse Fourier transformation. (*From* Vigen KK, Daniel BL, Pauly JM, et al. Triggered, navigated, multi-baseline method for proton resonance frequency temperature mapping with respiratory motion. Magn Reson Med 2003;50(5):1003–10. © 2003 Wiley-Liss, Inc. Reprinted with permission from Wiley-Liss, Inc., a subsidiary of John Wiley & Sons, Inc.)

Pulse sequences used to estimate temperature changes based on the PRF phenomenon must be velocity compensated to prevent misinterpreting phase distortion from flowing blood as temperature variations [30]. Another modification that must be made to pulse sequences to avoid erroneous temperature mapping is suppression of the fat signal because fat and water precess at different resonant frequencies and fat does not have a temperature-dependent frequency shift [23,29].

Another recent advancement in the path toward completely noninvasive therapy has been the combined use of MR imaging and focused ultrasound therapy [32,33]. Initially MR imaging is used to locate the target location and to plan the course of treatment. Then, during focused ultrasound thermotherapy, PRF techniques are used to monitor temperature changes in the target tissue

and to prevent damage to surrounding healthy tissue. In this way, the accumulated thermal dose can be monitored and adjusted to ensure tissue necrosis. One benefit of focused ultrasound compared with other methods of achieving hyperthermia is the ability to heat an irregularly shaped lesion (other methods are restricted to a roughly ellipsoidal temperature contour) [23].

Summary

The motivations for developing MR–guided minimally invasive therapy include its excellent soft tissue contrast, tomographic imaging in any direction (as opposed to projection imaging as in fluoroscopy), the absence of ionizing radiation, the abundance of contrast mechanisms (including bright blood pulse sequences that lead to excellent vessel conspicuity without exogenous contrast agent injection), the ability to obtain physiologic information such as perfusion, and an overall excellent safety profile.

The main pulse sequences used today for interventional MR imaging are T1/T2-weighted FISP and TrueFISP, T2-weighted turbo spin-echo, and T1-weighted FLASH. The specific clinical question, the underlying pathophysiology, and the procedure to be performed dictate which sequence is used. Each of these sequences has been written to acquire data in conventional rectilinear trajectories, radial k-space paths, or even spirals. In many ways, the questions being researched in interventional MR imaging have been dictated by the primary issues in greatest need of resolution or that most directly facilitate new clinical development. A decade ago, research focused on exploration of new scan strategies for contrast and temporal resolution. Advancements in the last decade have made it possible to acquire and display greater than 10 images per second in real time with millimeter resolution in all three directions. This temporal and spatial resolution is considered high enough to guide most interventions. With this capability, other research has focused on instrument tracking. The field has gone from the capability to track a single coil and superimpose it on a previously acquired roadmap to systems that follow, adapt, and provide high-resolution images due to the advent of multichannel receiver systems, improved graphics, higher processor speeds, and increases in speed and quantity of memory. Hence, instruments can be reliably identified and tracked and the information can be used to update pulse sequence parameters in real time, thereby opening new opportunities for interventional MR imaging that extend from biopsy and thermal therapy to image-guided vascular and cardiac procedures. Today, we see such issues as RF heating of wires used for device localization and the noise generated by rapid switching of MR gradients being significant obstacles yet to overcome to allow the full strength of MR–guided interventions to be realized clinically. It is anticipated that these topics will emerge as critical concepts in the next decade of interventional MR imaging research.

References

[1] Duerk JL, Butts K, Hwang KP, et al. Pulse sequences for interventional magnetic resonance imaging. Top Magn Reson Imaging 2000;11(3):147–62.

[2] Boll DT, Lewin JS, Duerk JL, et al. Comparison of MR imaging sequences for liver and head and neck interventions: is there a single optimal sequence for all purposes? Acad Radiol 2004;11(5):506–15.

[3] Zangos S, Eichler K, Engelmann K, et al. MR-guided transgluteal biopsies with an open low-field system in patients with clinically suspected prostate cancer: technique and preliminary results. Eur Radiol 2005;15(1):174–82.

[4] Markl M, Alley MT, Pelc NJ. Balanced phase-contrast steady-state free precession (PC-SSFP): a novel technique for velocity encoding by gradient inversion. Magn Reson Med 2003;49(5):945–52.

[5] Deshpande VS, Chung YC, Zhang Q, et al. Reduction of transient signal oscillations in true-FISP using a linear flip angle series magnetization preparation. Magn Reson Med 2003;49(1):151–7.

[6] Guttman MA, Dick AJ, Raman VK, et al. Imaging of myocardial infarction for diagnosis and intervention using real-time interactive MRI without ECG-gating or breath-holding. Magn Reson Med 2004;52(2):354–61.

[7] Guttman MA, Kellman P, Dick AJ, et al. Real-time accelerated interactive MRI with adaptive TSENSE and UNFOLD. Magn Reson Med 2003;50(2):315–21.

[8] Peters DC, Guttman MA, Dick AJ, et al. Reduced field of view and undersampled PR combined for interventional imaging of a fully dynamic field of view. Magn Reson Med 2004;51(4):761–7.

[9] Roberts TP, Hassenzahl WV, Hetts SW, et al. Remote control of catheter tip deflection: an opportunity for interventional MRI. Magn Reson Med 2002;48(6):1091–5.

[10] Miquel ME, Hegde S, Muthurangu V, et al. Visualization and tracking of an inflatable balloon catheter using SSFP in a flow phantom and in the heart and great vessels of patients. Magn Reson Med 2004; 51(5):988–95.

[11] Martin AJ, Weber OM, Saeed M, et al. Steady-state imaging for visualization of endovascular interventions. Magn Reson Med 2003;50(2):434–8.

[12] Razavi R, Hill DL, Keevil SF, et al. Cardiac catheterisation guided by MRI in children and adults with congenital heart disease. Lancet 2003; 362(9399):1877–82.

[13] Eggers H, Weiss S, Boernert P, et al. Image-based tracking of optically detunable parallel resonant circuits. Magn Reson Med 2003;49(6):1163–74.

[14] Green JD, Omary RA, Finn JP, et al. Passive catheter tracking using MRI: comparison of conventional and magnetization-prepared FLASH. J Magn Reson Imaging 2002;16(1):104–9.

[15] Yeung CJ, Susil RC, Atalar E. RF safety of wires in interventional MRI: using a safety index. Magn Reson Med 2002;47(1):187–93.

[16] Quick HH, Zenge MO, Kuehl H, et al. Interventional magnetic resonance angiography with no

strings attached: wireless active catheter visualization. Magn Reson Med 2005;53(2):446–55.

[17] Wong EY, Zhang Q, Duerk JL, et al. An optical system for wireless detuning of parallel resonant circuits. J Magn Reson Imaging 2000;12(4):632–8.

[18] Buecker A, Adam GB, Neuerburg JM, et al. Simultaneous real-time visualization of the catheter tip and vascular anatomy for MR-guided PTA of iliac arteries in an animal model. J Magn Reson Imaging 2002;16(2):201–8.

[19] Bock M, Volz S, Zuhlsdorff S, et al. MR-guided intravascular procedures: real-time parameter control and automated slice positioning with active tracking coils. J Magn Reson Imaging 2004;19(5):580–9.

[20] Elgort DR, Wong EY, Hillenbrand CM, et al. Real-time catheter tracking and adaptive imaging. J Magn Reson Imaging 2003;18(5):621–6.

[21] Susil RC, Yeung CJ, Atalar E. Intravascular extended sensitivity (IVES) MRI antennas. Magn Reson Med 2003;50(2):383–90.

[22] Hillenbrand CM, Elgort DR, Wong EY, et al. Active device tracking and high-resolution intravascular MRI using a novel catheter-based, opposed-solenoid phased array coil. Magn Reson Med 2004;51(4):668–75.

[23] Schulz T, Puccini S, Schneider JP, et al. Interventional and intraoperative MR: review and update of techniques and clinical experience. Eur Radiol 2004;14(12):2212–27.

[24] Zhu Y, Dumoulin CL. Extended field-of-view imaging with table translation and frequency sweeping. Magn Reson Med 2003;49(6):1106–12.

[25] Goyen M, Quick HH, Debatin JF, et al. Whole-body three-dimensional MR angiography with a rolling table platform: initial clinical experience. Radiology 2002;224(1):270–7.

[26] Polzin JA, Kruger DG, Gurr DH, et al. Correction for gradient nonlinearity in continuously moving table MR imaging. Magn Reson Med 2004;52(1):181–7.

[27] Shankaranarayanan A, Herfkens R, Hargreaves BM, et al. Helical MR: continuously moving table axial imaging with radial acquisitions. Magn Reson Med 2003;50(5):1053–60.

[28] Glover G, Pelc N. Method for correcting image distortion due to gradient nonuniformity United States patent no. 4,591,789;1986.

[29] Weidensteiner C, Quesson B, Caire-Gana B, et al. Real-time MR temperature mapping of rabbit liver in vivo during thermal ablation. Magn Reson Med 2003;50(2):322–30.

[30] Rieke V, Vigen KK, Sommer G, et al. Referenceless PRF shift thermometry. Magn Reson Med 2004;51(6):1223–31.

[31] Vigen KK, Daniel BL, Pauly JM, et al. Triggered, navigated, multi-baseline method for proton resonance frequency temperature mapping with respiratory motion. Magn Reson Med 2003;50(5):1003–10.

[32] McDannold N, Moss M, Killiany R, et al. MRI-guided focused ultrasound surgery in the brain: tests in a primate model. Magn Reson Med 2003;49(6):1188–91.

[33] Palussiere J, Salomir R, Le Bail B, et al. Feasibility of MR-guided focused ultrasound with real-time temperature mapping and continuous sonication for ablation of VX2 carcinoma in rabbit thigh. Magn Reson Med 2003;49(1):89–98.

ELSEVIER
SAUNDERS

Magn Reson Imaging Clin N Am
13 (2005) 431–439

MAGNETIC
RESONANCE
IMAGING CLINICS
of North America

MR-Guided Endovascular Interventions: Device Visualization, Tracking, Navigation, Clinical Applications, and Safety Aspects

Frank K. Wacker, MD[a,b,*], Claudia M. Hillenbrand, PhD[b],
Jeffrey L. Duerk, PhD[b], Jonathan S. Lewin, MD[c,d]

[a]Department of Radiology, Klinik und Hochschulambulanz für Radiologie und Nuklearmedizin,
Charité–Universitätsmedizin Berlin, Campus Benjamin Franklin, Hindenburgdamm 30,
12200 Berlin, Germany
[b]Department of Radiology, Case Western Reserve University, University Hospitals of Cleveland,
11100 Euclid Avenue, Cleveland, OH 44106, USA
[c]Office of the Chairman, Department of Radiology, The Johns Hopkins Outpatient Center,
The Johns Hopkins Hospital, 601 North Caroline Street, Room 4210, Baltimore, MD 21287-0842, USA
[d]The Russell H. Morgan Department of Radiology and Radiological Science,
The Johns Hopkins School of Medicine, Baltimore, MD, USA

As minimally invasive procedures become increasingly important in medicine, the need for more advanced and accurate methods for guiding and controlling these procedures continues to grow. MR imaging has many potential advantages that make it an attractive tool to guide diagnostic and therapeutic procedures, such as its high soft tissue contrast, unrestricted multiplanar imaging capabilities, lack of ionizing radiation, and the ability to provide functional information such as flow velocities, diffusion, and perfusion. General aspects of the technical development of MR imaging that have helped promote interventional MR imaging include more open magnet designs, faster imaging techniques, interactive imaging, fast image reconstruction, and improved MR angiography techniques.

The first MR–guided clinical procedures were diagnostic biopsies that were performed similarly to CT-guided biopsies. After more open MR imaging systems became available, continuous imaging of the needle advancement became possible [1–5]. More recently, percutaneous MR–guided thermal ablation has received increasing attention, and the ability of MR imaging to produce MR angiograms, MR cholangiograms, and MR urograms for diagnostic purposes has made MR imaging a potentially attractive tool to guide endoluminal and endovascular procedures. The first clinical endoluminal MR–guided applications that used MR cholangiography or MR urography sequences to control and guide catheters and guidewires endoluminally were percutaneous cholangiographies and nephrostomies [6–12]. A great advantage of the MR imaging guidance of both procedures is its lack of ionizing radiation because both methods expose the interventionalist and the patient to relatively high radiation doses [13].

Although the avoidance of radiation exposure is important for patients and interventionalists, the rationale for using MR imaging as an endovascular guidance tool is based primarily on its ability to add therapeutically relevant information to an interventional endovascular procedure. Unlike any other imaging modality, MR imaging is able to display functional information such as flow,

---

* Corresponding author. Department of Radiology, Klinik und Hochschulambulanz für Radiologie und Nuklearmedizin, Charité–Universitätsmedizin Berlin, Campus Benjamin Franklin, Hindenburgdamm 30, 12200 Berlin, Germany.

E-mail address: frank.wacker@charite.de (F.K. Wacker).

perfusion, or diffusion, which can greatly influence the end point of an endovascular therapy. MR imaging can also add new morphologic information in atherosclerotic arteries, where it visualizes not only the lumen of the vessel (as does conventional angiography) but also the vessel wall and the surrounding tissues. This visualization becomes especially important with the growing knowledge that the luminal appearance does not completely describe the progress and severity of atherosclerotic disease in vessels because narrowing does not correspond to the potential danger (also known as plaque vulnerability) associated with this devastating disease. In addition to the diagnostic benefits, MR–guided endovascular procedures can be performed without an iodinated contrast agent, making it an even more valuable imaging modality.

Tracking and navigation

To track endovascular devices, several methods have been suggested and shown to be valuable. In the so-called "passive approach," visualization relies on the local field distortions produced by paramagnetic rings or ferrite admixtures [14–16] that show up as areas of signal loss in gradient-echo images (Fig. 1). Alternatively, paramagnetic contrast agents within the lumen [17] (Fig. 2) or doped onto the surface of a catheter [18] are used in combination with a T1-weighted sequence. Such visualization techniques are well known with needle interventions but are also used for catheter-based interventions. In contrast to stiff, straight biopsy needles that can be completely visualized in a single image acquired along the needle shaft, angiographic catheters are much more flexible and allow perfect adjustment to tortuous vessels inside the human body. Therefore, it is impossible to visualize an entire angiographic catheter with an imaging technique based on a single slice. Although the catheter tip is the main target for tracking, the whole catheter must be visualized continuously during an intervention to exclude loops in the catheter shaft. A solution would be to use a projection technique in combination with a background suppression technique that allows selective visualization of the entire catheter [19–21]. The principal disadvantage of most of the passive tracking techniques, even if they come with automatic tracking based on pattern recognition [22], is that they are image-based, thereby necessitating a relatively time-consuming tracking scheme that makes it difficult to achieve fast and automatic scan plane adjustments relative to the catheter tip.

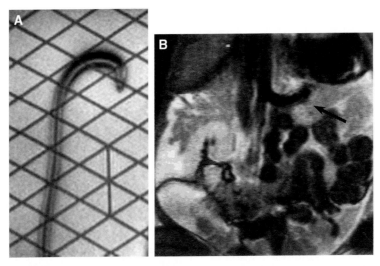

Fig. 1. Susceptibility artifact–based angiography catheter visualization. (*A*) MR image of a 5F C1-iron oxide containing a susceptibility artifact–inducing angiographic catheter in a gel phantom. Width of the artifact is 8 mm. (*B*) True fast imaging with steady-state precession images acquired in a 0.2-T open magnet during insertion of the iron oxide–containing angiographic catheter (*arrow*) shown in *A*. The catheter was advanced though the suprarenal aorta into the splenic artery. (*B, From* Wacker FK, Reither K, Branding G, et al. Magnetic resonance-guided vascular catheterization: feasibility using a passive tracking technique at 0.2 Telsa in a pig model. J Magn Reson Imaging 1999;10(5):843; with permission.)

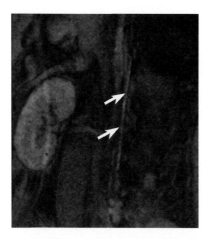

Fig. 2. Conventional angiographic catheter filled with 6% gadolinium diethylenetriamine pentaacetic acid solution. The catheter (*arrows*) is located in the aorta of a pig, with its tip in a suprarenal position.

In the "active approach" [23], small catheter-mounted receiver coils or antennas that are incorporated into the catheter (Fig. 3A, B) are used to determine the actual position of the catheter. The position of such coils within a two-dimensional projection slab can be visually monitored based on the strong signal generated by the radiofrequency microcoil when the transmit coil (in most cases the body coil) emits a nonselective radiofrequency pulse (see Fig. 3C, D). In contrast to this image-based approach, the MR imaging signal from the small tracking coils can be used to generate spatial coordinates for the catheter position in three-dimensional space. For this approach, only three gradient readouts are needed for localization of one coil, which makes this a very time-efficient method [24,25]. Based on the three-dimensional localization data of the coils, the position of the device inside the body is known without acquisition of an image. These localization data can be superimposed not only on MR roadmap images acquired before the intervention but also on images acquired in real time during the procedure (Fig. 4). In addition, automated scan plane adjustments based on the catheter position and automatic image parameter adaptation based on the catheter behavior inside the vessel [26,27] are easy to achieve (Fig. 5). With one single coil at the tip of the catheter, however, limited information is provided regarding the catheter shaft. One solution is to use a guidewire antenna in combination with a tip-marked catheter, each connected to a separate receiver channel [28,29]. With multiple receiver channels available, one can even use multiple microcoils along an angiographic catheter, each connected to a separate channel [30]. This system has the advantage of having peak unambiguity by applying the major three projections in x-, y-, and z-direction only. Another tracking technique is based on low flip angle amplification [13,31,32]. The main reason this technique was developed was to overcome the substantial drawback of excessive heat occurring around metallic devices in tracking approaches that use metallic wires or connecting signal cables inside the body to connect the antennas or coils to the MR scanner. To avoid the connecting cables, a coil or antenna tuned to the Larmor frequency of the scanner is attached to the tip of the catheter. This antenna couples the MR signal inductively into a surface coil. At low flip angles, the signal of resonant spins within the sensitive area of the catheter coil is amplified and couples into the surface coil. These spins appear bright due to the resonance in the coils, whereas the surrounding tissue gives a relatively low signal that is almost indistinguishable from sample noise. Such markers can be made switchable, without raising safety issues that result from metallic connecting cables, by using an optic fiber and a photo resistor within the circuit to detune the resonant circuit [33].

Applications

Shortly after the first interventional scanner became available, MR–guided catheter-based endovascular procedures were performed in animal models to test device visibility (see Fig. 1) and procedure feasibility [24,34–39]. More recently, complex procedures such as iliac and renal artery stenting (Fig. 6), coil embolization, septal occluder placement, and transjugular intrahepatic portosystemic shunt have been performed in preclinical settings [15,20,40–46]. Currently, there are only a few reports on MR–guided endovascular applications in patients [35,47–50]. These clinical applications are mainly feasibility studies that have not demonstrated the obvious additional benefit of MR imaging guidance for the specific procedure. Even with endovascular MR–guided procedures still in their infancy, however, the possibilities inherent in this technology offer completely new paradigms for almost any kind of intravascular therapy based on immediate functional information and more detailed morphologic information. It is fortunate that all major MR scanner manufacturers realize the potential of MR imaging to guide vascular

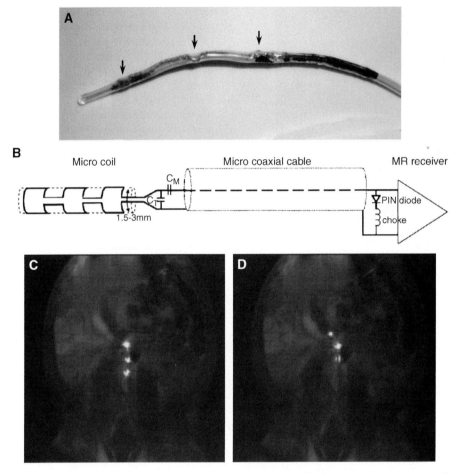

Fig. 3. Three-marker tracking coil. (*A*) Three geometrically separated microloops (*arrows*) are part of an active radiofrequency microantenna attached to the tip of a conventional angiographic catheter. (*B*) Schematic diagram of a three-element capacitively coupled tracking coil. The circuit is tuned to Larmor frequency of the MR scanner and matched to 50 Ω at the tip of catheter using capacitors C_T and C_M. Active detuning by way of positive-intrinsic-negative (PIN) diode and choke is accomplished remotely. Fifty-ohm microcoaxial cable is used to connect the tracking coil to an MR imaging receiver. (*C, D*) Images from a tracking experiment. The three-marker tracking coil is actively guided through the abdominal aorta (*C*) into the right renal artery (*D*) of a pig. (*B, Adapted from* Wacker FK, Elgort D, Hillenbrand CM, et al. The catheter-driven MR imaging scanner: a new approach to intravascular catheter tracking and imaging-parameter adjustment for interventional MRI. AJR Am J Roentgenol 2004;183(2):393; with permission.)

interventions so that shorter, more open MR scanners equipped with more flexible software, faster data transfer interfaces, and improved image reconstruction systems are being developed. Given the fact that interventional radiography units are highly specialized tools, it is nearly impossible to envision a multipurpose MR scanner that would allow all diagnostic procedures and any kind of MR–guided intervention.

As new scanner hardware is being developed, it is crucial for reliable tracking in delicate vessels to have imaging sequences that offer high temporal and spatial resolution for simultaneous device and anatomy visualization. An important obstacle in interventional MR imaging is that increased spatial resolution is often obtained at the cost of decreased temporal resolution. Techniques such as undersampled projection reconstruction [51], radial imaging [40], keyhole imaging [39], and parallel imaging [52] might become important as MR–guided endovascular applications evolve. It is beyond the scope of this article, however, to review technologies for fast MR imaging in more detail.

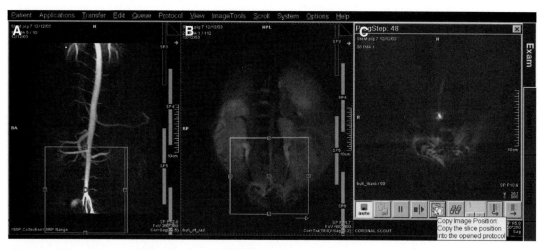

Fig. 4. Microcoil-based catheter tracking. Simultaneous display of the catheter tip position based on the three-dimensional localization data of the microcoil. The position is superimposed on an MR angiography roadmap image (*A*) and a single-slice MR image (*B*) acquired before the catheter insertion. In a separate window (*C*), the catheter localization can be controlled on images acquired in real time during the procedure.

Another crucial step for the further evolution of interventional MR imaging is to develop and manufacture MR-compatible, MR-visible, and MR-safe devices such as guidewires, diagnostic catheters, stents, and other interventional instruments. Without such dedicated instruments, no responsible interventionalist will risk performing clinical studies; however, these studies are necessary to demonstrate the benefits of MR imaging guidance for the patient and the interventionalist.

Radiation exposure and safety aspects of MR-guided vascular interventions

It is well known that MR–guided interventions do not involve ionizing radiation exposure. One might argue that stochastic radiation damage might not be relevant in elderly patients who often have high mortality, multimorbidity, and a low 10-year survival rate, but this argument does not hold true for the physicians and assistants present in the angiography suite during many interventions on a daily basis. Radiation exposure is also relevant for younger patients who are treated using an endovascular approach for heart disease, intracranial aneurysms, or intracranial arteriovenous malformations. Reducing radiation exposure is especially important for long-lasting, complex vascular interventions such as embolization procedures, percutaneous placement of transjugular portosystemic shunts, angioplasty, and stent placement and for cardiac

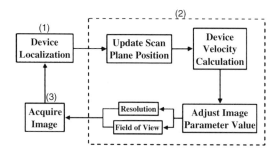

Fig. 5. Scheme of a catheter tracking system that facilitates automated scan plane adjustments and automatic image parameter adaptation based on the catheter behavior inside the vessel. System architecture includes three main components: (1) a localization technique, (2) data processing software, and (3) a fast imaging technique. (*From* Elgort DR, Wong EY, Hillenbrand CM, et al. Real-time catheter tracking and adaptive imaging. J Magn Reson Imaging 2003;18(5):622; with permission.)

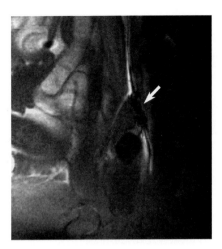

Fig. 6. MR–guided iliac artery stent placement in a pig. True fast imaging with steady-state precession image acquired in a 1.5-T short-bore magnet during insertion of a vascular stent (*arrow*) in the iliac arteries of a pig. The size of the stent artifact allows excellent visualization of the stent, but the vessel cannot be delineated.

electrophysiologic testing and ablation, for which deterministic radiation damage such as erythema and hair loss have been described in multiple reports [53–55]. Such damage is intolerable in any patient, regardless of age and life expectancy, and must therefore be prevented.

Although MR imaging does not have the risk of ionizing radiation, there are some hazards that must be accounted for when using interventional MR imaging [56]. Patients and medical staff who are present in the magnet room during data acquisition are exposed to static and dynamic magnetic fields and radiofrequency energy. For the diagnostic use of MR imaging, thresholds are defined that make adverse biologic effects unlikely; however, it remains unclear whether these values can also be used for longer-lasting and repeated exposure during MR–guided interventional procedures. Although there is no evidence of any direct biologic effect related to the use of interventional MR imaging, the pertinent literature does not include information derived from carefully controlled studies to unequivocally demonstrate the absolute safety of continued exposure to powerful magnetic fields [56]. This important question must therefore be explored more thoroughly. A well-known risk, especially for endovascular procedures, is the use of long metallic wires or cables used for signal transmission inside the magnet. As local temperature differences up to 44°C at 1.5 T

were observed [57–59], this potential risk must be addressed before routine clinical use of the active tracking technique in high-field systems [38,60].

Another important aspect of MR–guided interventions is acoustic noise. Fast and strong gradients that arise from real-time MR imaging sequences can approach the noise level of an airplane. The simplest and least expensive protective tools for patients are disposable earplugs that can decrease this noise by 10 to 30 dB, which usually affords adequate protection for MR-generated noise levels [56]. For the staff inside the magnet room, communication is essential during an intervention. Although the speech intelligibility is improved when wearing earplugs [61], headphones that allow effortless communication inside the scanner room can provide a significant benefit in an interventional MR environment (Fig. 7).

Another potential risk of interventional MR imaging is attributable to the fact that the magnetic field of an MR scanner attracts all ferromagnetic objects in immediate proximity to the scanner. It is not uncommon for accidents to occur as a result of surgical and other such instruments flying inside the magnet room. To

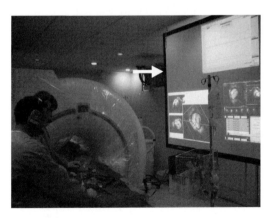

Fig. 7. Image from inside an interventional MR scanner suite during an MR–guided intervention. Interventionalists inside the magnet room are equipped with custom-made headsets that facilitate unimpaired communication during the intervention. The ceiling-mounted screen (*arrow*) shows three video streams back-projected from liquid crystal display–projectors presenting hemodynamics (*top*), interactive scanner control (*lower right*), and real-time interventional images (*lower left*). (*From* Dick AJ, Raman VK, Raval AN, et al. Invasive human magnetic resonance imaging during angioplasty: feasibility in a combined X-ray/MRI suite. Cathet Cardiovasc Intervent 2005;64(3):269.)

reduce this risk, ferromagnetic devices should not be allowed inside the magnet room. If it is necessary to use ferromagnetic objects during a procedure, they must be kept outside the 5-G line, and staff training in this respect is required. Even if expert users might know what can be used and what should kept outside the fringe field, a less experienced physician or assistant might not be aware of the risk associated with such instruments.

Summary

Reliable visualization and tracking are essential for guiding endovascular devices within blood vessels. The most commonly used methods are susceptibility artifact–based tracking that relies on the artifact created within the image by the device and microcoil- or antenna-based tracking that uses the high signal generated by small MR endovascular receive coils when the transmit coil emits a nonselective radiofrequency pulse. To date, the use of endovascular MR–guidance techniques has primarily been confined to animal experiments. There are only a few reports on MR–guided endovascular applications in patients. Therefore, access to the patient within the scanner, dedicated devices, and safety issues remain major challenges. To face these challenges, attention from all radiologists, especially interventional radiologists, is required to make MR–guided endovascular procedures a clinical reality.

References

[1] Silverman SG, Collick BD, Figueira MR, et al. Interactive MR-guided biopsy in an open-configuration MR imaging system. Radiology 1995;197(1):175–81.

[2] Frahm C, Gehl HB, Weiss HD, et al. [Technique of MRI-guided core biopsy in the abdomen using an open low-field scanner: feasibility and initial clinical results.]. Rofo Fortschr Geb Rontgenstr Neuen Bildgeb Verfahr 1996;164(1):62–7.

[3] Lu DS, Lee H, Farahani K, et al. Biopsy of hepatic dome lesions: semi-real-time coronal MR guidance technique. AJR Am J Roentgenol 1997;168(3):737–9.

[4] Lewin JS, Petersilge CA, Hatem SF, et al. Interactive MR imaging-guided biopsy and aspiration with a modified clinical C-arm system. AJR Am J Roentgenol 1998;170(6):1593–601.

[5] Zangos S, Kiefl D, Eichler K, et al. [MR-guided biopsies of undetermined liver lesions: technique and results.]. Rofo Fortschr Geb Rontgenstr Neuen Bildgeb Verfahr 2003;175(5):688–94.

[6] Faiss S, Zeitz M, Wolf KJ, et al. Magnetic resonance-guided biliary drainage in a patient with malignant obstructive jaundice and thrombocytopenia. Endoscopy 2003;35(1):89–91.

[7] Wacker F, Branding G, Wagner A, et al. MRI-guided cholangiography and drainage: assessment of passive catheter tracking in an animal model. Presented at the Sixth Scientific Meeting and Exhibition of the International Society for Magnetic Resonance in Medicine. Sydney, (Australia), April 18–24, 1998.

[8] Gohde SC, Pfammatter T, Steiner P, et al. MR-guided cholecystostomy: assessment of biplanar, real-time needle tracking in three pigs. Cardiovasc Intervent Radiol 1997;20(4):295–9.

[9] Hagspiel KD, Kandarpa K, Silverman SG. Interactive MR-guided percutaneous nephrostomy. J Magn Reson Imaging 1998;8(6):1319–22.

[10] Wacker FK, Faiss S, Reither K, et al. [MR imaging-guided biliary drainage in an open low-field system: first clinical experiences.]. Rofo Fortschr Geb Rontgenstr Neuen Bildgeb Verfahr 2000;172(9):744–7.

[11] Merkle EM, Hashim M, Wendt M, et al. MR-guided percutaneous nephrostomy of the nondilated upper urinary tract in a porcine model. AJR Am J Roentgenol 1999;172(5):1221–5.

[12] Nolte-Ernsting CC, Bucker A, Neuerburg JM, et al. MR imaging-guided percutaneous nephrostomy and use of MR-compatible catheters in the nondilated porcine urinary tract. J Vasc Interv Radiol 1999;10(10):1305–14.

[13] Williams JR. The interdependence of staff and patient doses in interventional radiology. Br J Radiol 1997;70(833):498–503.

[14] Rubin DL, Ratner AV, Young SW. Magnetic susceptibility effects and their application in the development of new ferromagnetic catheters for magnetic resonance imaging. Invest Radiol 1990;25(12):1325–32.

[15] Wacker FK, Reither K, Ebert W, et al. MR image-guided endovascular procedures with the ultrasmall superparamagnetic iron oxide SH U 555 C as an intravascular contrast agent: study in pigs. Radiology 2003;226(2):459–64.

[16] Bakker CJ, Hoogeveen RM, Weber J, et al. Visualization of dedicated catheters using fast scanning techniques with potential for MR-guided vascular interventions. Magn Reson Med 1996;36(6):816–20.

[17] Unal O, Korosec FR, Frayne R, et al. A rapid 2D time-resolved variable-rate k-space sampling MR technique for passive catheter tracking during endovascular procedures. Magn Reson Med 1998;40(3):356–62.

[18] Frayne R, Weigel C, Yanng Z, et al. MR evaluation of signal emitting coatings. In: Proceedings of the Seventh Scientific Meeting and Exhibition of the International Society for Magnetic Resonance in

Medicine. Berkeley (CA): International Society for Magnetic Resonance in Medicine; 1999. p. 580.

[19] Bakker CJ, Seppenwoolde JH, Bartels LW, et al. Adaptive subtraction as an aid in MR-guided placement of catheters and guidewires. J Magn Reson Imaging 2004;20(3):470–4.

[20] Omary RA, Frayne R, Unal O, et al. MR-guided angioplasty of renal artery stenosis in a pig model: a feasibility study. J Vasc Interv Radiol 2000;11(3): 373–81.

[21] Serfaty JM, Atalar E, Declerck J, et al. Real-time projection MR angiography: feasibility study. Radiology 2000;217(1):290–5.

[22] van der Weide R, Bakker CJ, Viergever MA. Localization of intravascular devices with paramagnetic markers in MR images. IEEE Trans Med Imaging 2001;20(10):1061–71.

[23] Dumoulin CL, Souza SP, Darrow RD. Real-time position monitoring of invasive devices using magnetic resonance. Magn Reson Med 1993;29(3): 411–5.

[24] Wacker FK, Reither K, Branding G, et al. Magnetic resonance-guided vascular catheterization: feasibility using a passive tracking technique at 0.2 Telsa in a pig model. J Magn Reson Imaging 1999;10(5): 841–4.

[25] Flask C, Elgort D, Wong E, et al. A method for fast 3D tracking using tuned fiducial markers and a limited projection reconstruction FISP (LPR-FISP) sequence. J Magn Reson Imaging 2001; 14(5):617–27.

[26] Elgort DR, Wong EY, Hillenbrand CM, et al. Real-time catheter tracking and adaptive imaging. J Magn Reson Imaging 2003;18(5):621–6.

[27] Wacker FK, Elgort D, Hillenbrand CM, et al. The catheter-driven MRI scanner: a new approach to intravascular catheter tracking and imaging-parameter adjustment for interventional MRI. AJR Am J Roentgenol 2004;183(2):391–5.

[28] Dick AJ, Guttman MA, Raman VK, et al. Magnetic resonance fluoroscopy allows targeted delivery of mesenchymal stem cells to infarct borders in swine. Circulation 2003;108(23):2899–904.

[29] Quick HH, Kuehl H, Kaiser G, et al. Interventional MR angiography with a floating table. Radiology 2003;229(2):598–602.

[30] Hillenbrand CM, Elgort DR, Wong EY, et al. Active device tracking and high-resolution intravascular MRI using a novel catheter-based, opposed-solenoid phased array coil. Magn Reson Med 2004;51(4):668–75.

[31] Burl M, Coutts GA, Young IR. Tuned fiducial markers to identify body locations with minimal perturbation of tissue magnetization. Magn Reson Med 1996;36(3):491–3.

[32] Quick HH, Zenge MO, Kuehl H, et al. Interventional magnetic resonance angiography with no strings attached: wireless active catheter visualization. Magn Reson Med 2005;53(2):446–55.

[33] Wong EY, Zhang Q, Duerk JL, et al. An optical system for wireless detuning of parallel resonant circuits. J Magn Reson Imaging 2000;12(4):632–8.

[34] Adam G, Glowinski A, Neuerburg J, et al. [Catheter visualization in MR-tomography: initial experimental results with field-inhomogeneity catheters.]. Rofo Fortschr Geb Rontgenstr Neuen Bildgeb Verfahr 1997;166(4):324–8.

[35] Bakker CJ, Hoogeveen RM, Hurtak WF, et al. MR-guided endovascular interventions: susceptibility-based catheter and near-real-time imaging technique. Radiology 1997;202(1):273–6.

[36] Glowinski A, Kursch J, Adam G, et al. Device visualization for interventional MRI using local magnetic fields: basic theory and its application to catheter visualization. IEEE Trans Med Imaging 1998;17(5):786–93.

[37] Ladd ME, Zimmermann GG, McKinnon GC, et al. Visualization of vascular guidewires using MR tracking. J Magn Reson Imaging 1998;8(1):251–3.

[38] Leung DA, Debatin JF, Wildermuth S, et al. Intravascular MR tracking catheter: preliminary experimental evaluation. Am J Roentgenol 1995;164(5): 1265–70.

[39] Wendt M, Busch M, Wetzler R, et al. Shifted rotated keyhole imaging and active tip-tracking for interventional procedure guidance. J Magn Reson Imaging 1998;8(1):258–61.

[40] Bücker A, Neuerburg JM, Adam G, et al. [MR-guided coil embolisation of renal arteries in an animal model.]. Rofo Fortschr Geb Rontgenstr Neuen Bildgeb Verfahr 2003;175(2):271–4.

[41] Kee ST, Rhee JS, Butts K, et al. Gary J, Becker Young Investigator Award. MR-guided transjugular portosystemic shunt placement in a swine model. J Vasc Interv Radiol 1999;10(5):529–35.

[42] Serfaty JM, Yang X, Foo TK, et al. MRI-guided coronary catheterization and PTCA: a feasibility study on a dog model. Magn Reson Med 2003; 49(2):258–63.

[43] Strother CM, Unal O, Frayne R, et al. Endovascular treatment of experimental canine aneurysms: feasibility with MR imaging guidance. Radiology 2000; 215(2):516–9.

[44] Yang X, Atalar E. Intravascular MR imaging-guided balloon angioplasty with an MR imaging guide wire: feasibility study in rabbits. Radiology 2000;217(2):501–6.

[45] Fink C, Bock M, Umathum R, et al. Renal embolization: feasibility of magnetic resonance-guidance using active catheter tracking and intraarterial magnetic resonance angiography. Invest Radiol 2004; 39(2):111–9.

[46] Rickers C, Jerosch-Herold M, Hu X, et al. Magnetic resonance image-guided transcatheter closure of atrial septal defects. Circulation 2003;107(1):132–8.

[47] Manke C, Nitz WR, Djavidani B, et al. MR imaging-guided stent placement in iliac arterial stenoses: a feasibility study. Radiology 2001;219(2):527–34.

[48] Manke C, Nitz WR, Lenhart M, et al. [Stent an-gioplasty of pelvic artery stenosis with MRI con-trol: initial clinical results.]. Rofo Fortschr Geb Rontgenstr Neuen Bildgeb Verfahr 2000;172(1): 92–7.

[49] Razavi R, Hill DL, Keevil SF, et al. Cardiac cathe-terisation guided by MRI in children and adults with congenital heart disease. Lancet 2003; 362(9399):1877–82.

[50] Paetzel C, Zorger N, Bachthaler M, et al. Feasibility of MR-guided angioplasty of femoral artery steno-ses using real-time imaging and intraarterial contrast-enhanced MR angiography. Rofo 2004; 176(9):1232–6.

[51] Peters DC, Lederman RJ, Dick AJ, et al. Under-sampled projection reconstruction for active cathe-ter imaging with adaptable temporal resolution and catheter-only views. Magn Reson Med 2003; 49(2):216–22.

[52] Guttman MA, Kellman P, Dick AJ, et al. Real-time accelerated interactive MRI with adaptive TSENSE and UNFOLD. Magn Reson Med 2003;50(2): 315–21.

[53] Miller DL, Balter S, Cole PE, et al. Radiation doses in interventional radiology procedures: the RAD-IR study: part I: overall measures of dose. J Vasc Interv Radiol 2003;14(6):711–27.

[54] Wong L, Rehm J. Images in clinical medicine. Radi-ation injury from a fluoroscopic procedure. N Engl J Med 2004;350(25):e23.

[55] Mooney RB, McKinstry CS, Kamel HA. Absorbed dose and deterministic effects to patients from inter-ventional neuroradiology. Br J Radiol 2000;73(871): 745–51.

[56] Shellock FG, Crues JV. MR procedures: biologic effects, safety, and patient care. Radiology 2004; 232(3):635–52.

[57] Konings MK, Bartels LW, Smits HF, et al. Heating around intravascular guidewires by resonating RF waves. J Magn Reson Imaging 2000;12(1):79–85.

[58] Liu CY, Farahani K, Lu DS, et al. Safety of MRI-guided endovascular guidewire applications. J Magn Reson Imaging 2000;12(1):75–8.

[59] Nitz WR, Oppelt A, Renz W, et al. On the heating of linear conductive structures as guide wires and cath-eters in interventional MRI. J Magn Reson Imaging 2001;13(1):105–14.

[60] Ladd ME, Quick HH. Reduction of resonant RF heating in intravascular catheters using coaxial chokes. Magn Reson Med 2000;43(4):615–9.

[61] Moelker A, Maas RA, Pattynama PM. Verbal com-munication in MR environments: effect of MR sys-tem acoustic noise on speech understanding. Radiology 2004;232(1):107–13.

Magn Reson Imaging Clin N Am
13 (2005) 441–464

MAGNETIC
RESONANCE
IMAGING CLINICS
of North America

Percutaneous Biopsy from Blinded to MR Guided: An Update on Current Techniques and Applications

Sherif Gamal Nour, MD[a,b,c,]*, Jonathan S. Lewin, MD[d,e]

[a]Department of Radiology, University Hospitals of Cleveland, 11100 Euclid Avenue, Cleveland, OH 44106, USA
[b]Departments of Radiology and Biomedical Engineering, Case Western Reserve University School of Medicine,
319 Wickenden Building, Cleveland, OH 44106, USA
[c]Department of Diagnostic Radiology, Cairo University Hospitals, Cairo, Egypt
[d]Department of Radiology, The Johns Hopkins Hospital, 600 North Wolfe Street,
Baltimore, MD 21287, USA
[e]The Russell H. Morgan Department of Radiology and Radiological Science,
The Johns Hopkins University School of Medicine, 720 Rutland Avenue, Baltimore, MD 21205, USA

Paul Ehrlich was studying the postprandial glycogen content of the liver in healthy subjects and diabetics when he performed the first known percutaneous living human biopsy (Greek: *bios*, life; *opsi*s, sight) in 1883 at the Charité Hospital in Berlin [1–3] more than a decade before Roentgen discovered x-rays in 1895. A quote from a description of this procedures reads: "…after withdrawing the stylus, there entered into the bore of the trocar sometimes a few drops of blood but usually, in addition, some liver cells either isolated or in groups; occasionally a larger worm-like portion of liver tissue would be found in the trocar, which was (then) hardened in alcohol, and sectioned after embedding in Celluloidin" [1]. Later, in France (1907), Schupfer [4] published the first series of percutaneous biopsies for the diagnosis of cirrhosis and hepatic tumors.

The reports of percutaneous biopsies that followed in the early 1900s generated much dispute within the medical community, with grave reservations over the reported mortalities [5,6] and skepticism regarding the diagnostic value of these tiny pieces of tissue among pathologists whose primary function at that time was the study of death through necropsy (Greek: *necros*, corpse) rather than biopsy [3].

By the middle of the 1900s, the development of histopathologic techniques, the increasing familiarity of pathologists with the interpretation of biopsies [7], and the collected experience of physicians [8–10] were met by an increasing interest in tissue diagnosis prompted by the World War II epidemics of hepatitis, which created an environment in which the practice of percutaneous biopsies, especially of the liver, began to thrive [3].

Physicians have since been practicing percutaneous biopsies and aspirations of palpable pathologic findings [11,12], superficial body parts [13–15], and deep organs [16–23] using surface anatomy landmarks without image guidance.

The subsequent incorporation of image guidance while attempting percutaneous tissue diagnosis has been a milestone that has changed the face of the practice of these procedures. During the 1960s, reports began to emerge that described the improved puncture using "modern radiological techniques" under x-ray fluoroscopy [24–27]. Soon after, during the 1970s, the techniques of biopsy as practiced today began to materialize and to blossom as a result of the pioneering work of Holm and Goldberg and their colleagues [28,29] in ultrasound (US)-guided interventions

* Corresponding author. Department of Radiology, University Hospitals of Cleveland, 11100 Euclid Avenue, Cleveland, OH 44106.
   E-mail address: nour@uhrad.com (S.G. Nour).

and of Haaga and his colleagues [30–32] in CT-guided interventions.

The scene of patients transferred from hospital wards to radiology departments to undergo percutaneous biopsy or aspiration has gradually become customary, with the expectations from these procedures raised well beyond "obtaining tissue and avoiding mortality." Procedural complications became readily identifiable and manageable, thereby increasing the procedure safety, minimizing periprocedural patient discomfort, and providing an insight into the effects of instrument placement in tissue. Additionally, image guidance has led to improvement of the diagnostic yield of obtained specimens, to the ability to target focal disease processes rather than diffuse organ pathologic findings under direct visualization, and, in some cases, to the avoidance of invasive surgical biopsies and drains by allowing access to anatomic locations that could not be approached using the blind techniques.

MR imaging era

Since its inception for clinical diagnostic scanning in the early 1980s, MR imaging has brought new dimensions to the realm of diagnostic imaging with an unprecedented level of soft tissue contrast and clarity of anatomic details, but it was not until turn of the decade before investigators began to explore the possibility of using this robust imaging modality to guide percutaneous procedures [33–39].

The term *interventional MR imaging* was then introduced into the medical terminology to describe the use of MR imaging techniques for rapid guidance and/or monitoring of minimally invasive diagnosis or therapy, with the entire procedure performed in the interventional MR imaging suite in a manner analogous to conventional angiographic or sonographically guided interventions.

Early efforts in this field focused on designing new MR imaging–compatible biopsy needles [32,33,36], on performing simple needle navigations in the MR imaging environment [35,37–39], and, subsequently, on studying the various parameters that affect device visibility during interventional MR imaging procedures [40,41]. The enthusiasm of radiologists to take advantage of the superb image quality of MR imaging to perform safer interventions was, however, significantly hampered by their inability to access the patients located within the long closed bores of superconducting magnets and by the long image acquisition times that precluded timely updates of device position during navigation.

MR imaging scientists have since been striving to facilitate patient access through the introduction of open scanners and the development of what is now referred to as "MR fluoroscopy" through the innovation of rapid gradient echo pulse sequences that would allow time-effective acquisition, reconstruction, and display of MR imaging scans in near real-time. These arms of development, "open scanning" and "rapid scanning," were confounded by the associated significant loss of signal-to-noise ratio that would deprive MR imaging of its basic advantage of unparalleled clarity of anatomic details and would thereby place the whole notion of MR imaging guidance into question.

The era of the 1990s witnessed the development of the core technology, including fast efficient magnetic gradients and high-quality low-noise receiver chains that allowed rapid acquisition of high signal-to-noise ratio images in the open low-field environment and therefore rendered interventional MR imaging a viable branch of the current clinical radiologic practice, with a growing sector of radiologists and scientists being actively involved in practicing and refining its technology [42–49]. Currently, interventional MR imaging has moved from the laboratory to the clinic, with many academic radiology departments inside and outside the United States having interventional MR imaging capabilities and routinely scheduling patients for MR-guided procedures.

Interventional MR imaging suites

Interventional MR imaging suites share three fundamental requirements: the availability of an open-field scanner configuration to facilitate patient access, the ability to implement rapid pulse sequences to ensure safe device placement, and the ability to operate the scanner and to review updated images at the patient's bedside without having to remove the operator's hand at any time from the interventional device. The designs of this equipment do, however, vary according to the manufacturer, nature of procedures performed, and user preferences, for example. Most of the open scanners use low- or middle-field magnets. A few institutions have recently installed newer generations of open-bore high-field scanners. Other institutions are implementing hybrid systems that incorporate conventional x-ray fluoroscopic units into the interventional MR imaging suite. See the article by Merkle and colleagues elsewhere in this issue for further exploration of interventional MR imaging equipment.

The advantages of using MR imaging for biopsy and/or aspiration guidance are related to several inherent features of this imaging technique and can be outlined as follows [50–53]:

1. The unparalleled high soft tissue contrast allows confident needle navigation in areas of complex anatomy and permits visualization of some lesions that are not resolved on US or CT scanning.
2. The ability to shift between T1- and T2-weighted contrast during the procedure allows maximization of the anatomic and/or pathologic conspicuity. For example, T2-weighted techniques allow sampling of the nonnecrotic regions of complex masses, thereby increasing the diagnostic tissue yield. T2 weighting is also helpful in delineating submucosal pharyngeal and laryngeal lesions that are often difficult to define on CT and may be hidden by normal overlying mucosa on endoscopic examination.
3. The multiplanar imaging capabilities ensure precise centralization of the biopsy needle along the axial as well as the craniocaudad dimension in the anatomy of interest. In addition, imaging in any arbitrary plane allows the device trajectory to be tailored according to the individual case.
4. The ability to visualize vascular structures continuously during the entire procedure without contrast administration is ensured. The high vascular conspicuity is attributable to flow-related enhancement effects characteristic of the gradient echo sequences used for procedure guidance. This feature is particularly helpful when advancing a needle in the vicinity of vital vascular structures, such as in the suprahyoid neck and in the retroperitoneum.

Needle visualization in the MR imaging environment

Unlike guidance using US or x-ray–based techniques, such as fluoroscopy and CT, there are a number of user-defined imaging parameters and needle trajectory decisions that can markedly alter device visibility and therefore affect the accuracy and safety of MR-guided biopsy and aspiration [40].

Pulse sequence–dependent factors

Sequence design (spin echo, turbo spin echo, and rapid gradient echo)

The most important pulse sequence issue with regard to needle visibility is the sensitivity of the sequence to magnetic susceptibility effects [40]. The commonly used rapid gradient echo (GRE) sequences (fast imaging with steady-state precession [FISP], true FISP, and mirrored fast imaging with steady-state precession [PSIF]) are associated with more prominent susceptibility artifacts from needles than are the relatively slower spin echo (SE) or turbo spin echo (TSE) sequences. Therefore, to reduce artifactual needle widening, the use of TSE imaging for position confirmation or primary guidance should be strongly considered when needle placement within 5 mm of major neurovascular structures is contemplated rather than relying on the more rapid GRE sequences for guidance of the entire procedure [50,51].

Field strength

The higher the MR imaging field strength, the larger is the apparent width of the needles and other interventional devices used (Fig. 1). On the low-field (0.2-T) system, the apparent needle width under GRE image guidance ranges from approximately 4 mm for smaller gauges to 9 mm for larger gauges [40]. Although this degree of artifactual widening is acceptable for larger lesions in areas of low neurovascular density, such as the abdomen and extremities, it is clearly unacceptable for lesions located in complex anatomic regions or adjacent to major vessels. The degree of artifactual widening can be reduced by approximately a factor of 2 by using a TSE pulse sequence or higher sampling bandwidth [40].

Pulse sequence sampling bandwidth

The higher the sampling bandwidth, the less apparent is the needle and/or interventional device widening [40].

Frequency-encoding direction

When frequency encoding is perpendicular to the needle, it results in artifactual widening. When parallel to the needle, it results in less obvious artifact at the tip and hub of the needle. Depending on needle composition and orientation, swapping the frequency- and phase-encoding axes relative to the needle shaft can reduce or increase

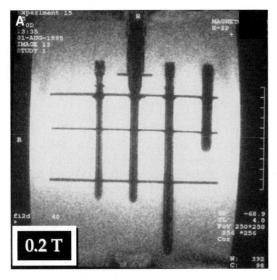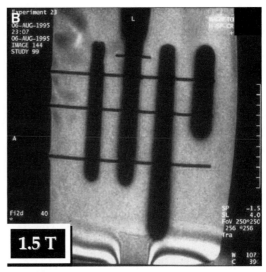

Fig. 1. Effect of magnetic field strength on needle visualization. MR imaging scans of the same set of various needles were taken at 0.2 T (*A*) and 1.5 T (*B*). Both sets were imaged with a fast gradient echo sequence commonly used to guide interventions (fast imaging with steady-state free precession), with the shafts of needles perpendicular to the static magnetic field. Note the marked artifactual widening of the needles caused by the higher magnetic field strength in (*B*). (*From* Lewin JS, Duerk JL, Jain VR, et al. Needle localization in MR-guided biopsy and aspiration: effects of field strength, sequence design, and magnetic field orientation. AJR Am J Roentgenol 1996;166(6):1337–45; with permission.)

the apparent needle width by a factor of 0.33 to 2.5 for TSE sequences [40] (Fig. 2). This effect can be used to decrease the apparent needle width when the needle artifact obscures adjacent anatomic structures by setting the frequency-encoding axis of the image parallel to the needle shaft [50,51]. In the presence of even mild respiratory motion, the needle tip for thinner (eg, 22-gauge) needles can be difficult to visualize with certainty in tissue. Therefore, in our experience, this effect is usually more useful to identify the needle tip location more confidently on TSE images by maximizing the needle artifact through frequency encoding the image in a direction perpendicular to the needle shaft.

Needle-dependent factors

Needle composition

The optimal material for needle fabrication varies with MR imaging system field strength. Relatively less expensive materials, such as high-nickel high-chromium stainless steel, may be adequate at 0.2 T but may give rise to unacceptable artifact at 1.5 T [40,41]. Conversely, small-caliber needles constructed from low-artifact materials, such as titanium, may be difficult to identify in certain clinical settings at low field strength.

Needle orientation relative to the main magnetic field

The apparent needle diameter diminishes markedly from a decrease in artifact as the needle shaft approaches the axis of the static magnetic field (Fig. 3) [33,40,41]. Artifacts resulting from field distortion arise most significantly where the field enters and exits objects of differing magnetic susceptibilities, such as the needle and surrounding tissue.

When the needle is parallel to the field, distortion of the field (and therefore image artifact) occurs mostly at the tip and hub and, to a lesser extent, along the needle shaft. The field is increased within the needle shaft. Because there are no protons to image within the needle, however, no image distortion occurs. The field is also distorted slightly adjacent to the shaft. At low fields, this distortion is much less than the effect of the applied imaging gradients; therefore, little mismapping occurs with the artifact along the shaft, related primarily to mild signal loss caused by decreased T2*. When the needle is perpendicular to the main magnetic field (B_0), the field enters and exits throughout the length of the shaft. Local field distortion, and thus more prominent artifact, can thus be observed along the entire needle.

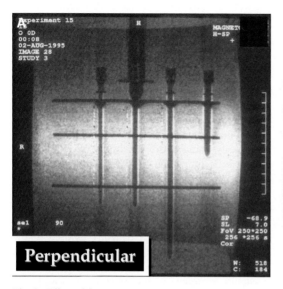
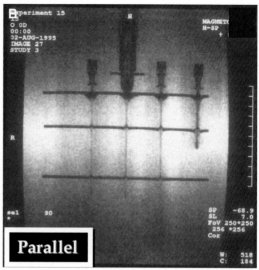

Fig. 2. Effect of frequency-encoding direction on needle visualization. Spin echo MR imaging scans of the same set of needles as in Fig. 7 were obtained with the frequency-encoding direction perpendicular to needle shafts (*A*) and parallel to needle shafts (*B*). The sequence used in (*A*) resulted in more artifactual needle widening than that used in (*B*) yet rendered the needle tip more visible. (*From* Lewin JS, Duerk JL, Jain VR, et al. Needle localization in MR-guided biopsy and aspiration: effects of field strength, sequence design, and magnetic field orientation. AJR Am J Roentgenol 1996;166(6):1337–45; with permission.)

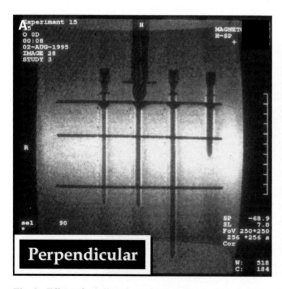
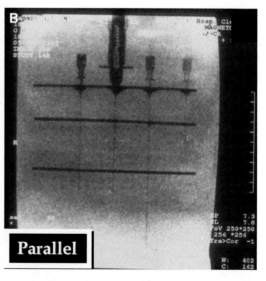

Fig. 3. Effect of needle orientation relative to visualization of the main magnetic field (B_0). Spin echo MR imaging scans of the same set of needles as in Figs. 7 and 8 were obtained with needle shafts perpendicular (*A*) and parallel (*B*) to a static magnetic field at 0.2 T. Note the marked reduction in artifactual needle widening when needles are parallel to the static magnetic field. This effect can render smaller needles invisible during interventions. (*From* Lewin JS, Duerk JL, Jain VR, et al. Needle localization in MR-guided biopsy and aspiration: effects of field strength, sequence design, and magnetic field orientation. AJR Am J Roentgenol 1996;166(6):1337–45; with permission.)

Although the apparent needle width decreases as it is positioned parallel to the static magnetic field (vertically for most biplanar magnets and along the long axis of cylindrical or "double-donut" systems), artifact at the device tip blooms and obscures the true tip position. Steep needle trajectories may be more familiar from experience with CT or US guidance or may seem to be advantageous in some anatomic locations but may not be appropriate because of poor needle conspicuity and loss of tip position information.

Interactive MR imaging guidance techniques

Several methods may be used to guide interactive near–real-time needle navigation toward the target pathologic finding under MR imaging. The choice among these techniques is based on several factors, including the level of comfort of the interventionalist with a particular method, the availability of the technology, and the nature of the procedure.

Freehand technique

This is the simplest and the most commonly used technique of MR imaging guidance because it does not involve further equipment in addition to the basic interventional package and because it fits the skill set developed by radiologists during

their earlier use of more conventional image guidance under fluoroscopy, US, and CT scanning (Fig. 4).

The skin entry point may be located using a fingertip [54] or a syringe filled with water for T2-weighted image guidance [53] or with dilute gadolinium for a T1-weighted approach [55]. The needle is then advanced into the targeted pathologic finding under MR "fluoroscopic" guidance, generally using short repetition time (TR) and short echo time (TE) GRE sequences. The choice of tissue contrast weighting during the guidance phase depends on the organ and the lesion attempted, as discussed in the section on current applications. Such choice is, however, a largely flexible process and is frequently tailored to the best individual conspicuity of a particular lesion as it appears on preprocedural imaging. We thus usually examine the conspicuity of the target lesion on a group of preset "biopsy sequences" and assess the optimal needle trajectory and patient position during or before the procedure.

The guidance phase itself consists of a continuous imaging mode that allows automated sequential acquisition, reconstruction, and in-room display of multiple sets of three contiguous, parallel, thin slices centered on the needle position. Image sets in two orthogonal scan planes oriented along the shaft of the needle are used during this continuous imaging mode to guide its

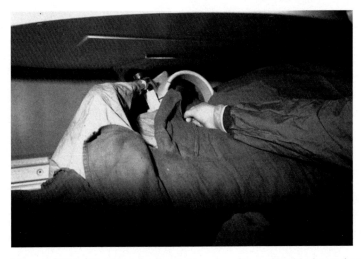

Fig. 4. Freehand technique for MR-guided biopsy and aspiration. A surface coil is placed over the area of interest, and the biopsy needle is inserted under interactive MR imaging guidance while the MR imaging scans are reconstructed and displayed on the in-room radiofrequency-shielded monitor shown in Fig. 5 or on a large free-standing screen. The system enables the interventionalist to operate the scanner and to replot the scan plane as desirable at the patient's bedside. This method permits an unrestricted approach to the target anatomy. The belt-shaped surface coil provides depth coverage approximately equal to the diameter of the closed ring.

insertion with respect to the three-dimensional (3D) geometry of the target. In this process, the scan plane is plotted manually by the operator and must be readjusted whenever the needle trajectory is modified.

Stereotactic techniques

Frame-based stereotaxy systems

These systems use MR imaging–compatible versions of the traditional external stereotactic frames that enable calculation of target location based on Cartesian coordinates and allow needle advancement along a set of predetermined trajectories. They have long been used in neurosurgery, although they involve mounting cumbersome rigid frames to the patient's head. They also suffer the limitations of their inability to navigate beyond fixed trajectories and of not compensating for intraprocedural tissue shift. MR-guided intracranial biopsies and aspirations are therefore largely performed with one of the frameless stereotaxy methods described below or using the freehand technique. Frame-based stereotaxy remains, however, the mainstay of MR-guided breast biopsies at most institutions, as detailed in the section on breast applications.

Frameless stereotaxy systems

These systems offer the accuracy of a measured stereotactic approach while maintaining the convenience of a liberal freehand technique and allowing navigation in unlimited trajectories because they are not restricted by fixed local coordinate systems. They do, however, involve additional equipment and/or software and may possibly add an element of complexity when used during otherwise straightforward procedures.

Optically linked stereotaxy. This technique is based on actively coupling the scan plane to the orientation of the interventional device. This is facilitated by mounting light-emitting diodes (LEDs) or small reflective balls to the interventional device and installing an infrared camera that continuously monitors the emitted or reflected light. This data is constantly fed to a 3D digitizer, thereby updating the information about the spatial orientation of the device. This information is shared through a common interface with the measurement control software of the MR imager, which is then enabled to execute a scan automatically along the new orientation of the interventional device.

Previously, frameless stereotactic systems had been used primarily for surgical guidance based on historic imaging data sets. The ability to acquire MR images rapidly and interactively in an arbitrary plane determined by a handheld sterilizable probe or other interventional device allows rapid planning and confirmation of complex trajectories for rigid instruments. This type of interactive image guidance system was first described as a component (Flashpoint; Image Guided Technologies, Boulder, Colorado) of the double-donut system (SIGNA SP; General Electric Medical Systems, Milwaukee, Wisconsin) and has subsequently been applied for guidance of image acquisition on C-arm systems (developed in collaboration with Radionics, Burlington, Massachusetts and Siemens Medical Systems, Erlangen, Germany) (Fig. 5) [50,51,56–59].

Active tracking. This is another technique for automatic scan position and/or plane readjustment during freehand navigation that is based on the same idea of actively linking the image plane to the orientation of the interventional device. The link does not, however, use infrared light as in the optical tracking system and thereby eliminates the need for expensive stereotactic cameras and other added equipment.

Rather, this versatile system replaces the hardware equipment with a software interface that was developed in our laboratory and serves to link the measurement unit of the imager with prototype wireless fiducial markers tuned to the resonance frequency of the scanner and mounted to biopsy needles or to other interventional devices. The active tracking technology has been successfully validated on an experimental basis [60]; however, no clinical data are yet available using this system. The method has also been effectively used to drive image acquisition during intravascular flexible catheter and coil tracking under MR imaging, where tracking markers are also used for high-resolution catheter-based vessel wall imaging [61]. An "adaptive image parameters" software has also been reported [62,63] that can be used in conjunction with active tracking to allow automated intraoperative adjustments of imaging parameters other than scan plane position and/ or orientation, such as field of view (FOV), temporal resolution, and tissue contrast.

Prospective stereotaxy. In contrast to optically linked and adaptive tracking frameless stereotaxy that is based on continuously updating the scan

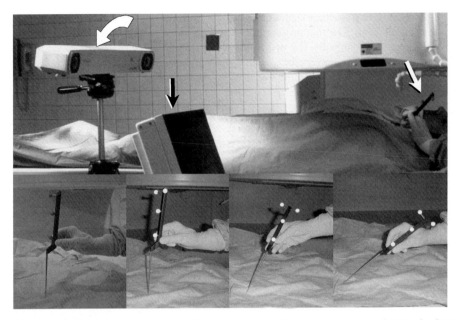

Fig. 5. Optical tracking system. A two-camera video sensor array (*curved white arrow*) detects the location and orientation of a handheld probe or needle guide (*straight white arrow and lower row*). The system automatically acquires continuous MR imaging based on the probe position and automatically updates a display of three images on a shielded liquid crystal display monitor adjacent to the scanner (*straight black arrow*). It is essential to maintain a clear line of sight between the camera system and the probe for this tracking mechanism to function. (Courtesy of Siemens Medical Systems, Erlangen, Germany; with permission.)

plane to match needle orientation until the target is located, Truwit and Liu [64] have described a prospective frameless stereotaxy method to guide neuronavigation, which basically works in the reverse. It starts by locating the target, which is then aligned with a pivot point, where a trajectory guide (Navigus; Image-guided Neurologics, Melbourne, Florida) is secured to the patient's skull. The needle trajectory is subsequently aligned on a virtual line in the space along the extension of these two points: the intracranial target and the skull pivot point (Fig. 6). Once the needle is aligned along the correct trajectory, the pivot is locked and repeated fluoroscopic MR imaging scans can be obtained to monitor needle advancement toward the target in near real-time (Fig. 7) [65,66].

Augmented reality techniques

These systems are intended to facilitate quick and accurate targeting for needle biopsies outside the closed bores of superconducting magnets while taking advantage of the image quality of high-field scanners. The patient is first scanned in the usual fashion, and the MR imaging table is then moved outside the scanner, where a 3D display mounted to the radiologist's head and using the augmented reality system maps the acquired data into the patient's body space, thus enabling in situ perception of MR imaging (Fig. 8) [67–70]. These systems provide a time-efficient approach with intuitive hand-eye coordination while eliminating the spatial restrictions imposed by factors like needle length and geometry of the closed-bore scanners during high-field interventions, because the actual procedure is performed outside the magnet. Additionally, there are no restrictions on the choice of the skin entry point or the patient's position during the intervention, because the preprocedural MR imaging data set can be acquired and reformatted in any plane.

The major limitation of augmented reality systems is, however, the fact that image plane calibration is based on the assumption that no patient or internal organ movement occurred between the time of the preprocedural scan and the time of actual needle insertion. These systems are therefore more suitable for targeting lesions that do not suffer respiratory motion, such as those within the pelvis, retroperitoneum, and musculoskeletal system, while ensuring adequate

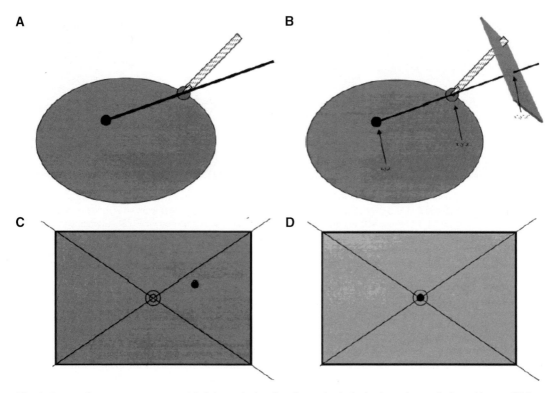

Fig. 6. Prospective stereotaxy system. (*A*) Schematic drawing shows the desired orientation, as indicated by a solid line connecting the target point and the pivot point. (*B*) Schematic drawing shows an imaging plane that is placed approximately perpendicular to the solid line and intersects the MR imaging–visible alignment stem. (*C*) Schematic drawing shows a cross-sectional view of the alignment stem (*black dot*) before the ideal position of the alignment stem (center of donut). (*D*) Alignment stem now is perfectly coincident with the ideal position. (*Adapted from* Truwit CL, Liu H. Prospective stereotaxy: a novel method of trajectory alignment using real-time image guidance. J Magn Reson Imaging 2001;13(3):452–7; with permission.)

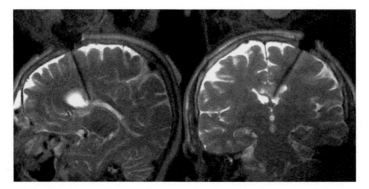

Fig. 7. Brain biopsy using prospective stereotaxy. MR imaging performed during brain biopsy using the trajectory guide and method confirms perfect placement of the biopsy needle within the target lesion (proven astrocytoma) in sagittal and coronal planes. (*Adapted from* Truwit CL, Liu H. Prospective stereotaxy: a novel method of trajectory alignment using real-time image guidance. J Magn Reson Imaging 2001;13(3):452–7; with permission.)

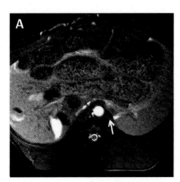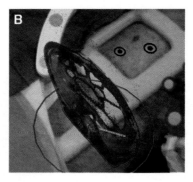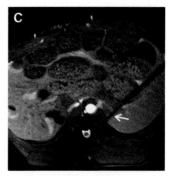

Fig. 8. Augmented reality (AR)–guided MR imaging–based biopsy. (*A*) Baseline true fast imaging with steady-state precession (FISP) image (TR/TE: 3.03/1.52 milliseconds, flip angle of 70°, 6-mm slice thickness) is used for target (*arrow*) selection in a swine model. The same MR imaging scan is used to create the augmented view. (*B*) Augmented view of the needle placement as shown by the AR guidance system. The needle (*blue*) as well as its projected forward extension (*yellow*) is visualized as a thin cylinder. The target structure is represented by the central green disk; the outer rings merge as the operator advances the needle. In contrast to this two-dimensional impression, the user is provided with a stereoscopic view of the augmented scene. (*C*) MR imaging control scan (true FISP) after AR-guided puncture demonstrating the needle (*arrow*) in position. (*From* Wacker FK, Vogt V, Khamene A, et al. An augmented reality system for MRI-guided needle biopsies. Stud Health Technol Inform 2003;94:151 7; with permission.)

immobilization of the patient's entire body. To target liver lesions that move during the breathing cycle, a breathing motion correction must be implemented.

Similarly, adjustments to needle trajectory during advancement spoils needle calibration and results in missing the targeted lesion [67]. Rather, the needle should be advanced on a predetermined path along a virtual line extending from the skin entry point to the target.

Image fusion techniques

These methods aim to maximize the information content provided to the interventionalist during the procedure by integrating functional and/or metabolic data into the usual anatomic images while the latter are being interactively updated to reflect the temporal position of the interventional device and its relation to vital structures. These techniques are still largely investigational, although a few groups have reported on clinical applications almost exclusively in guiding neurologic procedures [71–75]. The freehand and stereotactic techniques of guidance are applicable using these methods.

The ability to register data, such as functional MR imaging data, to the corresponding anatomic volume during neuronavigation can clearly contribute to a more favorable procedure outcome by enabling the salvage of critical areas (eg, eloquent cortex) via direct visualization rather than by relying on knowledge of their expected locations.

Likewise, the fusion of positron emission tomography (PET) and MR imaging scans augments the morphologic data with an insight into metabolic activity of the tissues, thereby helping to direct biopsy needles or other interventional devices to areas of viable tumor cells (Fig. 9). This approach can be particularly helpful to enhance the target definition in some territories, such as the prostate gland, where visualization of small tumors remains a significant challenge. Similarly, multimodal image fusion can incorporate a wide array of preprocedural data sets, such as MR angiograms, CT, or single photon emission computed tomography (SPECT) images, to provide a "road map" that fits the particular needs during an MR-guided procedure.

With the ongoing exciting advancements in the entire field of medical imaging, embracing the technology of multimodal image fusion seems to hold a strong potential to revolutionize MR-guided diagnostic and therapeutic interventions so that the future may witness the incorporation of data from such technologies as cellular and molecular imaging into a working paradigm of interventional MR imaging.

Current applications

Percutaneous biopsy and/or aspiration was the first reported use of MR imaging to guide interventional procedures. Much of the early work in this field has revolved around sampling

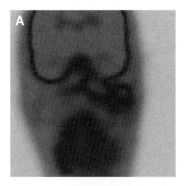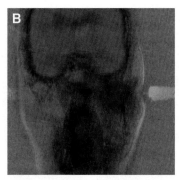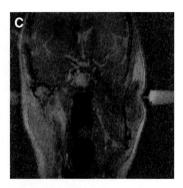

Fig. 9. Multimodal image fusion during biopsy guidance. Fluorodeoxyglucose positron emission tomography scan before (*A*) and after (*B, C*) fusion with a coronal MR imaging scan demonstrates a large area of increased tracer uptake at the left side of upper neck corresponding to an ill-defined soft tissue mass lesion centered on the ipsilateral masticator space, encroaching on the parapharyngeal space, and extending superiorly to erode the skull base. Such integration of metabolic information into the anatomic data set helps to enhance the accuracy of targeting and thereby the diagnostic yield, particularly in small or necrotic tumors located within complex anatomic territories.

head and neck lesions [35,50,51]. The rapid acceptance of MR imaging guidance among the radiologic community and the increasing awareness among clinicians of its benefits have subsequently encouraged several investigators to explore further applications in which this technique may have potential benefits. Currently, numerous published reports are available reflecting the developed experience in many institutions that use MR imaging to guide biopsies and aspiration in various body organs and highlighting the contribution of interventional MR imaging to the expanding scope of percutaneous procedures performed in radiology departments.

Obviously, MR imaging guidance is not intended to be a substitute for other less expensive and relatively simpler modes of biopsy and/or aspiration guidance whenever their use is appropriate. Rather, interventional MR imaging procedures assume a role when the patient would otherwise be subjected to surgical exploration or open biopsy performed solely for the purpose of tissue diagnosis or when procedure safety under the more conventional methods of guidance is considered less than optimal.

Head and neck and neuroradiology applications

As indicated previously, this subset of applications has enjoyed the greatest deal of expertise that has developed over the years in the field of interventional MR imaging. The original work of Lufkin and other investigators [34–36,38] laid the foundation for subsequent exploration of the full

potential of these applications, exploiting the concurrent technical innovations that facilitated the generation of rapid high-quality images in an open-field environment, as noted earlier in this article. Fried et al [76] reported in 1998 on head and neck image-guided biopsies performed within a "new, investigational, open configuration" intraoperative MR imaging scanner using the double-donut middle-field scanner (SIGNA SP). Lewin et al [51] simultaneously published their early large series evaluating 106 MR-guided procedures performed on a biplanar low-field scanner (Magnetom Open, Siemens Medical Systems). They concluded that the use of MR imaging for guidance of biopsies and aspirations was most advantageous for sampling suprahyoid neck lesions (Fig. 10). Similarly, several investigators later demonstrated the feasibility and safety of the MR-guided approach to biopsy retropharyngeal [77,78] and other masses within the deep head and neck spaces [79–83]. The use of MR imaging to guide thyroid gland biopsies [84] did not, however, gain popularity, because the use of high-frequency US transducers provides excellent visualization of subcentimeter thyroid nodules and is efficiently used to guide biopsies of this subcutaneous organ in a simple, quick, and cost-effective manner.

Lesions of the skull base and high cervical spine are particularly well suited to MR-guided biopsy [50,51] because of the lack of beam-hardening artifacts associated with CT imaging of this area. Masses at the root of the neck, particularly those encroaching on the brachial

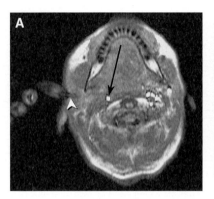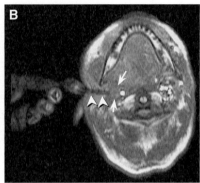

Fig. 10. A 50-year-old man with small recurrent squamous cell carcinoma of the oropharynx adjacent to the right internal carotid artery. MR imaging scans obtained from a continuous series obtained at 1.7 seconds per frame with a fast imaging with steady-state precession sequence (TR/TE: 18/7 milliseconds, one acquisition, flip angle of 90°) during insertion of the needle show the operator's hand directing the needle (*arrowheads*) into the small mass. With two-dimensional gradient echo techniques such as those used here, bright vessels from inflow help to avoid critical structures, such as the internal carotid artery (*arrow, A*). Tissue contrast characteristics are poor, however, with the mass (*arrows, B*) being poorly defined. The location of the mass was better seen on prior T2-weighted images (not shown). The external carotid artery in this patient had been previously occluded with Gianturco coils to control oropharyngeal bleeding. The coils did not result in significant image distortion and did not preclude biopsy. (*From* Lewin JS, Petersilge CA, Hatem SF, et al. Interactive MR imaging-guided biopsy and aspiration with a modified clinical C-arm system. AJR Am J Roentgenol 1998;170(6):1593–601; with permission.)

plexus, have also offered an excellent application, using the multiplanar capabilities, tissue contrast, vascular conspicuity, and spatial resolution of MR imaging to allow confident tissue sampling adjacent to the neurovascular structures of the thoracic inlet (Fig. 11) [50,51]. For biopsies and aspiration procedures within the spinal canal, GRE T2-weighted images have proven helpful because they offer a clear distinction between cerebrospinal fluid (CSF) or cyst contents and the adjacent spinal cord, thus allowing confident needle navigation and ensuring procedure safety (Fig. 12) [51,53,85].

Open-configuration MR imaging systems have been used to guide fine aspiration and cutting biopsy needles into brain tumors interactively [50,58,86–90], including transnasal and transsphenoidal MR-guided tissue sampling of petroclival lesions [91]. Minimally invasive aspiration of intracranial cysts and abscesses has also been reported to be feasible and safe and to result in complete drainage, thereby obviating the need for open surgical procedures [92,93]. Monitoring the procedures using near–real-time MR imaging provides immediate feedback on the associated intracranial dynamic tissue changes, such as the degree of cyst or abscess aspiration and the presence or absence of hemorrhage or induced brain edema secondary to decompression of the

adjacent brain parenchyma and the ventricular system. Bernays et al [94] reported on a significantly favorable neurologic outcome after MR-guided evacuation of hypertensive hematomas in the basal ganglia. A detailed review of the full spectrum and future perspectives of intraoperative MR-guided procedures is available in the article by Jolesz [95] and elsewhere in the current issue (see the article by Hall and Truwit).

Abdominal and pelvic applications

The rationale for using interactive MR imaging to guide abdominal and other body soft tissue biopsies and aspirations is quite different from that in head and neck or neurologic applications. In the latter, MR imaging guidance exploits the superb level of anatomic visualization that has rendered MR imaging the imaging modality of choice in head and neck and neurologic diagnostic imaging, thereby clearly providing a minimally invasive alternative to open surgical procedures. Conversely, body interventions have long been practiced using well-established, more conventional, and often successful modes of guidance, such as CT and US, with most radiologists acquiring a fair level of expertise in their use during their early years of training. It is therefore imperative to recognize that the role of MR-

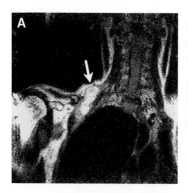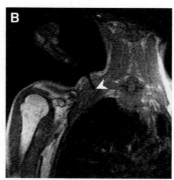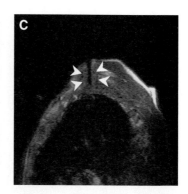

Fig. 11. Right supraclavicular fullness in a 52-year-old man who previously underwent a left lung resection for carcinoma. The surgeon's physical examination revealed generalized fullness but no discrete mass. (*A*) Turbo spin echo T2-weighted image (TR/TE: 2000/105 milliseconds, number of signal averages [NSA] = 2, 59-second scanning time) reveals a focal mass displacing the brachial plexus (*arrow*). (*B*) Single frame from a continuous series of fast imaging with steady-state precession (FISP) images (TR/TE: 18/7 milliseconds, NSA = 2, flip angle of 90°, 3.5-second scanning time) shows an 18-gauge side-notch cutting needle (*arrowhead*) inserted into the dominant mass. (*C*) Oblique parasagittal FISP image orthogonal to and with the same parameters as in (*B*) reveals a needle centered within the mass (*arrowheads*) with the central stylet extended. The continuous imaging sequence allowed the mass to be separated from adjacent vessels as well as from the adjacent portion of the brachial plexus. The pathologic diagnosis from the biopsy was poorly differentiated large cell carcinoma. (*From* Lewin JS. Interventional MR imaging: concepts, systems, and applications in neuroradiology. AJNR Am J Neuroradiol 1999;20:735–48; with permission.)

guided tissue sampling of abdominal and/or body pathologic findings is to expand the minimally invasive diagnostic options currently available to the patients through the appropriate and cost-effective use of this technology in selected cases.

In our experience [51,53], as in that of others [96,97], interactive MR imaging guidance offers unequivocal advantages in terms of procedure safety and diagnostic yield in cases in which the target lesions are not sufficiently visualized on CT or US scans (Fig. 13). The flexibility to obtain unlimited combinations of T1- and T2-weighted tissue contrast through the implementation of a wide array of near–real-time MR fluoroscopy sequences allows the operator to maximize the lesion's contrast-to-noise ratio while navigating the biopsy and/or aspiration device. For example, PSIF [98] and fast low angle shot (FLASH) [99] sequences have demonstrated their superiority in optimizing hepatic tumor conspicuity in most lesions sampled under MR imaging guidance. Other investigators [100] and the authors have also found the use of gadolinium-enhanced T1-weighted FLASH sequences during needle advancement to be helpful in delineating some otherwise inconspicuous liver lesions. TSE T2-weighted images are also advantageous in mapping out the areas of tumor necrosis, thereby helping to guide the biopsy needle into viable tumor tissue. Alternation between different image

weightings is a simple task that can be achieved in a time-effective manner during MR imaging guidance.

MR imaging guidance has also proven helpful in sampling transiently enhancing lesions, such as hepatocellular carcinoma and hypervascular metastases, by using the same concept of multiple contrast weightings and taking advantage of the high soft tissue contrast to assign tissue landmarks along the needle path and around the target pathologic finding. Another indication that is well suited for MR imaging guidance in the abdomen is when the frequent shift between various scan planes during interactive needle advancement is believed to provide additional procedure safety because of the complex anatomic location of the target lesion, such as within the dome of the liver (Fig. 14) [101], in the subphrenic regions [102], in the pancreas [103], and in the adrenal glands [104,105]. We have also found the high vascular conspicuity associated with the flow enhancement phenomenon inherent in gradient echo sequences to aid in obtaining a more confident sampling of retroperitoneal lesions abutting the aorta or the inferior vena cava (IVC) (Fig. 15).

The use of interactive MR imaging to guide prostate gland biopsy and to place brachytherapy seeds is an emerging new application of body interventional MR imaging, with a few recent reports available in the literature from a handful

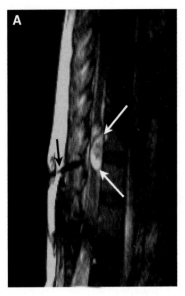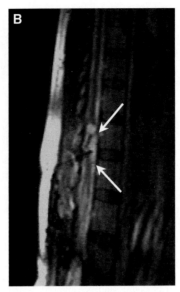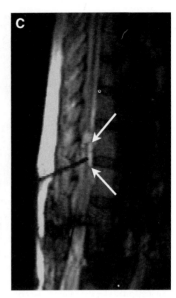

Fig. 12. A 36-year-old woman with paraparesis and pain after a motor vehicle accident with recent worsening of symptoms. (*A*) True fast imaging with steady-state precession (FISP) sagittal image (TR/TE: 11.7/5.9 milliseconds) during posterior interlaminar 22-gauge needle placement (*black arrow*) into a large posttraumatic subarachnoid cyst (*white arrows*). A posterior approach was used with the patient placed in the decubitus position. The procedure was performed to see if cyst decompression would be beneficial before definitive open surgical repair. (*B*) True FISP sagittal image (TR/TE: 11.7/5.9 milliseconds) after needle placement and partial aspiration of cyst (*arrows*). A smaller cyst can also be seen immediately superior as the larger cyst is decompressed. (*C*) True FISP sagittal image (TR/TE: 11.7/5.9 milliseconds, number of signal averages = 3, flip angle of 90°) at the end of the aspiration procedure demonstrates a small residual cyst (*arrows*) with re-expansion of the thoracic spinal cord. (*From* Lewin JS, Petersilge CA, Hatem SF, et al. Interactive MR imaging-guided biopsy and aspiration with a modified clinical C-arm system. AJR Am J Roentgenol 1998;170(6):1593–601; with permission.)

of research groups practicing the technique via transrectal [106], transgluteal [107], and transperineal [108–111] approaches. Because clinical data are currently sparse, further evaluation of the merits of the technique and assessment of its safety, diagnostic yield, and cost-effectiveness compared with the standard transrectal US-guided approach are still warranted.

Breast applications

This is another area of intervention in which MR-guided biopsy and aspiration have been gaining an increasing interest since the early literature started to evaluate the potential of this technique almost a decade ago [112–116].

The high sensitivity of MR imaging in detecting mammographically, sonographically, and clinically occult breast lesions [112] is frequently restricted by its limited specificity, which results from the overlap between the enhancement characteristics of benign and malignant lesions. Although the recent application of dynamic

contrast-enhanced (DCE) MR imaging techniques has improved the sensitivity of MR imaging in characterizing malignant breast lesions to reach values between 90% and 100% [112,114,117], the specificity of DCE MR imaging has been inconsistent and often moderate in the literature, ranging between 75% and 85% [115,118], with a recent large series reporting specificity as low as 59.4% [114,117]. The mounting number of indeterminate lesions detected exclusively on breast MR imaging therefore remains a clinical dilemma that is expected to amplify, as does the use of DCE MR imaging of the breast. The ability to perform fine needle aspiration or core biopsy of these lesions under MR imaging guidance implies a reduction in the number of surgical excisions of potentially benign lesions. Additionally, in the subset of these patients who are scheduled for surgical intervention, MR imaging would be the only imaging modality available to guide preoperative hookwire placement.

MR-guided biopsy and/or hookwire placement procedures are usually performed using a "dead-

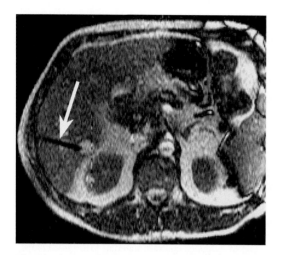

Fig. 13. A 38-year-old man with pancreatic carcinoma and a liver mass with a previous unsuccessful CT-guided biopsy attempt. Liver masses, in particular, are typically difficult to visualize without T2-weighted images. Guidance of a 22-gauge needle (*arrow*) was provided in this case, with a 1-second per frame true fast imaging with steady-state precession sequence (TR/TE: 11.7/5.9 milliseconds, number of signal averages = 1, flip angle of 90°), with a series of 9 to 12 images obtained with a continuous update during each breath hold. The pathologic diagnosis was a simple hepatic cyst. (*From* Lewin JS, Petersilge CA, Hatem SF, et al. Interactive MR imaging-guided biopsy and aspiration with a modified clinical C-arm system. AJR Am J Roentgenol 1998;170(6):1593–601; with permission.)

reckoning navigation" technique in a fashion analogous to that which mammographers use during stereotactic breast biopsies [119]. Multiple prototype stereotactic devices for MR imaging guidance have been described in the literature, with the technology being commercially available only in the past few years. The common theme of these devices is providing sufficient breast tissue immobilization and accurate stereotaxy while being integrated into an imaging coil. Tissue immobilization is achieved via compression plates while the patient is in the prone [113,114,120–122], semiprone [122,123], supine [122,124], lateral [114,125], or sitting [118,125] position. Attention should be given to applying moderate rather than strong compression so as not to impede enhancement of the target lesion [126]. Stereotaxy is accomplished by designing the coil and/or compression plates as a fenestrated grid with built-in or added MR imaging–visible fiducial markers that serve as coordinates to calculate lesion location (Fig. 16).

Currently, most of these procedures are performed on the same closed-bore scanner where diagnostic breast imaging takes place. This implies that confirmation of needle position relative to the target lesion is the only step that is controlled by MR imaging guidance, whereas the actual needle placement is performed when the patient is withdrawn from the bore of the magnet based on the coordinates' calculations.

A few reports have described an interactive approach to MR-guided biopsy and/or wire placement through the use of open-configuration

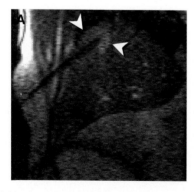
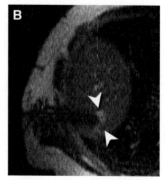

Fig. 14. Coronal (*A*) and axial (*B*) rapid true fast imaging with steady-state precession images acquired during needle insertion into a metastatic lesion (*arrowheads*) located in segment 7 within the posterior aspect of the dome of the right lobe of the liver. Sampling liver dome lesions is a typical indication for the use of MR imaging to guide biopsy or aspiration procedures. The multiplanar imaging capability provides a clear advantage because it allows safe needle insertion without risking pleural puncture. This patient subsequently underwent radiofrequency ablation of this metastatic lesion under MR imaging guidance and monitoring in the same session.

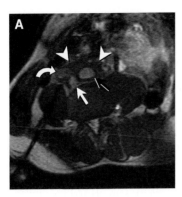 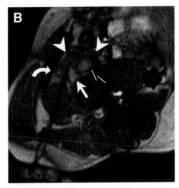 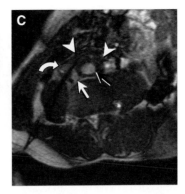

Fig. 15. Another example illustrating the value of MR-guided biopsy within the abdomen and pelvis in this 50-year-old man with retroperitoneal fibrosis. A retroperitoneal soft tissue mantle (*arrowheads*) is seen encasing the aorta (*black arrows*) and IVC (*white arrows*) and entrapping the dilated right ureter (*curved arrows*) at the level of L4 vertebral body. Renal function was impaired, precluding intravenous administration of iodinated contrast material. MR-guided biopsy was performed using true fast imaging with steady-state precession guidance. The flow enhancement phenomenon inherent in this gradient echo sequence facilitated a clear delineation of the aorta and IVC throughout the procedure without the need for contrast administration. Additionally, the T2 weighting provided by this sequence helped visualization of the dilated ureter as a rather hyperintense structure. (*A*) Biopsy needle is introduced through a transpsoas approach. (*B*) Needle is safely advanced between the IVC and the dilated right ureter. (*C*) Cutting notch is deployed further into the retroperitoneal abnormal tissues anterolateral to the abdominal aorta.

low-field [128] and middle-field [118,127,129] MR imaging scanners to allow real-time updating of needle position and timely adjustments of trajectory as needed. The interactive approach may be implemented with the same stereotactic devices described previously or with a freehand technique while the breast is immobilized within a thermoplastic mesh or between a belt-shaped coil and a fixation plate [118,127–129]. Such a freehand

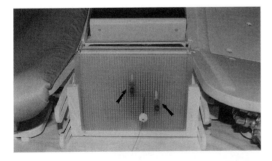

Fig. 16. MR-guided breast biopsy and localization device. The breast is compressed between a fixed medial plate and a mobile lateral plate. The lateral plate, made of polycarbonate plastic (Lexan; GE Plastics, Pittsfield, Massachusetts), is removable and can be sterilized. Copper sulfate reference markers (*arrows*) are placed arbitrarily into holes in the plate. (*From* Orel SG, Schnall MD. MR imaging of the breast for the detection, diagnosis, and staging of breast cancer. Radiology 2001;220(1):13–30; with permission.)

approach helps to avoid the dead spaces between the holes of perforated compression plates, thereby enabling unrestricted access to virtually every location within the breast at any arbitrary trajectory. The technique is, however, associated with a higher rate of manipulations and a higher rate of wire displacement [122]. The augmented reality system described previously in the section on interactive MR imaging guidance techniques may potentially be used to guide breast biopsies using a freehand approach along a straight augmented needle path to reduce manipulations. It also allows the use of high-field MR imaging quality while performing the actual procedure outside the narrow bore of the magnet. Such an approach, however, has not yet been reported in the literature.

An in vivo proof-of-principle for a prototype MR imaging–compatible robotic system has recently been reported, where the radiologist can remotely guide a manipulator operating within a high-field closed-bore scanner to obtain large core breast biopsies [130].

Musculoskeletal applications

In the diagnostic arena, MR imaging has become the primary imaging modality routinely pursued after plain radiography to investigate musculoskeletal abnormalities, with CT scans being regarded as a problem-solving tool to assess subtle osseous abnormalities primarily in trauma patients. Nevertheless, the use of MR imaging to guide percutaneous diagnostic interventions in the musculoskeletal system has not gained the same level of popularity that it has achieved in the field of neuroradiology.

Literature reports do exist describing the application of interventional MR imaging techniques to guide musculoskeletal aspirations, core biopsies, and transcortical trephine biopsies using open biplanar (low-field, 0.2-T) [51,131–133] or double-donut (middle-field, 0.5-T) [134,135] scanners or using a hybrid system combining a high-field (1.5-T) closed-bore scanner with a C-arm conventional fluoroscopic unit [136]. These are predominantly feasibility studies investigating the utility of the current technology to guide safe musculoskeletal tissue sampling and evaluating the diagnostic yield of tissue samples retrieved under MR imaging.

For most primary soft tissue neoplasms and bone tumors that breach the cortex to extend into the adjacent soft tissues, the principal challenge for MR imaging to attain a genuine role in biopsy guidance is the remarkably high tissue sampling success rates of US and CT guidance, which reach up to 98% for each modality [137,138]. For this particular indication, the window for MR-guided intervention is in those lesions that are deeply seated in complex locations such that a double-oblique approach (Fig. 17) or precise vascular localization is considered necessary for a safer procedure. In these cases, MR imaging may offer an additional advantage of guiding the biopsy needle into nonnecrotic parts of a tumor through

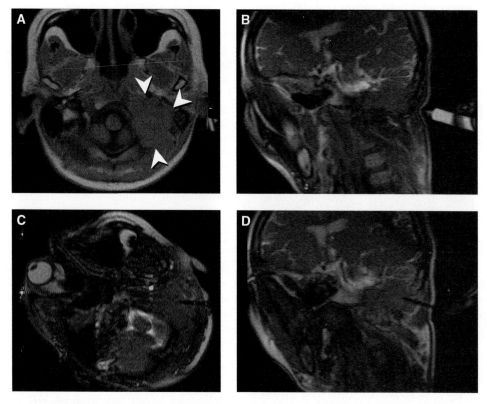

Fig. 17. A 71-year-old man with a plasmacytoma centered on the skull base, destroying the left occipital condyle and extending superiorly into the ipsilateral posterior cranial fossa. (*A*) Axial T1-weighted spin echo image demonstrates the aggressive isointense mass lesion (*arrowheads*). (*B*) Coronal oblique T2-weighted true fast imaging with steady-state precession was performed when planning the skin entry point. (*C, D*) Double-oblique T2-weighted images obtained in orthogonal planes demonstrate the biopsy needle within the targeted tumor mass. This retromastoid approach benefits from the oblique scan planes achieved with MR imaging, enabling imaging of the entire craniad and anteriorly angled needle.

the use of T2 contrast weighting, as described earlier in the section on abdominal and soft tissue applications. It has been reported that TSE T2-weighted sequences are more reliable for depicting areas of tumor necrosis compared with GRE T2*-weighted sequences [133].

The core contribution of interventional MR imaging technology to musculoskeletal diagnosis stems from its ability to target lesions that are poorly delineated with other imaging modalities. In addition to occasional ill-defined soft tissue lesions, infiltrative bone marrow processes that remain within the cortical confines seem to represent an excellent scenario for MR-guided intervention. Generally, unenhanced T1-weighted GRE sequences, such as FISP or FLASH, are well suited for this purpose and can clearly outline the extent of marrow-replacing pathologic change, which appears as a hypointense signal amid the surrounding normal hyperintense and predominantly fat-containing adult bone marrow (Fig. 18). Conversion of red to fatty marrow normally progresses from the peripheral to the axial skeleton and is complete by approximately 25 years of age. A

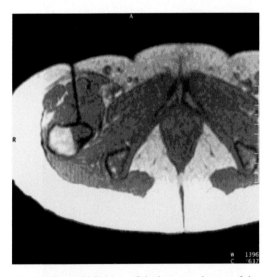

Fig. 18. Desmoid fibroma of the lesser trochanter of the right femur. Unenhanced T1-weighted fast low-angle shot (TR/TE: .50/9 milliseconds, number of signal averages = 2, flip angle of 70°, two acquisitions) imaging before drilling shows an 11-gauge trephine resting on the intact cortical bone overlying the lesion. The extent of the marrow abnormality can be accurately delineated in contrast to the normal bright fatty marrow. (*From* Koenig CW, Duda SH, Truebenbach J, et al. MR-guided biopsy of musculoskeletal lesions in a low-field system. J Magn Reson Imaging 2001;13(5):761–8; with permission.)

reconversion process may occur with illness, stress, or anemia in which hematopoietic marrow is recruited back in a reverse order (ie, from the axial to the peripheral skeleton) [139–141]. It is therefore necessary to add T2 weighting when attempting MR-guided sampling of lesions within expected areas of red marrow, where pathologic areas demonstrate higher signal compared with the intact intermediate-signal red marrow.

A variety of MR imaging–compatible biopsy needles and coaxial drill systems powered by hand, by a motor [142], or piezoelectrically [135] are presently available for sampling skeletal lesions.

Percutaneous sampling of lesions in the vicinity of nonferromagnetic hardware is another situation in which MR imaging guidance may assume a role in musculoskeletal system biopsy or aspiration [133]. A recent report has also described the use MR imaging guidance for preoperative coil marking of musculoskeletal tumors, where MR imaging–compatible titanium coils were interactively placed to aid in definitive delineation of soft tissue or bone marrow tumor margins during subsequent surgery in a manner analogous to preoperative wire placement in breast lesions [143].

The scope of interventional MR imaging applications in the musculoskeletal system extends to include several therapeutic procedures, such as guidance of perineural injections and ablations. Discussion of these procedures is beyond the intent of this article but may be reviewed in detail elsewhere in this issue (see the article by Blanco Sequeiros and Carrino).

Pediatric applications

Although the application of interactive MR imaging to guide interventional procedures in the pediatric age group seems to be of particular relevance because of the lack of ionizing radiation, especially when repeated interventions are required, the experience in this field is still in its infancy, with only a few groups recently reporting on dedicated pediatric work on small numbers of children [144].

The apparent reluctance to adopt pediatric applications by the interventional MR imaging community is, in part, attributable to the more demanding setup for interventions in children compared with those for adults. General anesthesia and/or sedation is required during virtually all types of pediatric procedures, thereby placing an increased emphasis on issues like the availability of MR imaging–compatible anesthesia and monitoring equipment and on the ability to coordinate a multidisciplinary system of staff, nursing personnel, and technologists with a fair understanding of the concepts, approaches, and limitations of interventional MR imaging. Maintaining scan times at a minimum and securing ready access for close monitoring and for handling emergency situations in the anesthetized child are other factors that must be stressed while attempting pediatric interventions using MR imaging.

Such a complex setup, although in many ways similar to the requirements for intraoperative MR-guided neurointerventions, implies the added sensitivity of pediatric monitoring and, for some applications, lacks the robust justification recognized for MR-guided neurologic procedures. As such, neurologic interventions have dominated the sparse data available thus far in the literature regarding pediatric applications of interventional MR imaging. Successful tumor biopsies, intracranial cyst aspirations, and stereotactic catheter placements have been reported using frameless stereotaxy in children between 6 weeks and 18 years of age employing a vertically open (double-donut) scanner [145]. A few other reports describing MR-guided neurosurgery to evaluate the extent of tumor resection in the pediatric population [146–149] are also available, although such discussion is beyond the "biopsy and aspiration" topic of this article.

A few musculoskeletal biopsies have also been reported in pediatric patients [150,151] during recent years. The rationale is similar to that in the adult population as outlined in the section on musculoskeletal applications.

The authors are not aware of any group that is currently performing pediatric abdominal biopsies or aspirations under MR imaging guidance. This is probably an area where an expanding role of MR imaging guidance is difficult to foresee in the near future in light of the existing equipment and interventional setup, as indicated previously. Conversely, the ease of use of US at the child's bedside, along with the fully controlled access, easy monitoring, and standard anesthesia and/or sedation equipment, remains an attractive choice to guide these procedures at the present time.

Summary

The advent of interventional MR imaging techniques as well as their adoption to guide percutaneous biopsies and aspirations has served as a further step along a series of technical refinements that commenced with the implementation of image-guided approaches for tissue sampling. Nowadays, the practice of and the expectations from these procedures are quite different from those of the blind percutaneous thrusts performed in the late nineteenth and early twentieth centuries. As the field of interventional MR imaging continues to flourish and to attract more radiologists who realize the many opportunities that this technology can offer to their patients, there is a need for a full comprehension of the concepts, techniques, limitations, and cost-effectiveness of MR imaging guidance to present this service to clinical partners in the appropriate setting. Radiologists should also recognize the need for their significant involvement in the technical aspects of MR-guided procedures, because several user-defined parameters and trajectory decisions can alter device visualization in the MR imaging environment and hence affect procedure safety.

Acknowledgments

The authors acknowledge the members of the Interventional MR Imaging Research Program at the University Hospitals of Cleveland/Case Western Reserve University for their ongoing commitment to the development of interventional MR imaging techniques. The authors also thank Bonnie Hami for her invaluable editorial assistance.

References

[1] Frerichs FT. Üeber den Diabetes. Berlin: Hirschwald; 1884 [in German].

[2] Levy H. Liver biopsy. Lancet 1945;2:480.

[3] Reuben A. Just a second. Hepatology 2003;38(5): 1316–20.

[4] Schupfer F. De la possibilité de faire "intra vitam" un diagnostic précis des maladies du foie et de la rate. Semin Méd 1907;27:229–30 [in French].

[5] Bingel A. Üeber der Parenchympunktion der Leber. Verhandl d. Deutsch. Gesellsch f. Inn Med 1923;35:210–2 [in German].

[6] Olivet J. Die diagnostiche Leberparenchympunction. Med Klin 1926;22:1440–3 [in German].

[7] Weed LA, Dahlin DC. Bacteriologic examination of tissue removed for biopsy. Am J Clin Pathol 1950;20(2):116–32.

[8] Iverson P, Roholm K. On aspiration biopsy of the liver, with remarks on its diagnostic significance. Acta Med Scand 1939;102:116.

[9] Terry R. Liver biopsy. St Bartholomews Hosp J 1949;53(10):202–4.

[10] Weisbrod FG, Schiff L, et al. Needle biopsy of the liver; experiences in the differential diagnosis of jaundice. Gastroenterology 1950;14(1):56–72.

[11] Brower AB. Relationship of nodular goiter to thyroid carcinoma; brief review with a note on the diagnostic role of needle biopsy. Ann West Med Surg 1949;3(11):395–7.

[12] Sainani GS, Malani BS. The value of percutaneous thyroid biopsy. J Assoc Physicians India 1972; 20(10):733–6.

[13] Telkka A. Bone marrow biopsy. Duodecim 1950; 66(10):789–92.

[14] Priessnitz O. Diagnostic value of biopsy in diseases of the muscles. Z Orthop Ihre Grenzgeb 1950;79(4): 726–31.

[15] Hendricks FB, Lambird PA, Murph GP. Percutaneous needle biopsy of the testis. Fertil Steril 1969;20(3):478–81.

[16] Ghobrial F, Guirguis S. The value of aspiration biopsy in the diagnosis of tumours. J Egypt Med Assoc 1950;33(10–11):890–900.

[17] Cioni A. Transparietal puncture biopsy of tumors of the lung by the Condorelli technique. J Fr Med Chir Thorac 1950;4(5):417–23.

[18] Menghini G. One-second needle biopsy of the liver. Gastroenterology 1958;35(2):190–9.

[19] Menghini G. One-second biopsy of the liver—problems of its clinical application. N Engl J Med 1970;283(11):582–5.

[20] Menghini G, Lauro G, Caraceni M. Some innovations in the technic of the one-second needle biopsy of the liver. Am J Gastroenterol 1975;64(3):175–80.

[21] Kark RM, Muehrcke RC. Biopsy of kidney in prone position. Lancet 1954;266(6821):1047–9.

[22] Brun C, Raaschou F. Complications of 500 performances of percutaneous renal biopsy. Ugeskr Laeger 1958;120(46):1513–6.

[23] De La Pena A, Cavanaugh RJ, Ballard LG. Prostatic percutaneous biopsy. Urol Int 1961;12:1–5.

[24] Krokowski E, Kollwitz AA. Roentgenological localization of percutaneous needle biopsy of the kidneys. Fortschr Geb Rontgenstr Nuklearmed 1960; 93:613–6 [in German].

[25] Miller FL. Percutaneous needle biopsy in clinically inoperable pulmonary tumors. US Armed Forces Med J 1960;11:858–71.

[26] Stein HL, Evans JA. Percutaneous transthoracic lung biopsy utilizing image amplification. Radiology 1966;87(2):350.

[27] Laubenberger T, Jahnecke J. Percutaneous radioscopic kidney biopsy. The improvement of the renal puncture by the introduction of modern radiological media. Dtsch Med Wochenschr 1967;92(3): 104–6 [in German].

[28] Holm HH, Kristensen JK, Rasmussen SN, et al. Ultrasound as a guide in percutaneous puncture technique. Ultrasonics 1972;10(2):83–6.

[29] Goldberg BB, Pollack HM. Ultrasonic aspiration transducer. Radiology 1972;102(1):187–9.

[30] Haaga JR, Alfidi RJ. Precise biopsy localization by computer tomography. Radiology 1976;118(3): 603–7.

[31] Haaga JR, Alfidi RJ, Havrilla TR, et al. CT detection and aspiration of abdominal abscesses. AJR Am J Roentgenol 1977;128(3):465–74.

[32] Haaga JR, Reich NE, Havrilla TR, et al. Interventional CT scanning. Radiol Clin N Am 1977;15(3): 449–56.

[33] Mueller PR, Stark DD, Simeone JF, et al. MR-guided aspiration biopsy: needle design and clinical trials. Radiology 1986;161(3):605–9.

[34] Lufkin R, Teresi L, Hanafee W. New needle for MR-guided aspiration cytology of the head and neck. AJR Am J Roentgenol 1987;149(2):380–2.

[35] Lufkin R, Teresi L, Chiu L, et al. A technique for MR-guided needle placement. AJR Am J Roentgenol 1988;151(1):193–6.

[36] Trapp T, Lufkin R, Abemayor E, et al. A new needle and technique for MRI-guided aspiration cytology of the head and neck. Laryngoscope 1989; 99(1):105–8.

[37] Mueller PR, Stark DD, Simeone JF, et al. Clinical use of a nonferromagnetic needle for magnetic resonance-guided biopsy. Gastrointest Radiol 1989; 14(1):61–4.

[38] Duckwiler G, Lufkin RB, Teresi L, et al. Head and neck lesions: MR-guided aspiration biopsy. Radiology 1989;170(2):519–22.

[39] Duckwiler G, Lufkin RB, Hanafee WN. MR-directed needle biopsies. Radiol Clin N Am 1989; 27(2):255–63.

[40] Lewin JS, Duerk JL, Jain VR, et al. Needle localization in MR-guided biopsy and aspiration: effects of field strength, sequence design, and magnetic field orientation. AJR Am J Roentgenol 1996; 166(6):1337–45.

[41] Frahm C, Gehl HB, Melchert UH, et al. Visualization of magnetic resonance-compatible needles at 1.5 and 0.2 Tesla. Cardiovasc Intervent Radiol 1996;19(5):335–40.

[42] Duerk JL, Lewin JS, Wu DH. Application of keyhole imaging to interventional MRI: a simulation study to predict sequence requirements. J Magn Reson Imaging 1996;6(6):918–24.

[43] Mahfouz AE, Rahmouni A, Zylbersztejn C, et al. MR-guided biopsy using ultrafast T1- and T2- weighted reordered turbo fast low-angle shot sequences: feasibility and preliminary clinical applications. AJR Am J Roentgenol 1996; 167(1):167–9.

[44] Duerk JL, Lewin JS, Wendt M, et al. Remember true FISP? A high SNR, near 1-second imaging method for T2-like contrast in interventional

MRI at .2 T. J Magn Reson Imaging 1998;8(1): 203–8.

[45] Chung YC, Merkle EM, Lewin JS, et al. Fast T(2)-weighted imaging by PSIF at 0.2 T for interventional MRI. Magn Reson Med 1999;42(2): 335–44.

[46] Wendt M, Wacker F, Wolf KJ, et al. Keyhole-true FISP: fast T2-weighted imaging for interventional MRT at 0.2 T. Rofo Fortschr Geb Rontgenstr Neuen Bildgeb Verfahr 1999;170(4):391–3 [in German].

[47] Duerk JL, Butts K, Hwang KP, et al. Pulse sequences for interventional magnetic resonance imaging. Top Magn Reson Imaging 2000;11(3):147–62.

[48] Busch M, Bornstedt A, Wendt M, et al. Fast "real time" imaging with different k-space update strategies for interventional procedures. J Magn Reson Imaging 1998;8(4):944–54.

[49] Daniel BL, Butts K. The use of view angle tilting to reduce distortions in magnetic resonance imaging of cryosurgery. Magn Reson Imaging 2000;18(3): 281–6.

[50] Lewin JS. Interventional MR imaging: concepts, systems, and applications in neuroradiology. AJNR Am J Neuroradiol 1999;20:735–48.

[51] Lewin JS, Petersilge CA, Hatem SF, et al. Interactive MR imaging-guided biopsy and aspiration with a modified clinical C-arm system. AJR Am J Roentgenol 1998;170(6):1593–601.

[52] Merkle EM, Lewin JS, Aschoff AJ, et al. Percutaneous magnetic resonance image-guided biopsy and aspiration in the head and neck. Laryngoscope 2000;110:382–5.

[53] Lewin JS, Nour SG, Duerk JL. Magnetic resonance image-guided biopsy and aspiration. Top Magn Reson Imaging 2000;11:173–83.

[54] Genant JW, Vandevenne JE, Bergman AG, et al. Interventional musculoskeletal procedures performed by using MR imaging guidance with a vertically open MR unit: assessment of techniques and applicability. Radiology 2002;223(1):127–36.

[55] Neuerburg JM, Adam G, Buecker A, et al. MRI-guided biopsy of bone in a hybrid system. J Magn Reson Imaging 1998;8(1):85–90.

[56] Silverman SG, Collick BD, Figueira MR, et al. Interactive MR-guided biopsy in an open-configuration MR imaging system. Radiology 1995;197(1):175–81.

[57] Ojala R, Sequeiros RB, Klemola R, et al. MR-guided bone biopsy: preliminary report of a new guiding method. J Magn Reson Imaging 2002;15(1):82–6.

[58] Schneider JP, Dietrich J, Lieberenz S, et al. Preliminary experience with interactive guided brain biopsies using a vertically opened 0.5-T MR system. Eur Radiol 1999;9(2):230–6.

[59] Jolesz FA, Kikinis R, Talos IF. Neuronavigation in interventional MR imaging. Frameless stereotaxy. Neuroimaging Clin N Am 2001;11(4):685–93.

[60] Flask C, Elgort D, Wong E, et al. A method for fast 3D tracking using tuned fiducial markers and a limited projection reconstruction FISP (LPR-FISP) sequence. J Magn Reson Imaging 2001;14(5): 617–27.

[61] Hillenbrand CM, Elgort DR, Wong EY, et al. Active device tracking and high-resolution intravascular MRI using a novel catheter-based, opposed-solenoid phased array coil. Magn Reson Med 2004;51(4):668–75.

[62] Elgort DR, Wong EY, Hillenbrand CM, et al. Real-time catheter tracking and adaptive imaging. J Magn Reson Imaging 2003;18(5):621–6.

[63] Wacker FK, Elgort D, Hillenbrand CM, et al. The catheter-driven MRI scanner: a new approach to intravascular catheter tracking and imaging-parameter adjustment for interventional MRI. AJR Am J Roentgenol 2004;183(2):391–5.

[64] Truwit CL, Liu H. Prospective stereotaxy: a novel method of trajectory alignment using real-time image guidance. J Magn Reson Imaging 2001;13(3): 452–7.

[65] Liu H, Hall WA, Truwit CL. Neuronavigation in interventional MR imaging. Prospective stereotaxy. Neuroimaging Clin N Am 2001;11(4): 695–704.

[66] Samset E, Hirschberg H. Image-guided stereotaxy in the interventional MRI. Minim Invasive Neurosurg 2003;46(1):5–10.

[67] Wacker FK, Vogt V, Khamene A, et al. An augmented reality system for MRI-guided needle biopsies. Stud Health Technol Inform 2003;94: 151–7.

[68] Wendt M, Sauer F, Khamene A, et al. A head-mounted display system for augmented reality: initial evaluation for interventional MRI. Rofo Fortschr Geb Rontgenstr Neuen Bildgeb Verfahr 2003;175(3):418–21 [in German].

[69] Rosenthal M, State A, Lee J, et al. Augmented reality guidance for needle biopsies: an initial randomized, controlled trial in phantoms. Med Image Anal 2002;6(3):313–20.

[70] Iseki H, Masutani Y, Iwahara M, et al. Volumegraph (overlaid three-dimensional image-guided navigation). Clinical application of augmented reality in neurosurgery. Stereotact Funct Neurosurg 1997;68(1–4 Part 1):18–24.

[71] Jannin P, Fleig OJ, Seigneuret E, et al. A data fusion environment for multimodal and multiinformational neuronavigation. Comput Aided Surg 2000;5(1):1–10.

[72] Rohlfing T, West JB, Beier J, et al. Registration of functional and anatomical MRI: accuracy assessment and application in navigated neurosurgery. Comput Aided Surg 2000;5(6):414–25.

[73] Gering DT, Nabavi A, Kikinis R, et al. An integrated visualization system for surgical planning and guidance using image fusion and an open MR. J Magn Reson Imaging 2001;13(6):967–75.

[74] Moche M, Busse H, Dannenberg C, et al. Fusion of MRI, fMRI and intraoperative MRI data. Methods and clinical significance exemplified by neurosurgical interventions. Radiologe 2001;41(11): 993–1000 [in German].

[75] Moche M, Schmitgen A, Schneider JP, et al. First clinical experience with extended planning and navigation in an interventional MRI unit. Rofo Fortschr Geb Rontgenstr Neuen Bildgeb Verfahr 2004;176(7):1013–20 [in German].

[76] Fried MP, Hsu L, Jolesz FA. Interactive magnetic resonance imaging-guided biopsy in the head and neck: initial patient experience. Laryngoscope 1998;108(4 Part 1):488–93.

[77] Maghami EG, Bonyadlou S, Larian B, et al. Magnetic resonance imaging–guided fine-needle aspiration biopsies of retropharyngeal lesions. Laryngoscope 2001;111(12):2218–24.

[78] Lai A, Maghami E, Borges A, et al. MRI-guided access to the retropharynx. J Magn Reson Imaging 2003;17(3):317–22.

[79] Davis SP, Anand VK, Dhillon G. Magnetic resonance navigation for head and neck lesions. Laryngoscope 1999;109(6):862–7.

[80] Merkle EM, Lewin JS, Aschoff AJ, et al. Percutaneous magnetic resonance image-guided biopsy and aspiration in the head and neck. Laryngoscope 2000;110(3 Part 1):382–5.

[81] Wang SJ, Sercarz JA, Lufkin RB, et al. MRI-guided needle localization in the head and neck using contemporaneous imaging in an open configuration system. Head Neck 2000;22(4): 355–9.

[82] He Y, Zhang Z, Tian Z, et al. The application of magnetic resonance imaging-guided fine-needle aspiration cytology in the diagnosis of deep lesions in the head and neck. J Oral Maxillofac Surg 2004; 62(8):953–8.

[83] Sack MJ, Weber RS, Weinstein GS, et al. Image-guided fine-needle aspiration of the head and neck: five years' experience. Arch Otolaryngol Head Neck Surg 1998;124(10):1155–61.

[84] Kacl GM, Bicik I, Schonenberger AW, et al. Interactive MR-guided biopsies of the thyroid gland: validation of a new method. Eur Radiol 1998; 8(7):1173–8.

[85] Takahashi S, Morikawa S, Egawa M, et al. Magnetic resonance imaging-guided percutaneous fenestration of a cervical intradural cyst. Case report. J Neurosurg Spine 2003;99(3):313–5.

[86] Kollias SS, Bernays R, Marugg RA, et al. Target definition and trajectory optimization for interactive MR-guided biopsies of brain tumors in an open configuration MRI system. J Magn Reson Imaging 1998;8(1):143–59.

[87] Bernays RL, Kollias SS, Khan N, et al. Histological yield, complications, and technological considerations in 114 consecutive frameless stereotactic biopsy procedures aided by open intraoperative magnetic resonance imaging. J Neurosurg 2002; 97(2):354–62.

[88] Lewin JS, Metzger A, Selman WR. Intraoperative magnetic resonance image guidance in neurosurgery. J Magn Reson Imaging 2000;12(4): 512–24.

[89] Lewin JS, Metzger AK. Intraoperative MR systems. Low-field approaches. Neuroimaging Clin N Am 2001;11(4):611–28.

[90] Fenchel S, Boll DT, Lewin JS. Intraoperative MR imaging. Magn Reson Imaging Clin N Am 2003; 11(3):431–47.

[91] Schulz T, Schneider JP, Bootz F, et al. Transnasal and transsphenoidal MRI-guided biopsies of petroclival tumors. J Magn Reson Imaging 2001;13(1): 3–11.

[92] Kollias SS, Bernays RL. Interactive magnetic resonance imaging-guided management of intracranial cystic lesions by using an open magnetic resonance imaging system. J Neurosurg 2001;95(1):15–23.

[93] Bernays RL, Kollias SS, Yonekawa Y. Dynamic changes during evacuation of a left temporal abscess in open MRI: technical case report. Neuroradiology 2002;44(5):438–42.

[94] Bernays RL, Kollias SS, Romanowski B, et al. Near-real-time guidance using intraoperative magnetic resonance imaging for radical evacuation of hypertensive hematomas in the basal ganglia. Neurosurgery 2000;47(5):1081–9 [discussion: 1089–90].

[95] Jolesz FA. Future perspectives for intraoperative MRI. Neurosurg Clin N Am 2005;16(1):201–13.

[96] Lu DS, Silverman SG, Raman SS. MR-guided therapy. Applications in the abdomen. Magn Reson Imaging Clin N Am 1999;7(2):337–48.

[97] Rofsky NM, Yang BM, Schlossberg P, et al. MR-guided needle aspiration biopsies of hepatic masses using a closed bore magnet. J Comput Assist Tomogr 1998;22(4):633–7.

[98] Boll DT, Lewin JS, Duerk JL, et al. Comparison of MR imaging sequences for liver and head and neck interventions: is there a single optimal sequence for all purposes? Acad Radiol 2004;11(5):506–15.

[99] Zangos S, Kiefl D, Eichler K, et al. MR-guided biopsies of undetermined liver lesions: technique and results. Rofo Fortschr Geb Rontgenstr Neuen Bildgeb Verfahr 2003;175(5):688–94 [in German].

[100] Konig CW, Trubenbach J, Fritz J, et al. Contrast enhanced MR-guided biopsy of hepatocellular carcinoma. Abdom Imaging 2004;29(1):71–6.

[101] Schmidt AJ, Kee ST, Sze DY, et al. Diagnostic yield of MR-guided liver biopsies compared with CT- and US-guided liver biopsies. J Vasc Interv Radiol 1999;10(10):1323–9.

[102] Adam G, Bucker A, Nolte-Ernsting C, et al. Interventional MR imaging: percutaneous abdominal and skeletal biopsies and drainages of the abdomen. Eur Radiol 1999;9(8):1471–8.

[103] Kariniemi J, Blanco Sequeiros R, Ojala R, et al. MRI-guided abdominal biopsy in a 0.23-T open-

configuration MRI system. Eur Radiol 2005;15(6): 1256–62.

[104] Frahm C, Gehl HB, Weiss HD, et al. Technique of MRT-guided core biopsy in the abdomen using an open low-field scanner: feasibility and initial clinical results. Rofo Fortschr Geb Rontgenstr Neuen Bildgeb Verfahr 1996;164(1):62–7 [in German].

[105] Konig CW, Pereira PL, Trubenbach J, et al. MR imaging-guided adrenal biopsy using an open low-field-strength scanner and MR fluoroscopy. AJR Am J Roentgenol 2003;180(6):1567–70.

[106] Beyersdorff D, Winkel A, Hamm B, et al. MR imaging-guided prostate biopsy with a closed MR unit at 1.5 T: initial results. Radiology 2005; 234(2):576–81.

[107] Zangos S, Eichler K, Engelmann K, et al. MR-guided transgluteal biopsies with an open low-field system in patients with clinically suspected prostate cancer: technique and preliminary results. Eur Radiol 2005;15(1):174–82.

[108] Kooy HM, Cormack RA, Mathiowitz G, et al. A software system for interventional magnetic resonance image-guided prostate brachytherapy. Comput Aided Surg 2000;5(6):401–13.

[109] Menard C, Susil RC, Choyke P, et al. MRI-guided HDR prostate brachytherapy in standard 1.5T scanner. Int J Radiat Oncol Biol Phys 2004;59(5): 1414–23.

[110] Susil RC, Krieger A, Derbyshire JA, et al. System for MR image-guided prostate interventions: canine study. Radiology 2003;228(3):886–94.

[111] Susil RC, Camphausen K, Choyke P, et al. System for prostate brachytherapy and biopsy in a standard 1.5 T MRI scanner. Magn Reson Med 2004;52(3): 683–7.

[112] Harms SE, Flamig DP, Hesley KL, et al. MR imaging of the breast with rotating delivery of excitation off resonance: clinical experience with pathologic correlation. Radiology 1993;187(2): 493–501.

[113] Orel SG, Schnall MD, Newman RW, et al. MR imaging-guided localization and biopsy of breast lesions: initial experience. Radiology 1994;193(1): 97–102.

[114] Heywang-Kobrunner SH, Huynh AT, Viehweg P, et al. Prototype breast coil for MR-guided needle localization. J Comput Assist Tomogr 1994;18(6): 876–81.

[115] Schnall MD, Orel SG, Connick TJ. MR guided biopsy of the breast. Magn Reson Imaging Clin N Am 1994;2(4):585–9.

[116] Fischer U, Vosshenrich R, Keating D, et al. MR-guided biopsy of suspect breast lesions with a simple stereotaxic add-on-device for surface coils. Radiology 1994;192(1):272–3.

[117] Teifke A, Hlawatsch A, Beier T, et al. Undetected malignancies of the breast: dynamic contrast-enhanced MR imaging at 1.0 T. Radiology 2002; 224(3):881–8.

[118] Schneider JP, Schulz T, Horn LC, et al. MR-guided percutaneous core biopsy of small breast lesions: first experience with a vertically open 0.5T scanner. J Magn Reson Imaging 2002;15(4):374–85.

[119] Orel SG, Schnall MD. MR imaging of the breast for the detection, diagnosis, and staging of breast cancer. Radiology 2001;220(1):13–30.

[120] Wald DS, Weinreb JC, Newstead G, et al. MR-guided fine needle aspiration of breast lesions: initial experience. J Comput Assist Tomogr 1996; 20(1):1–8.

[121] Heywang-Kobrunner SH, Heinig A, Schaumloffel U, et al. MR-guided percutaneous excisional and incisional biopsy of breast lesions. Eur Radiol 1999;9(8):1656–65.

[122] Helbich TH. Localization and biopsy of breast lesions by magnetic resonance imaging guidance. J Magn Reson Imaging 2001;13(6):903–11.

[123] Kuhl CK, Elevelt A, Leutner CC, et al. Interventional breast MR imaging: clinical use of a stereotactic localization and biopsy device. Radiology 1997;204(3):667–75.

[124] Fischer U, Vosshenrich R, Doler W, et al. MR imaging-guided breast intervention: experience with two systems. Radiology 1995;195(2):533–8.

[125] deSouza NM, Kormos DW, Krausz T, et al. MR-guided biopsy of the breast after lumpectomy and radiation therapy using two methods of immobilization in the lateral decubitus position. J Magn Reson Imaging 1995;5(5):525–8.

[126] Perlet C, Schneider P, Amaya B, et al. MR-guided vacuum biopsy of 206 contrast-enhancing breast lesions. Rofo Fortschr Geb Rontgenstr Neuen Bildgeb Verfahr 2002;174(1):88–95 [in German].

[127] Thiele J, Schneider JP, Franke P, et al. New method of MR-guided mammary biopsy. Rofo Fortschr Geb Rontgenstr Neuen Bildgeb Verfahr 1998; 168(4):374–9 [in German].

[128] Sittek H, Perlet C, Herrmann K, et al. MR mammography. Preoperative marking of non-palpable breast lesions with the Magnetom open at 0.2 T. Radiologe 1997;37(9):685–91 [in German].

[129] Daniel BL, Birdwell RL, Ikeda DM, et al. Breast lesion localization: a freehand, interactive MR imaging-guided technique. Radiology 1998;207(2): 455–63.

[130] Pfleiderer SO, Reichenbach JR, Azhari T, et al. A manipulator system for 14-gauge large core breast biopsies inside a high-field whole-body MR scanner. J Magn Reson Imaging 2003;17(4):493–8.

[131] Blanco Sequeiros R, Klemola R, Ojala R, et al. MRI-guided trephine biopsy and fine-needle aspiration in the diagnosis of bone lesions in low-field (0.23 T) MRI system using optical instrument tracking. Eur Radiol 2002;12(4):830–5.

[132] Parkkola RK, Mattila KT, Heikkila JT, et al. Dynamic contrast-enhanced MR imaging and MR-guided bone biopsy on a 0.23 T open imager. Skeletal Radiol 2001;30(11):620–4.

[133] Koenig CW, Duda SH, Truebenbach J, et al. MR-guided biopsy of musculoskeletal lesions in a low-field system. J Magn Reson Imaging 2001; 13(5):761–8.

[134] Genant JW, Vandevenne JE, Bergman AG, et al. Interventional musculoskeletal procedures performed by using MR imaging guidance with a vertically open MR unit: assessment of techniques and applicability. Radiology 2002;223(1):127–36.

[135] Fritzsch D, Scholz R, Werner A, et al. Use of a newly developed piezoelectrically driven drilling machine for MR-guided bone biopsies. Rofo Fortschr Geb Rontgenstr Neuen Bildgeb Verfahr 2002;174(10):1309–12 [in German].

[136] Neuerburg JM, Adam G, Buecker A, et al. MRI-guided biopsy of bone in a hybrid system. J Magn Reson Imaging 1998;8(1):85–90.

[137] Logan PM, Connell DG, O'Connell JX, et al. Image-guided percutaneous biopsy of musculoskeletal tumors: an algorithm for selection of specific biopsy techniques. AJR Am J Roentgenol 1996; 166(1).137–41.

[138] Rubens DJ, Fultz PJ, Gottlieb RH, et al. Effective ultrasonographically guided intervention for diagnosis of musculoskeletal lesions. J Ultrasound Med 1997;16(12):831–42.

[139] Andrews CL. From the RSNA Refresher Courses. Radiological Society of North America. Evaluation of the marrow space in the adult hip. Radiographics 2000;20(Suppl):S27–42.

[140] Levine CD, Schweitzer ME, Ehrlich SM. Pelvic marrow in adults. Skeletal Radiol 1994;23(5): 343–7.

[141] Jaramillo D, Laor T, Hoffer FA, et al. Epiphyseal marrow in infancy: MR imaging. Radiology 1991; 180(3):809–12.

[142] Neuerburg J, Adam G, Bucker A, et al. A new MR- (and CT-) compatible bone biopsy system:

first clinical results. Rofo Fortschr Geb Rontgenstr Neuen Bildgeb Verfahr 1998;169(5):515–20 [in German].

[143] Pereira PL, Fritz J, Koenig CW, et al. Preoperative marking of musculoskeletal tumors guided by magnetic resonance imaging. J Bone Joint Surg Am 2004;86-A(8):1761–7.

[144] Schulz T, Trobs RB, Schneider JP, et al. Pediatric MR-guided interventions. Eur J Radiol 2005; 53(1):57–66.

[145] Vitaz TW, Hushek SG, Shields CB, et al. Interventional MRI-guided frameless stereotaxy in pediatric patients. Stereotact Funct Neurosurg 2002; 79(3–4):182–90.

[146] Hall WA, Martin AJ, Liu H, et al. High-field strength interventional magnetic resonance imaging for pediatric neurosurgery. Pediatr Neurosurg 1998;29(5):253–9.

[147] Lam CH, Hall WA, Truwit CL, et al. Intra-operative MRI-guided approaches to the pediatric posterior fossa tumors. Pediatr Neurosurg 2001;34(6): 295–300.

[148] Nimsky C, Ganslandt O, Gralla J, et al. Intraoperative low-field magnetic resonance imaging in pediatric neurosurgery. Pediatr Neurosurg 2003;38(2): 83–9.

[149] Vitaz TW, Hushek S, Shields CB, et al. Intraoperative MRI for pediatric tumor management. Acta Neurochir Suppl (Wien) 2003;85:73–8.

[150] Ueno S, Yokoyama S, Hirakawa H, et al. Use of real-time magnetic resonance guidance to assist bone biopsy in pediatric malignancy. Pediatrics 2002;109(1):E18.

[151] Schulz T, Bennek J, Schneider JP, et al. MRI-guided pediatric interventions. Rofo Fortschr Geb Rontgenstr Neuen Bildgeb Verfahr 2003; 175(12):1673–81 [erratum: 2004;176(2):266] [in German].

ELSEVIER
SAUNDERS

Magn Reson Imaging Clin N Am
13 (2005) 465–479

**MAGNETIC
RESONANCE
IMAGING CLINICS**
of North America

Cardiovascular Interventional MR Imaging:
A New Road for Therapy and Repair in the Heart

Carsten Rickers, MD[a],[*], Dara Kraitchman, VMD, PhD[b],
Gunther Fischer, MD[a], Hans Heiner Kramer, MD[a],
Norbert Wilke, MD[c], Michael Jerosch-Herold, PhD[d]

[a]*Department of Pediatric Cardiology, University Hospital Schleswig-Holstein, Campus Kiel,
Brunswiker Strasse 10, 24105 Kiel, Germany*
[b]*The Russell H. Morgan Department of Radiology and Radiological Science, The Johns Hopkins University,
601 North Caroline Street, JHOC 4231, Baltimore, MD 21287-0845, USA*
[c]*Health Science Center, University of Florida, 655 West Eighth Street, Jacksonville, FL 32209-6511, USA*
[d]*Advanced Imaging Research Center, Oregon Health and Science University, Mailcode L452,
3181 SW Sam Jackson Park Road, Portland, OR 97239, USA*

Within the last decade, cardiovascular MR imaging has made rapid progress. Developments in scanner technology and pulse sequence design have resulted in exquisite capabilities for imaging cardiac anatomy, function, and perfusion, including new capabilities for real-time imaging. MR imaging is now recognized, among other cardiovascular applications, as an excellent tool for assessment of congenital cardiac malformations and for accurate quantification of blood flow. The introduction of 1.5-T short-bore magnets to allow access to the groin area for catheter-based procedures, flat-panel display technology compatible with high magnetic fields, and improvements in the hardware of the magnetic field gradient systems for faster image acquisitions have catalyzed progress in interventional MR imaging. Real-time imaging and the development of catheter-based MR imaging antennas for localized intravascular signal reception and high-resolution imaging have been key ingredients of these developments. This article provides an overview of the technical aspects of cardiovascular interventional MR imaging. The authors present important applications such as repair of congenital defects and injection of stem cells under MR imaging guidance and review

several pioneering studies that have proved the feasibility of these applications.

Cellular and gene therapeutics have seen an enormous growth in potential applications in recent years; however, the demonstration of efficacy has hinged in most preclinical studies on postmortem histologic analysis to validate gene transfection or stem cell/progenitor cell engraftment. MR imaging offers the potential to provide high-resolution anatomic detail for precise targeting of the therapeutics. The recent ability to label cells with MR contrast agents or to demonstrate selective contrast uptake with gene expression offers a method to serially study the distribution of stem cells or longevity of gene transfection. Moreover, clinical trials require methodologies that can be used to noninvasively and serially assess the presence of stem cells or gene expression, which in turn helps to determine the safety and efficacy of these therapies. Thus, the introduction of MR clinical scanners with real-time imaging capabilities has expanded the use of MR imaging from diagnostic tool to interventional application.

Setup for interventional MR imaging

Although conventional MR scanners have been used for MR-guided interventional studies,

---

* Corresponding author.
E-mail address: c_rickers@hotmail.com (C. Rickers).

there is a clear trend toward the development of MR imaging equipment and facilities specifically tailored for interventional procedures. Fig. 1 shows one of the first facilities in the United States built expressly for interventional cardiovascular MR-guided studies. At least in the near future, it is likely that investigators in this field will not rely exclusively on MR imaging as the imaging modality for interventional studies but will prefer a hybrid setup with an MR imaging scanner and x-ray fluoroscopy equipment in close proximity and a movable patient table that allows unfettered movement of the patient between the two types of equipment.

Numerous aspects need to be considered in the design of such a facility. The x-ray–shielded and radiofrequency (RF)-shielded suite should include MR-compatible anesthesia and monitoring equipment. The image intensifier of the x-ray unit needs to be magnetically shielded to avoid disturbing the homogeneity of the magnetic field in the MR imaging magnet. Liquid crystal displays are installed next to the magnet bore, often suspended from the ceiling on articulated arms so that an operator manipulating catheters can see the MR images that are being acquired or can control the MR imaging acquisition parameters. Due to the

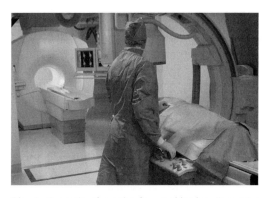

Fig. 1. Example of a suite for combined radiography and MR imaging studies (in this case, the UCSF Interventional XMR Suite (University of California, San Francisco). A patient can be moved rapidly and without repositioning on the patient table between the C-arm in the foreground (used for x-ray fluoroscopy) and the MR scanner in the background. The C-arm can be used for initial positioning of catheters, whereas the MR scanner is used for MR-guided procedures. Flat-panel displays suspended from the ceiling next to the bore of the MR magnet can be used for simultaneous display of MR and radiographic images for procedure guidance. (Courtesy of A. Martin, PhD, San Francisco, California.)

possibly high levels of acoustic noise during MR scanning, operators often wear special headphone/ microphone sets to communicate with each other and with personnel outside the suite. An interesting design feature of an installation in the United Kingdom [1] is the use of a scrub room as an "RF airlock" (ie, personnel can enter or leave the main MR imaging suite during scanning without causing interference with image acquisitions).

Real-time MR imaging

Continuous advances in the development of MR gradient systems have been crucial for enabling high-speed MR imaging, with image acquisition times sufficiently short to allow real-time imaging, as required for image-guided interventions. With standard gradient-echo imaging, the signal-to-noise ratio and the image quality often become suboptimal when the receiver bandwidth exceeds approximately 100 to 200 kHz. Gradient-echo imaging with steady-state free precession has circumvented this limitation and provides images with excellent signal-to-noise ratio and mixed T1 and T2 contrast while maintaining short image acquisition times (~ 250 milliseconds for 128 phase encodings). In their simplest embodiments, these techniques sample the image data on a Cartesian grid (in k-space). To speed-up the image acquisition in fluoroscopic applications, the central part of k-space, which defines the most prominent image features, can be updated more frequently than the outer edges. For example, while acquiring all phase encodings for the first image, all subsequent images use some k-space lines from previous acquisitions to fill the outer portions of k-space, and only the central approximately 30% to 50% of k-space is refreshed during each image acquisition. This technique is appropriately referred to as "key-hole" imaging [2–4]. An interesting alternative is reduced field-of-view imaging, which can be thought of as imaging through a "key-hole" in real space instead of k-space [5].

More recently, the parallel acquisition of image data with arrays of coils has led to the development of techniques such as MR imaging with sensitivity encoding [6] and MR imaging with simultaneous acquisition of spatial harmonics [7]. MR imaging with sensitivity encoding and with simultaneous acquisition of spatial harmonics reduce scan time by taking advantage of the local spatial information that can be obtained from each coil. Sensitivity profiles are obtained for each coil and a full field-of-view image is obtained by combining the intermediate images obtained in parallel from each coil, thereby reducing the number of phase-encoding steps while maintaining spatial in-plane resolution. These parallel imaging techniques can provide speed-up factors (R) of approximately two to three for real-time cardiovascular imaging with four- to eight-element phased-array coils [8,9]. If the coil sensitivity profiles do not overlap, then the signal-to-noise ratio would drop by a factor that is proportional to the square root of the speed-up factor ($\propto \sqrt{R}$) compared with nonparallel imaging (ie, adding signals from each coil before image reconstruction). In real-world settings, the sensitivity profiles of coil elements overlap, and the decrease in signal-to-noise ratio is then even higher. Speed-up factors higher than two to three can be obtained, in principle, with arrays that have higher numbers of coil elements, but for real-time imaging in particular, image speed-up factors higher than approximately two to three prove impractical or suboptimal.

Alternatively or in combination with parallel imaging, techniques such as spiral or echoplanar scanning are used to scan k-space efficiently after each RF excitation. Conventional scanning on a Cartesian grid is done by acquiring one line of data at a time, whereas spiral and echoplanar scanning acquire several lines of data or data along a spiral that start at the center of k-space after each RF excitation. Spiral [10,11] and echoplanar [12] imaging have been successfully applied for real-time imaging of the heart, and probably work best at field strengths of 1.5 T or lower, although one recent report indicated success by using echoplanar imaging with spectral-spatial excitation pulses for real-time imaging at 3 T [13]. An interesting combination of echotrain readouts along radial trajectories, with steady-state free precession, was demonstrated by Larson and Simonetti [14] to achieve a temporal resolution of 45 milliseconds, which would translate into a fluoroscopic frame rate of 20 frames per second.

For fluoroscopic imaging applications, frame rates on the order of 10 to 20 frames per second can readily be achieved with the currently available technology. The slice plane can be continuously adjusted by the operator with interactive mouse or track-ball control of the slice position and orientation and without interruption of the scan. Current state-of-the-art scanners have sufficiently fast reconstruction and display processors to allow fluoroscopic imaging with latency times on the order of 1 second or shorter.

Catheter tracking

Methods for catheter tracking can be roughly divided into two categories, namely, passive [15–17] and active [18] tracking. The difference is based mainly on whether the catheter functions as a receive antenna or whether its detection is based on a characteristic "signature" on images acquired with external coils. Catheter tips, not designed for receiving an MR signal, can cause signal loss around the catheter ("susceptibility artifacts") that can be accentuated by impregnating the catheter with paramagnetic substances such as dysprosium oxide [19]. Alternatively, bright signal spots (T1-based enhancement) can be created by loading the catheter with contrast agent [20]. Both methods can be used to recognize the position of a catheter during an endovascular procedure in a passive manner.

The high signal intensity areas around metallic components in a conventional radiographic catheter or guidewire are the result of "focusing" RF energy by the metallic components in the catheter tip, with subsequent localized heating. These signal "hot spots" in metallic devices have raised safety concerns [21] about active MR catheters and devices that are non–MR compatible. Nevertheless, certain passive features of catheters and guidewires can be exploited (albeit with considerable care) for detection of the catheter position on the MR imaging images. Taking this one step further, some sort of resonant circuit can be incorporated in the catheter tip, which can be optically detuned over a fiber-optic link so that the appearance of high signal intensities around the catheter tip can be controlled by the operator [22]. The use of a fiber-optic link rather than an electrical connection reduces the risk to the patient of excessive local heating.

Of the two tracking methods, active tracking is the more versatile because it allows a signal to be received from tissue and blood in the immediate vicinity of the catheter, in parallel to the acquisition of images with the customary external coils. The catheter simply constitutes one additional coil element with its own receive channel, and the image from the catheter can be reconstructed separately. For tracking, the image from the catheter can be color encoded and superimposed on the gray-scale MR image acquired with the external coils. The spatial sensitivity range of the catheter coil is relatively short and strongly peaked around the catheter tip. A color-encoded image from the catheter coil, with its steep drop-off of signal intensity with increasing distance from the catheter tip, facilitates the localization of the tip. In many cases, the image obtained from the catheter tip is of low quality and used only to update information about the position of the catheter tip and to display this information as a small graphic overlay (eg, a "catheter tip icon") on the images acquired with the external coils.

Although the use of passive or active tracking addresses the localization of the catheter tip on the MR images, it still leaves the user with the variably challenging task of continuously adjusting the image slice so that the catheter tip can be seen at all times while the catheter is advanced. In initial studies, the bright signal from the catheter antenna allowed the clinician to use relatively thick slices, similar to the approach of using high intravascular contrast enhancement and maximum intensity projection to see vessel segments in a thick slab. The resulting MR image would allow reasonably accurate localization of the catheter within the slice plane, but at the price of drastically reduced resolution in the slice direction. More novel imaging protocols incorporate a set of projection scouts to detect the catheter location or use multiple tracking coils on the catheter, and then an MR image with adequate resolution in a slice plane that tracks the catheter tip is obtained [23]. This methodology results in minimal disturbance of the normal imaging protocol, and the additional encoding steps for catheter tip detection take no more than 20 to 30 milliseconds and can be interleaved with normal anatomic imaging.

User interfaces

By its very nature, interventional MR imaging requires a more interactive approach than is required for diagnostic studies. Clinicians would like to have multiple views of the target area with adequate resolution, updated at high speed (ie, short latency times); however, these requirements cannot all be reconciled to achieve uniformly optimal settings. Rather, a balance needs to be struck between the requirements of spatial resolution, temporal resolution, and signal-to-noise ratio. The development of graphic user interfaces can go a long way toward alleviating some of the repercussions from these constraints by allowing a switch between rapid, real-time imaging during catheter movement and high-resolution scanning while the catheter remains stationary. Fig. 2 shows an example of a user interface designed for interventional MR imaging studies.

Intravascular antennas

Catheters and guidewires can be designed such that they also function as receiving devices to pick up an MR signal from surrounding tissue. Designs with wire loops and loopless designs have been proposed to accommodate the requirements of miniaturizing an MR receiving antenna without disrupting the functionality of the catheter or guidewire. Examples of both designs are shown in Fig. 3, including the opposed solenoid design [24] and a design based on twisted wire pairs [25]. Intravascular catheter-based MR antennas with wire loops (eg, in the form of opposed solenoids as initially proposed by Hurst and colleagues [24]) were introduced first, whereas the loopless designs are more recent [26]. The opposed solenoid–based design offers the advantage of some intrinsic isolation from RF excitation by an external coil [27]. Compared with solenoid-based configurations, the key advantages of the loopless designs are their compactness, their lack of orientation dependence on antenna performance with respect to the static main magnetic field in the magnet, and the slower drop-off of receiver sensitivity with distance [28]. Recently, it was also shown that a vascular stent could be designed such that the stent becomes an inductive component of an intravascular RF resonator that could be inductively coupled to an external antenna [29]. This type of stent-based resonator would allow localized MR imaging to assess patency of stented vessel segments.

Safety of interventional MR imaging devices

New safety concerns are raised when MR imaging is performed with intravascular coils. Such intravascular coils may be used, for example, to examine vulnerable plaque on vessel walls, and the resultant localized heating in the vicinity of the coil could disrupt the plaque with catastrophic consequences. Any MR receive-only antenna incorporated into a catheter can interact with the RF transmit coil, usually the body coil of an MR imaging scanner. The complexity of this

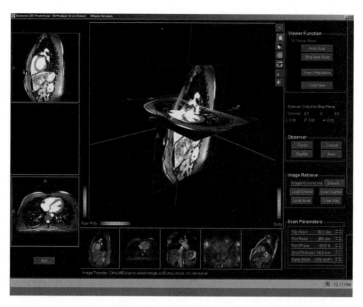

Fig. 2. Example of a user interface developed for real-time imaging and interactive scan control to facilitate MR-guided interventional procedures. In this screenshot, the interface is used to control the acquisition of images of the heart, including the standard short- and long-axis views, which are combined in the main viewing window to show the relative orientation of these two views, updated in real-time. This front-end can be operated in two modes. Mode 1 can be used to visualize cardiac motion while the image planes remain fixed. Mode 2 can be used for active slice manipulation so that slices can track catheter tip location. In mode 1, the application can also automatically extract image features (eg, volume time curves can be generated in the background). (Courtesy of C.H. Lorenz, PhD, Imaging and Visualization, Siemens Corporate Research, Princeton, New Jersey; with permission.)

interaction makes it difficult, in principle, to predict the RF specific absorption rate around the catheter antenna. The coupling between catheter antenna and body coil depends, among other factors, on the geometry of the coil, the position and orientation within the scanner, and the electrical properties of the patient. It is almost impossible to control all of these factors, so clinicians focus on effective decoupling of the two antennas. One possible solution is to use detuning circuits that switch off the resonant properties of the receive-only antenna while RF power is being transmitted.

Previous work has confirmed the possibility of substantial local heating with straight copper wires, tracking catheters, and guidewires in place. As already mentioned, such heating effects can be minimized or eliminated by incorporating decoupling circuitry into the device and thereby limiting the amount of energy transfer through the probe/wire by the transmit coil. The authors conducted temperature measurement of the heating effects in a gel phantom with a miniature, loopless intravascular antenna (Surgi-Vision, Marietta, Georgia). The 1-m loopless, coaxial (dipole)

antenna was connected to a decoupling, matching, and tuning interface. This interface contains an RF trap circuit and an active detuning circuit with an RF pin diode. During the transmit phase, the pin diode is activated and presents a short circuit for signals traveling on the inner conductor of the loopless antenna. The effectiveness of the decoupling mechanism was tested in an 8-in diameter and 20-in long cylindric gel phantom with a dielectric constant of 81 and a conductivity of 0.7 siemens per meter. Tests were performed to investigate the effect of antenna position within the phantom, the position of the phantom relative to the isocenter of the MR system, and the insertion depth of the antenna in the phantom. In all experiments, temperature-versus-time curves were obtained. In most cases, the temperature in the disconnected state remained below $1\,°C$, with the exception of the distal tip, the midcoil, the hypotube, and the entry point. These four positions typically showed a temperature rise of up to $7\,°C$ to $8\,°C$ for an RF field of 3.6 µT rms. The exact temperature varies as a function of insertion depth and coil position in the phantom and bore. In the connected state, the temperature rise never

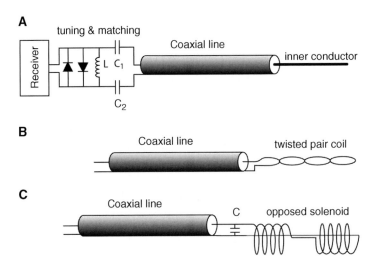

Fig. 3. Examples of intravascular antenna designs. (*A*) Loopless design. This design uses the internal conductor of a coaxial cable as dipole antenna and the relatively modest drop-off of receiver sensitivity ($\sim 1/r$) compared with $1/r^3$ for designs with wire loops. A further advantage of this loopless design is the flexibility of moving the circuits to tune the resonance frequency and match the impedance to the distal end of a coaxial cable (ie, to a location outside the body). (*B*, *C*) These designs use a twisted-pair coil (*B*) and a pair of solenoids in opposed orientations (*C*) for signal detection.

exceeded 4°C and, in most cases, remained below 1°C. In the absence of or with malfunction of the decoupling, matching, and tuning interface, however, a temperature increase on the order of 10°C to 20°C could be observed under worst-case circumstances with the antenna connected to the MR receiver.

Safety concerns have to be addressed conclusively before conducting clinical studies in humans and especially in pediatric patients. When standing waves form along the conductive catheter wires in the body, they can cause thermal injury [30,31]. Guidewires used in the studies should be connected to an RF decoupling/detuning box that limits the energy transferred by the RF pulses to the receive-only antenna [26,32].

MR-guided interventions in pediatric patients

Concerns exist about the long-term health effects of x-ray doses used in cardiac catheterization, in particular when ionizing radiation impinges on immature and proliferating tissue such as in infants or in developing breasts. For adults, the UK National Radiological Protection Board has calculated a mean risk of developing a solid tumor after one cardiac catheterization of about 1 in 2500 [33]. In children, however, there are two important additional factors to consider. First, the younger the patient, the higher the risk: for example, if exposure occurs at age 5 years, the risk

is about 1 in 1000. Second, because a substantial number of children with congenital heart disease undergo repeated fluoroscopically guided cardiac catheterizations, the risk is multiplied [34–36].

Transcatheter balloon dilatation with or without stent placement in aortic recoarctation as an alternative to surgical resection has seen widespread use in pediatric cardiology centers [37–39]. Recently, it has been demonstrated that MR-guided dilatation of artificially created coarctations of the aorta and stent placement using intravascular miniature antenna guidewires is feasible in a porcine model (Fig. 4) [40]. The results were directly compared with conventional x-ray–guided catheter interventions in the same clinical setting and showed that there was a better correlation of MR measurements of the diameters of the stenosis with intraoperative measurements than with stenosis diameter measurements obtained from radiographic images. There was no significant difference in pressure gradients across the stenosis calculated from velocity-encoded cine MR imaging and invasive measurements.

Dilatation of the aortic stenosis with an air-filled balloon can be well visualized under MR fluoroscopy (Fig. 5A). Furthermore, it was demonstrated that the nitinol stent could be connected to a loopless miniature antenna and therefore serve as an active receiver for high-resolution MR imaging. After decoupling of the stent from the wire, the stent was no longer actively visible and

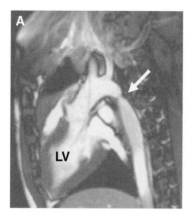

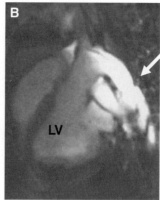

Fig. 4. (*A*) Sagittal view of the aortic arch and descending aorta obtained with a bright blood gradient echo cine sequence shows a severe coarctation of the aorta. A trigger catheter coming from the carotid artery was placed in the left ventricle (*LV*). (*B*) Image shows one frame acquired during guidewire tracking with real-time MR imaging using only a loopless miniature antenna wire. With the conventional external phased-array coils turned off, the short-range receiver profile predominantly shows structures in the near vicinity of the guidewire. Arrow shows coarctation of the aorta.

created only a passive artifact resulting from the nitinol mesh (see Fig. 5B, stent in aorta). This design was also adapted for improving visibility of other cardiovascular implants such as the Amplatzer ASD occluder (AGA Medical Corporation, Golden Valley, Minnesota) (Fig. 6A, B) or aortic stents (see Fig. 6C).

A different strategy to improve signal-to-noise ratio is to use inductive coupling to an endovascular stent [29]. This design has the potential advantage of providing increased local signal intensity even many years after its implantation for assessment of restenosis, without requiring an invasive electrical connection to the device. So far, this prototype has been used only in rabbit aorta, which unlike the

heart, is a fairly static organ. The use for coronary imaging has not yet been demonstrated.

Clinical implications

Currently for all age groups, radiography is the modality of choice for atrial septal defect closure and other cardiovascular catheter interventions [41–43]. Ionizing radiation, however, becomes an issue for radiographic imaging in more complex, lengthy procedures as opposed to relatively straightforward atrial septal defect closures [44]. MR imaging uses a noniodinated contrast agent (gadolinium) that has no adverse effects [45], which is especially appealing for use in patients

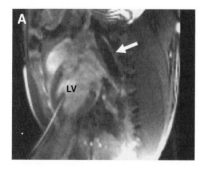

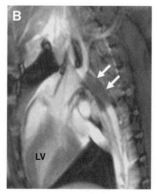

Fig. 5. (*A*) Dilatation of the coarctation was performed with an air-filled balloon under MR fluoroscopy with a true fast imaging with steady precession pulse sequence, with interactive control of scan plan by an assistant operator. The air-filled balloon (*arrow*) can be seen clearly as a dark structure in the lumen of the aorta, with excellent contrast against the bright blood. (*B*) The same view post dilatation and after placement of a nitinol stent (dark structure highlighted by *two arrows*). LV, left ventricle.

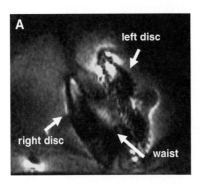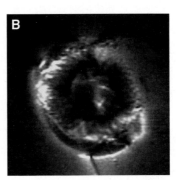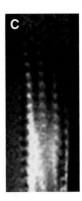

Fig. 6. Orthogonal views of customized Amplatzer septal occluder device (AGA Medical Corporation), implanted under MR imaging guidance in a porcine model with atrial septal defect. (*A*, *B*) Images acquired at the end of the procedure with a loopless catheter antenna (Surgi-Vision) using a gradient echo pulse sequence with steady-state free precession ("true FISP"). The septal occluder device was custom made out of nitinol. The nitinol mesh produced artifacts with acceptable characteristics for passive tracking at a field strength of 1.5 T. (*A*) Side view shows the left and right discs on the respective sides of the atrial wall and the "waist of the device" (ie, the part that passes through the atrial septal defect). (*C*) A nitinol stent in the aorta that is inductively coupled to a catheter antenna, resulting in signal enhancement in the proximity of the stent mesh.

with renal compromise. In addition, MR imaging is attractive because it allows for concurrent atrial septal defect sizing and measurements of right cardiac volume.

Practicality and ease of use are an important aspect in performing complex cardiovascular interventions. Interventional MR-guided percutaneous procedures require direct access to the groin and neck for manipulation of catheters and devices. In the authors' studies in a short-bore magnet, they were able to manipulate the catheters from the groin. Open-sided MR systems would be ideal but are limited by a low magnetic field strength (<1 T) that reduces the signal-to-noise ratio, making the resultant images often unacceptable for cardiac interventions [46,47]. Currently, widespread application of interventional MR imaging is hampered by the limited commercial availability of MR-compatible guidewires, delivery cables, and monitoring equipment.

Endovascular MR imaging and delivery techniques

Endovascular delivery offers a method to apply a high concentration of vectors in a localized region for gene therapy, thereby potentially avoiding the side effects associated with systemic administration. The earliest effort at MR-guided endovascular gene in vivo delivery was performed by Yang and colleagues [48]. A Remedy (SCIMED Remedy; Boston Scientific, Natick,

Massachusetts) gene delivery catheter was used, and the conventional guidewire was replaced with a loopless antenna [26] to create an active MR imaging guidewire. A lentiviral vector gene carrying green fluorescent protein was mixed with 6% gadolinium contrast agent, and delivery was monitored in real-time (Fig. 7) and confirmed by postmortem histology.

RF heating of imaging guidewires, which is normally of concern with active catheter systems, has been exploited in this application by Gao and colleagues [49] to enhance gene transfection rates. In a similar study to visualize gene delivery, Barbash and coworkers [50] used a percutaneous approach in a rat infarction model to deliver an adenoviral LacZ reporter gene mixed with gadolinium by way of a 22-gauge needle.

Transvenous and transesophageal approaches for vascular imaging have been successfully demonstrated in human clinical trials using an active MR-compatible imaging guidewire. The advantage of these techniques is that the higher signal-to-noise ratio that can be achieved compared with surface coils enables high-resolution imaging using a minimally invasive approach. Hofmann and Liddell [51] recently showed the ability to obtain high-resolution images of plaques in the common iliac artery using a transvenous approach in patients with claudication (Fig. 8). Because real-time MR imaging does not have the high temporal resolution of x-ray angiography, a transvenous approach enables imaging with sufficient

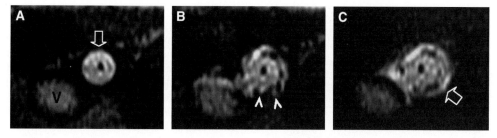

Fig. 7. High-resolution MR images of the gadolinium/green fluorescent protein–lentivirus transfer in the iliac artery of a pig. (*A*) Before gadolinium/green fluorescent protein–lentivirus infusion, the balloon is inflated with 3% gadopentetate dimeglumine. Open arrow indicates the artery; scale = 1 mm. (*B*) At 3 minutes after gadolinium/green fluorescent protein–lentivirus infusion, the arterial wall is enhanced by the gadolinium coming from the gene infusion channels (*arrowheads*) of the gene delivery catheter. (*C*) At 15 minutes post injection, the arterial wall is enhanced as a ring (*open arrow*). V, vein. (*Adapted from* Yang X, Atalar E, Li D, et al. Magnetic resonance imaging permits in vivo monitoring of catheter-based vascular gene delivery. Circulation 2001;104:1589; with permission.)

resolution and without risk of trauma to arterial plaques, which may occur using a direct transarterial approach without adequate visualization.

Another niche where interventional MR imaging is likely to see large growth is the application to interventions in which conventional x-ray fluoroscopy is poor at demonstrating soft tissue detail. Weiss and coworkers [52] developed a novel device and an MR fluoroscopy platform to create minimally invasive mesocaval shunts (ie, anastomoses between the portal mesenteric venous system and the inferior vena cava). Such procedures that alleviate portal hypertension in cirrhosis patients are currently performed surgically (ie, with end-to-side mesocaval shunts or by percutanous transjugular intrahepatic portosystemic shunts). Using a real-time steady-state free precession pulse sequence with interactive scan plan acquisition, the procedure was demonstrated in swine using an active MR imaging intravascular needle system, which was guided into the inferior vena cava. The needle was guided through the inferior vena cava into the superior mesenteric or portal vein, followed by an MR angiogram/venogram to confirm proper puncture location (Fig. 9). A nitinol needle was advanced into the portal venous system so that angioplasty with subsequent placement of an anastomostic device under x-ray fluoroscopy could be performed. Such puncture procedures are precluded by x-ray fluoroscopy alone due to the risk of puncturing adjacent structures that are invisible without the high spatial resolution and soft tissue detail of MR imaging.

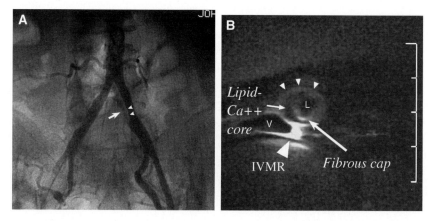

Fig. 8. Using a transvenous approach with an MR-compatible active imaging guidewire in the common iliac vein, a coronal x-ray angiogram (*A*) of a 61-year-old patient with bilateral claudication demonstrates a large plaque (*arrows, arrowheads*) in the common iliac artery. (*B*) An axial high-resolution T1-weighted axial MR image demonstrates the bright fibrous cap with the hypointense lipid calcium (Ca++) in the iliac artery. IVMR, MR-compatible active imaging guidewire; L, lumen; V, vein. (Courtesy of L.V. Hofmann, MD, Baltimore, Maryland.)

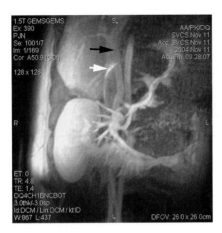

Fig. 9. MR angiogram/venogram demonstrates successful transcaval puncture of the portal vein in a swine
model. Active intravascular needle consisting of nitinol
hypotubings arranged in a loopless antenna configuration [26] appears hyperintense (*white arrow*) as it exits
the inferior vena cava and enters the portal venous
system (*black arrow*). An MR-compatible guidewire is
then advanced into the portal system for angioplasty and
placement of an anatomosis device under MR or x-ray
fluoroscopy. (Courtesy of A. Arepally, MD, Baltimore,
Maryland.)

Lederman, McVeigh, Raval, and coworkers
[52a,52b] have been developing devices for other,
novel interventional MR imaging applications
such as septal punctures and total vessel occlusion
recanalization.

Cellular labeling strategies for MR imaging delivery and tracking

Most cellular labeling strategies have been
directed toward labeling with ultrasmall superparamagnetic iron oxide (SPIO) compounds for in
vivo applications. The preferred method for cell
labeling by MR imaging is internalization of the
compound because surface labels may become
detached and transferred to other cells. Thus, the
primary advantages of SPIO labeling over paramagnetic labeling is that, even when internalized,
the large magnetic moment of the SPIO creates
a substantial disturbance in the local magnetic
field, leading to a rapid dephasing of protons
including those not directly in the vicinity of the
targeted cell. Consequently, picogram quantities
of iron per cell can lead to large hypointense
artifacts on T2*-weighted images that can be
easily visualized. In fact, several groups have
demonstrated the ability to image single cells
labeled with SPIOs [53,54].

SPIOs and ultrasmall SPIOs are readily taken
up by phagocytic cells. Hence, clinically approved
applications of these compounds are for tumor
detection in the liver where Kupffer cells (specialized macrophages in the liver) are replaced by
neoplastic cells that fail to phagocytize SPIOs.
Although many methods have been developed to
internalize SPIOs and ultrasmall SPIOs within
cells, methods using transfection agents, such as
poly-L-lysine [55–57] and protamine sulfate [58],
are rapidly becoming the preferred methods for
cellular labeling because these techniques are
non–species specific and use compounds that are
inexpensive and readily available. Another advantage of SPIO labeling is that when the cells are
lysed, the iron oxide is only taken up by phagocytic cells and ultimately recycled in the iron pool,
rendering the label nontoxic. Other groups have
used large, styrene/divinyl benzene-coated magnetic microspheres [59,60] called "Bang" particles,
but it remains to be determined whether a clinical
formulation can be achieved that is biocompatible.

The biggest potential problem with SPIO
labeling is that cells that are degraded can
potential release the SPIO, which may be incorporated by adjacent phagocytic cells. Thus,
hypointense artifacts in images at later time points
after cell delivery may represent cells other than
the original exogenously labeled cells. Therefore,
strict quantification of cell numbers based on the
change in the volume of the hypointense artifact is
difficult to determine.

Imaging stem cell delivery

Several cardiovascular applications have recently been explored that exploit the ability of
MR imaging to noninvasively demonstrate infarcted tissue from delayed-contrast MR imaging
[61] to target labeled stem cells to specific regions
of the heart [55,60,62,63]. Clinical trials with stem
cell therapeutics in the heart are underway in
Europe [64–66]. MR cellular labeling has the
potential to precisely target the cells and determine
the cellular engraftment by the persistence of
hypointense artifacts on follow-up examinations.

Using a real-time imaging platform, Lederman
and colleagues [67] were the first to demonstrate
the use of transendocardial injections of MR
contrast agents under MR fluoroscopy on a clinical 1.5-T scanner in swine. Injections were
performed through combined use of an interactive
custom software interface and a modified Boston
Scientific Stiletto (Boston Scientific) injection

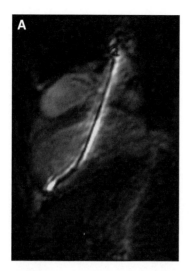
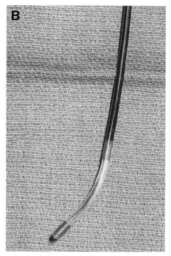

Fig. 10. (*A*) The distal tip of a custom MR-compatible loopless antenna [63] for transendocardial injection of genetic and cellular therapeutics appears as a bright signal at the distal tip and along a large portion of the in-plane length in a long-axis T1-weighted cardiac image. (*B*) The mechanical properties for steering and flexibility to reach all portions of the left ventricular endocardium are incorporated into a pull-wire. Approximately 25% deflection capability of the catheter tip is demonstrated.

catheter originally designed for x-ray fluoroscopy. Subsequently, the ability to track SPIO-poly-L-lysine (PLL)–labeled allogeneic mesenchymal stem cells (MSCs) as hypointense artifacts on T2*-weighted images in a clinically relevant swine model of acute myocardial infarction was demonstrated by Kraitchman and coworkers [68]. Follow-up MR imaging at several weeks after MSC injection showed changes in signal intensity and volume of the hypoenhancing artifact indicative of migration of the MSC within the myocardial infarction (Fig. 10). Delivery of the magnetically labeled MSCs was performed under x-ray fluoroscopy, with only approximately 70% of the injections visualized by MR imaging. Thus, the potential for enhanced injection success rate could be envisioned using MR delivery of magnetically labeled stem stells. Karmarkar and coworkers [63] designed an MR-compatible injection catheter specifically for cellular therapy applications that demonstrated enhanced steerability and, thus, the ability to target all areas of the ventricle (Fig. 11). In addition, this loopless antenna device was optimized to have high a signal-to-noise ratio along several centimeters of the length such that visualization could be achieved using standard vendor hardware and software. Modifications need to be made, however, to decrease heating of the device when the needle is deployed during therapeutic injections.

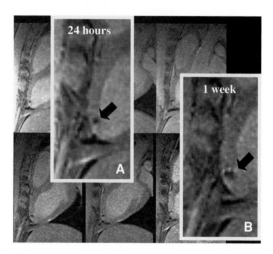

Fig. 11. Contiguous long-axis MR images acquired with a high-resolution, breath-hold ECG-gated fast gradient echo pulse ($500 \times 500 \times 5000 \ \mu m^3$ resolution) sequence show a hypointense lesion (*arrows*) caused by Feridex-PLL-labeled MSCs acquired within 24 hours (*A*) and 1 week (*B*) of injection in a pig with a myocardial infarction. The inset to right shows a magnified view from a single long-axis image demonstrating expansion of lesion over 1 week and a change in the shape of the hypointense lesion from an ovid shape to a shape with more irregular borders, suggesting migration of the MSCs. (*Adapted from* Kraitchman DL, Heldman AW, Atalar E, et al. In vivo magnetic resonance imaging of mesenchymal stem cells in myocardial infarction. Circulation 2003;107:2292; with permission.)

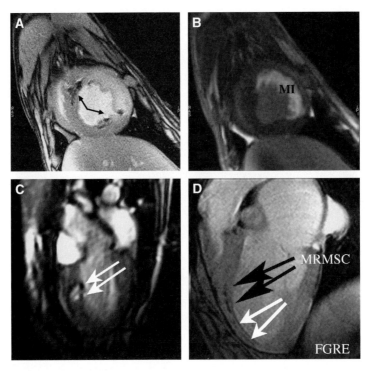

Fig. 12. Targeting of the autologous canine ferumoxides-poly-L-lysine–labeled MSCs (MRMSC) in a canine myocardial infarction (*MI*) model to the peri-infarction region using MR fluoroscopic delivery can be guided by delayed contrast-enhanced short-axis MR imaging, which shows infarcted myocardium (*B*). Stem cell placement was validated on high-resolution fast gradient echo (FGRE) short-axis images (*A*). Still-frame long-axis view from real-time MR imaging (*C*) demonstrate labeled MSCs as hypoenhancing artifacts (*arrows*) after initial two injections at 3 days post infarction. Top lesion is 7×10^6 Feridex-labeled MSCs; bottom lesion is 3×10^6 labeled MSCs with 4×10^6 unlabeled MSCs. At 2 months after injection, the initial two injections (*D, black arrows*) are still visible, as are additional injections (*D, yellow arrows*) with as low as 1×10^5 labeled MSCs at initial injection in high-resolution FGRE images. Hypoenhancing artifacts change from round lesions to linear lesions by 8 weeks. (*Adapted from* Bulte JW, Kraitchman DL. Monitoring cell therapy using iron oxide MR contrast agents. Curr Pharm Biotechnol 2004;5:579; with permission. *See the Web version for color.*)

Hill and colleagues [62] showed in a swine myocardial infarction model that as few as 10^5 labeled MSCs could be detected. Dick and co-workers [60] using Bang-labeled MSCs in this same swine myocardial infarction model were able to precisely target the magnetically labeled MSCs to the infarct with a 100% success rate using MR fluoroscopic delivery. In a dosing study in a canine model of myocardial infarction, Bulte and colleagues [55] demonstrated that 10^5 autologous SPIO-PLL–labeled MSCs injected under MR fluoroscopy were still visible by MR imaging at 2 months post injection and demonstrated precise targeting to the peri-infarction region (Fig. 12). Thus, magnetically labeled stem cells can be successfully delivered noninvasively using MR fluoroscopy with noninvasive serial follow-up of the persistence and, hence, engraftment of the MSCs.

Much of the thrust of SPIO-labeled cellular delivery with MR fluoroscopic guidance has been to perform studies in large animals in which the devices that are developed are similar to those that would be used in human trials. In addition, these imaging protocols were developed on 1.5-T MR clinical scanners for translation to clinical trials. Moreover, it can be expected that many of these studies with magnetically labeled stem cells will soon present results of the regional changes in infarction size, perfusion, and global and regional function using the inherent advantages of the high spatial resolution, and of the noninvasiveness of MR imaging techniques. In a dog model of chronic myocardial infarction, Rickers and colleagues [69] used MR imaging in this manner to assess improvements in myocardial perfusion reserve and regional myocardial function in animals that received unlabeled stem cells (eg, multipotent adult progenitor cells) compared with control animals that received sham intramyocardial injections by way of a surgical approach.

Another possible approach will be the use of hybrid x-ray/MR imaging systems. A prototypic steerable catheter with a nitinol needle for endovascular injections manufactured by Bioheart (Sunrise, Florida) is coated with gadolinium oxide markers for visualization under such a system [70]. As visualization and multimodality fusion tools improve, it can be envisioned that cardiac catheterization will be performed under radiographic guidance using delayed contrast-enhanced MR imaging roadmaps to precisely target infarcted myocardium because unlike other tissue, the heart does not tend to deform as greatly after cellular injections.

Gene and stem cell therapeutics for the heart have been advancing rapidly in the last few years. In concert, MR imaging methods and devices have been rapidly evolving to keep pace. Thus, it is likely that MR techniques for tracking gene expression and cellular labeling will provide noninvasive means to determine the success of these therapies as we move into clinical trials.

Summary

Over the last 5 years, interventional MR imaging has been fertile ground for research. Real-time MR imaging, combined with recent advances in other MR imaging modalities such as perfusion imaging and intravascular imaging, has opened up new paths for cardiac therapy. The recent reports on cardiac stem cell therapy guided and monitored by MR imaging suggest that we are already seeing the establishment of an important role for cardiac MR imaging in cardiac restoration. The collaborative effort from a multidisciplinary team of basic biologists, engineers, and clinicians will refine stem cell incubation and labeling for MR-guided transcatheter endomyocardial injections, and this in turn may facilitate new studies in humans.

Several groups have demonstrated in animal studies the feasibility of MR-guided catheter interventions for the treatment of congenital heart disease and arrythmia therapy. Hence, applications in humans remain the challenge for the next years. Although there have been first reports of cardiac catheterizations in humans by combined use of x-ray fluoroscopy and MR imaging, there are no reports in the literature suggesting that active tracking methods by MR imaging have been applied to humans. Safety issues (namely, heating of catheters and wires) hamper clinical use, particularly in infants and children. Current reports are promising that these limitations will be overcome in the near future and will eventually reduce x-ray usage during catheterization. In its current state, cardiac MR imaging offers a unique opportunity to investigate new therapeutic strategies for the treatment of congenital and acquired heart disease.

References

[1] Razavi R, Hill DL, Keevil SF, et al. Cardiac catheterisation guided by MRI in children and adults with congenital heart disease. Lancet 2003;362: 1877–82.

[2] van Vaals JJ, Brummer ME, Dixon WT, et al. "Keyhole" method for accelerating imaging of contrast agent uptake. J Magn Reson Imaging 1993;3: 671–5.

[3] Busch M, Bornstedt A, Wendt M, et al. Fast "real time" imaging with different k-space update strategies for interventional procedures. J Magn Reson Imaging 1998;8:944–54.

[4] Bakker CJ, Hoogeveen RM, Weber J, et al. Visualization of dedicated catheters using fast scanning techniques with potential for MR-guided vascular interventions. Magn Reson Med 1996;36:816–20.

[5] Hu X, Parrish T. Reduction of field of view for dynamic imaging. Magn Reson Med 1994;31:691–4.

[6] Pruessmann KP, Weiger M, Boesiger P. Sensitivity encoded cardiac MRI. J Cardiovasc Magn Reson 2001;3:1–9.

[7] Sodickson DK, Manning WJ. Simultaneous acquisition of spatial harmonics (SMASH): fast imaging with radiofrequency coil arrays. Magn Reson Med 1997;38:591–603.

[8] Weiger M, Pruessmann KP, Boesiger P. Cardiac real-time imaging using SENSE. SENSitivity Encoding scheme. Magn Reson Med 2000;43:177–84.

[9] Guttman MA, Kellman P, Dick AJ, et al. Real-time accelerated interactive MRI with adaptive TSENSE and UNFOLD. Magn Reson Med 2003;50:315–21.

[10] Rivas PA, Nayak KS, Scott GC, et al. In vivo real-time intravascular MRI. J Cardiovasc Magn Reson 2002;4:223–32.

[11] Buecker A, Spuentrup E, Grabitz R, et al. Magnetic resonance-guided placement of atrial septal closure device in animal model of patent foramen ovale. Circulation 2002;106:511–5.

[12] Plein S, Smith WH, Ridgway JP, et al. Qualitative and quantitative analysis of regional left ventricular wall dynamics using real-time magnetic resonance imaging: comparison with conventional breath-hold gradient echo acquisition in volunteers and patients. J Magn Reson Imaging 2001;14: 23–30.

[13] Nayak KS, Cunningham CH, Santos JM, et al. Real-time cardiac MRI at 3 tesla. Magn Reson Med 2004;51:655–60.

[14] Larson AC, Simonetti OP. Real-time cardiac cine imaging with SPIDER: steady-state projection imaging with dynamic echo-train readout. Magn Reson Med 2001;46:1059–66.

[15] Bakker CJ, Bos C, Weinmann HJ. Passive tracking of catheters and guidewires by contrast-enhanced MR fluoroscopy. Magn Reson Med 2001;45:17–23.

[16] Araki T, Aoki S, Ishigame K, et al. MR-guided intravascular catheter manipulation: feasibility of both active and passive tracking in experimental study and initial clinical applications. Radiat Med 2002;20:1–8.

[17] Saeed M, Saloner D, Weber O, et al. MRI in guiding and assessing intramyocardial therapy. Eur Radiol, in press.

[18] Zhang Q, Wendt M, Aschoff AJ, et al. Active MR guidance of interventional devices with target-navigation. Magn Reson Med 2000;44:56–65.

[19] Bakker CJ, Hoogeveen RM, Hurtak WF, et al. MR-guided endovascular interventions: susceptibility-based catheter and near-real-time imaging technique. Radiology 1997;202:273–6.

[20] Omary RA, Unal O, Koscielski DS, et al. Real-time MR imaging-guided passive catheter tracking with use of gadolinium-filled catheters. J Vasc Interv Radiol 2000;11:1079–85.

[21] Yeung CJ, Atalar E. RF transmit power limit for the barewire loopless catheter antenna. J Magn Reson Imaging 2000;12:86–91.

[22] Wong EY, Zhang Q, Duerk JL, et al. An optical system for wireless detuning of parallel resonant circuits. J Magn Reson Imaging 2000;12:632–8.

[23] Dumoulin CL, Souza SP, Darrow RD. Real-time position monitoring of invasive devices using magnetic resonance. Magn Reson Med 1993;29:411–5.

[24] Hurst GC, Hua J, Duerk JL, et al. Intravascular (catheter) NMR receiver probe: preliminary design analysis and application to canine iliofemoral imaging. Magn Reson Med 1992;24:343–57.

[25] Zuehlsdorff S, Umathum R, Volz S, et al. MR coil design for simultaneous tip tracking and curvature delineation of a catheter. Magn Reson Med 2004;52:214–8.

[26] Ocali O, Atalar E. Intravascular magnetic resonance imaging using a loopless catheter antenna. Magn Reson Med 1997;37:112–8.

[27] Crottet D, Meuli R, Wicky S, et al. Reciprocity and sensitivity of opposed-solenoid endovascular MRI probes. J Magn Reson 2002;159:219–25.

[28] Susil RC, Yeung CJ, Atalar E. Intravascular extended sensitivity (IVES) MRI antennas. Magn Reson Med 2003;50:383–90.

[29] Kivelitz D, Wagner S, Schnorr J, et al. A vascular stent as an active component for locally enhanced magnetic resonance imaging: initial in vivo imaging results after catheter-guided placement in rabbits. Invest Radiol 2003;38:147–52.

[30] Nitz WR, Oppelt A, Renz W, et al. On the heating of linear conductive structures as guide wires and catheters in interventional MRI. J Magn Reson Imaging 2001;13:105–14.

[31] Budinger TF. Nuclear magnetic resonance (NMR) in vivo studies: known thresholds for health effects. J Comput Assist Tomogr 1981;5:800–11.

[32] Atalar E, Bottomley PA, Ocali O, et al. High resolution intravascular MRI and MRS by using a catheter receiver coil. Magn Reson Med 1996;36:596–605.

[33] NRPB. Guidelines on patient dose to promote the optimisation of protection for diagnostic medical exposures. Chilton (UK): National Radiological Protection Board; 1999.

[34] Kovoor P, Ricciardello M, Collins L, et al. Risk to patients from radiation associated with radiofrequency ablation for supraventricular tachycardia. Circulation 1998;98:1534–40.

[35] Faulkner K, Love HG, Sweeney JK, et al. Radiation doses and somatic risk to patients during cardiac radiological procedures. Br J Radiol 1986;59:359–63.

[36] Modan B, Keinan L, Blumstein T, et al. Cancer following cardiac catheterization in childhood. Int J Epidemiol 2000;29:424–8.

[37] Duke C, Qureshi SA. Aortic coarctation and recoarctation: to stent or not to stent? J Interv Cardiol 2001;14:283–98.

[38] Forbes T, Matisoff D, Dysart J, et al. Treatment of coexistent coarctation and aneurysm of the aorta with covered stent in a pediatric patient. Pediatr Cardiol 2003;24:289–91.

[39] de Giovanni JV. Covered stents in the treatment of aortic coarctation. J Interv Cardiol 2001;14:187–90.

[40] Rickers C, Jerosch-Herold M, Murthy NS, et al. Magnetic resonance imaging guided dilation of aortic coarctation and stent placement: feasibility and comparison to x-ray guided catheter techniques. Circulation 2003;108:3195.

[41] Austin EH. Transcatheter closure of atrial septal defects [editorial]. J Thorac Cardiovasc Surg 2000;120:1032–3.

[42] Syamasundar Rao P, Sideris EB. Transcatheter closure of atrial septal defects. Heart 1999;82:644.

[43] Zahn EM, Wilson N, Cutright W, et al. Development and testing of the Helex septal occluder, a new expanded polytetrafluoroethylene atrial septal defect occlusion system. Circulation 2001;104:711–6.

[44] Nayak KS, Pauly JM, Kerr AB, et al. Real-time color flow MRI. Magn Reson Med 2000;43:251–8.

[45] Nelson KL, Gifford LM, Lauber-Huber C, et al. Clinical safety of gadopentetate dimeglumine. Radiology 1995;196:439–43.

[46] Lardo AC. Real-time magnetic resonance imaging: diagnostic and interventional applications. Pediatr Cardiol 2000;21:80–98.

[47] Kollias SS, Bernays R, Marugg RA, et al. Target definition and trajectory optimization for interactive MR-guided biopsies of brain tumors in an open configuration MRI system. J Magn Reson Imaging 1998;8:143–59.

[48] Yang X, Atalar E, Li D, et al. Magnetic resonance imaging permits in vivo monitoring of catheter-based vascular gene delivery. Circulation 2001; 104:1588–90.

[49] Gao F, Qui B, Kar S, et al. Intravascular MR/RF-enhanced VEFG gene therapy of atherosclerotic in-stent restenosis. In: Proceedings of the Twelfth Scientific Meeting and Exposition of the International Society of Magnetic Resonance in Medicine. Berkeley (CA): International Society of Magnetic Resonance in Medicine; 2004. p. 377.

[50] Barbash IM, Leor J, Feinberg MS, et al. Interventional magnetic resonance imaging for guiding gene and cell transfer in the heart. Heart 2004;90: 87–91.

[51] Hofmann LV, Liddell RP, Eng J, et al. Human peripheral arteries: feasibility of transvenous intravascular MR imaging of the arterial wall. Radiology 2005;235(2):617–22.

[52] Weiss CR, Karmarkar PV, Arepally A, et al. Real time MR guided meso-caval puncture: towards the development of a percutaneous MR guided mesocaval shunt. In: Proceedings of the Twelfth Scientific Meeting and Exposition of the International Society of Magnetic Resonance in Medicine. Berkeley (CA): International Society of Magnetic Resonance in Medicine; 2004. p. 962.

[52a] Raval AN, Karmarkar PV, Guttman MA, et al. Interactive real-time magnetic resonance-guided atrial septal puncture and atrial balloon saptostomy are feasible in swine. J Cardiovasc Magn Reson 2005;7(1):175.

[52b] Raval AN, Karmarkar PV, Ozturk C, et al. Chronic total peripheral artery occlusion recanalization using interactive real-time magnetic resonance imaging guidance is feasible in swine. J Cardiovasc Magn Reson 2005;7(1):176.

[53] Dodd SJ, Williams M, Suhan JP, et al. Detection of single mammalian cells by high-resolution magnetic resonance imaging. Biophys J 1999;76: 103–9.

[54] Foster-Gareau P, Heyn C, Alejski A, et al. Imaging single mammalian cells with a 1.5 T clinical MRI scanner. Magn Reson Med 2003;49:968–71.

[55] Bulte JW, Arbab AS, Douglas T, et al. Preparation of magnetically labeled cells for cell tracking by magnetic resonance imaging. Methods Enzymol 2004;386:275–99.

[56] Arbab AS, Bashaw LA, Miller BR, et al. Intracytoplasmic tagging of cells with ferumoxides and transfection agent for cellular magnetic resonance imaging after cell transplantation: methods and techniques. Transplantation 2003;76:1123–30.

[57] Frank JA, Miller BR, Arbab AS, et al. Clinically applicable labeling of mammalian and stem cells by combining superparamagnetic iron oxides and transfection agents. Radiology 2003;228:480–7.

[58] Arbab AS, Yocum GT, Kalish H, et al. Efficient magnetic cell labeling with protamine sulfate complexed to ferumoxides for cellular MRI. Blood 2004;104:1217–23.

[59] Hinds KA, Hill JM, Shapiro EM, et al. Highly efficient endosomal labeling of progenitor and stem cells with large magnetic particles allows magnetic resonance imaging of single cells. Blood 2003;102: 867–72.

[60] Dick AJ, Guttman MA, Raman VK, et al. Magnetic resonance fluoroscopy allows targeted delivery of mesenchymal stem cells to infarct borders in swine. Circulation 2003;108:2899–904.

[61] Judd RM, Lugo-Olivieri CH, Arai M, et al. Physiological basis of myocardial contrast enhancement in fast magnetic resonance images of 2-day-old reperfused canine infarcts. Circulation 1995;92: 1902–10.

[62] Hill JM, Dick AJ, Raman VK, et al. Serial cardiac magnetic resonance imaging of injected mesenchymal stem cells. Circulation 2003;108:1009–14.

[63] Karmarkar PV, Kraitchman DL, Izbudak I, et al. MR-trackable intramyocardial injection catheter. Magn Reson Med 2004;51:1163–72.

[64] Wollert KC, Meyer GP, Lotz J, et al. Intracoronary autologous bone-marrow cell transfer after myocardial infarction: the BOOST randomised controlled clinical trial. Lancet 2004;364:141–8.

[65] Assmus B, Schachinger V, Teupe C, et al. Transplantation of progenitor cells and regeneration enhancement in acute myocardial infarction (TOPCARE-AMI). Circulation 2002;106:3009–17.

[66] Schachinger V, Assmus B, Britten MB, et al. Transplantation of progenitor cells and regeneration enhancement in acute myocardial infarction: final one-year results of the TOPCARE-AMI Trial. J Am Coll Cardiol 2004;44:1690–9.

[67] Lederman RJ, Guttman MA, Peters DC, et al. Catheter-based endomyocardial injection with real-time magnetic resonance imaging. Circulation 2002;105:1282–4.

[68] Kraitchman DL, Heldman AW, Atalar E, et al. In vivo magnetic resonance imaging of mesenchymal stem cells in myocardial infarction. Circulation 2003;107:2290–3.

[69] Rickers C, Gallegos R, Seethamraju RT, et al. Applications of magnetic resonance imaging for cardiac stem cell therapy. J Interv Cardiol 2004; 17:37–46.

[70] Saeed M, Lee R, Martin A, et al. Transendocardial delivery of extracellular myocardial markers by using combination x-ray/MR fluoroscopic guidance: feasibility study in dogs. Radiology 2004;231: 689–96.

ELSEVIER
SAUNDERS

Magn Reson Imaging Clin N Am
13 (2005) 481–489

MAGNETIC
RESONANCE
IMAGING CLINICS
of North America

Intrabiliary MR Imaging

Aravind Arepally, MD*, Clifford R. Weiss, MD

*The Russell H. Morgan Department of Radiology and Radiological Science,
Division of Cardiovascular and Interventional Radiology, Johns Hopkins Medical Institutes,
Blalock 544, 600 North Wolfe Street, Baltimore, MD 21287, USA*

This article focuses on the technique of intra-biliary MR imaging (IBMR) and its potential clinical application in the setting of biliary obstruction. The biliary system is located in the central portion of the liver where multiple vascular structures are present in a tight, confined space. Because of this difficult anatomic location, assessment of the biliary tree has always been a diagnostic and therapeutic challenge. Most patients with bile duct obstruction undergo non-invasive imaging with ultrasound, CT, or MR imaging [1,2]. More often, additional invasive studies such as endoscopic retrograde cholangiopancreatography or percutaneous transhepatic cholangiography (PTC) are required for proper diagnosis and preoperative staging. Because these techniques are often inconclusive, obtaining tissue from the bile ducts using brush cytology or forceps biopsy is often needed to provide an accurate diagnosis. Each of these methods, however, has limited sensitivity and specificity and can result in false-negative examinations [3,4]. This complicated diagnostic process can cause treatment delays and force patients who have benign disease to undergo multiple unnecessary procedures.

Recent advances in coil designs have allowed for placement of MR receiver coils within vessels to enhance MR imaging. Intravascular MR imaging coils have already been described in atheromatous vessels and normal vasculature to obtain high-resolution imaging of the vessel wall [5–7]. This technique allows for superior spatial resolution and increased signal-to-noise ratio in the tissue immediately adjacent to the coil. By decreasing the field of view, 100- to 200-µm resolution of arterial wall pathology has been achievable [5]. For similar reasons, the authors hypothesized that similar coil technology could be adapted to the assessment of other, deep structures in the body such as the biliary tree where external coils are known to have limitations. Because involvement of the biliary tree can be subtle, high-resolution imaging would be vital to identify the presence of a malignant versus a benign obstruction. In addition, accurate depiction of tumor involvement could potentially assist in the stratification of patients who would benefit from resection.

To improve the accuracy of biliary diagnosis and staging, the authors implemented IBMR, a new technique in the assessment of patients who have biliary obstruction [8]. Although this technique holds promise to provide an alternative means to image the biliary tree, it is still in infancy with methodology and applications. This article focuses on the rationale for IBMR, the current techniques for performing IBMR, and the results from a pilot clinical trial in patients who have biliary obstruction.

Rationale for intrabiliary MR imaging

Biliary obstruction from a malignant or benign etiology occurs in three areas: intrahepatic, perihilar, and distal. Localized intrahepatic tumors can be treated (like hepatocellular carcinoma) with hepatectomy, when possible. The perihilar tumors are resected with reconstruction of biliary–enteric anastomosis. Distal tumors are managed similar to periampullary malignancies through surgical excision with pancreatoduodenectomy. Determining

---

* Corresponding author.
E-mail address: aarepal@jhmi.edu (A. Arepally).

1064-9689/05/$ - see front matter © 2005 Elsevier Inc. All rights reserved.
doi:10.1016/j.mric.2005.04.011

mri.theclinics.com

the preoperative factors of longitudinal and infiltrative extension of biliary malignancies is important in stratifying patients for surgery [9,10].

The Bismuth-Corlette classification is often used by many investigators to identify and describe biliary malignancies according to anatomic locations [11]. In this classification, type I tumors involve only the common hepatic duct and type II tumors extend to the bifurcation without involvement of secondary intrahepatic ducts. Types IIIa and IIIb tumors reach into the right and the left secondary intrahepatic ducts, respectively, and type IV tumors involve the secondary intrahepatic ducts on both sides. Therefore, the Bismuth-Corlette classification identifies the uppermost extent of the tumor to determine resectability.

In patients who have biliary obstruction, preoperative staging has been performed with standard imaging such as CT and MR imaging, with limited success. Despite advances in imaging technology, the overall accuracy for assessing resectability is 60% using multiphasic helical and MR imaging [12,13]. Multiple studies have shown that despite showing the presence of obstruction, precise localization with these conventional techniques has had only moderate agreement with direct cholangiography, especially with longitudinal tumor extension [14]. Another recurring problem with all of these techniques has been the overestimation of tumor extent, which has resulted in inaccurate classification [15,16].

The current "gold standard" for biliary imaging and staging is direct cholangiography, which is often performed with endoscopic retrograde cholangiopancreatography or PTC. At the authors' institution, most patients undergo PTC and percutaneous biliary drainage (PBD) in managing biliary obstruction. Percutaneous access can provide a number of advantages in the management of the patient who has malignant obstruction. First, the cholangiogram is important in staging the degree of tumor involvement of the biliary tree. Second, the biliary tube placed during the cholangiogram plays an important intraoperative role by providing an access for surgical anastomosis. This access allows the surgeon to evaluate the upper extent of tumor involvement and identify the limits of resectability. Third, having biliary diversion and decompression with a drainage catheter properly prepares the patient for surgery. Finally, in patients deemed unresectable, the use of the percutaneous access allows for palliative treatment of symptomatic patients who have obstructive jaundice. Because of these advantages and the low

sensitivity and specificity of noninvasive imaging tests, PTC (as opposed to noninvasive imaging) is used at the authors' institution for staging patients and managing patients who have malignant biliary obstruction.

Despite the excellent temporal and spatial resolution of cholangiography (endoscopic retrograde cholangiopancreatography or PTC), both techniques are only able to indirectly image biliary tumors. In fact, compared with direct surgical histopathology, cholangiography has been shown to be accurate in only approximately half of all patients. Even after optimum presurgical planning with cholangiography, at least 25% and up to 40% of patients who were deemed to be resectable were found to be unresectable during surgery [17]. Therefore, a technique that allows for visualization of the biliary wall and the adjacent liver parenchyma simultaneously provides a novel method for biliary imaging with the potential for more accurate diagnosis and staging. Because patients who have biliary tubes have a readily available conduit into the biliary system, the natural extension was to apply the emerging technology of intravascular MR imaging into the biliary system.

The placement of intravascular MR imaging receiver coils directly into the biliary system (IBMR) improves the imaging resolution of biliary tract by increasing the local signal in the biliary tree and the adjacent area of interest. The IBMR technique provides two advantages. First, by placing the receiver coil directly in the biliary system, the field of view can be decreased without significant phase-wrap artifact and still allow for high in-plane resolution. Second, the coil also produces increased signal in the biliary lumen, which provides contrast between the biliary lumen, biliary wall, and adjacent structures [8].

Technique of intrabiliary MR imaging

The purpose of IBMR is to create cross-sectional images of the bile duct wall and adjacent tissues (which cholangiography cannot do) and generate images with higher resolution than current ultrasound, CT, or MR imaging techniques. Compared with current MR imaging techniques, these coils are able to produce images with a very high spatial resolution for a small area adjacent to the coil.

To perform IBMR, all patients must have an existing PBD catheter. The technique of performing PTC/PBD has been well described and has a high success rate. With experienced interventional radiologists, this procedure can be performed with minimal complications and quickly in a patient with obstructive jaundice. The basics of a PTC/PBD procedure are briefly described so that the rationale and technique of IBMR may be further appreciated; however, a full elaboration of this procedure is beyond the scope of this article.

Percutaneous transhepatic cholangiogram/ percutaneous biliary drainage

In patients who are undergoing PBD, patient preparation is critical before the procedure. A history and physical examination are required to thoroughly access the physical status of the patient. Standard laboratory data include coagulation profile, liver function tests, and white blood cell and platelet counts. Coverage with a broad-spectrum antibiotic is required for all patients.

Insertion of a biliary tube is performed with full conscious sedation in a standard fashion under fluoroscopic visualization using a two-step technique. The procedure should be performed only by an experienced interventional radiologist. First, a 22-gauge Chiba needle (Cook, Bloomington, Indiana) is advanced into the liver from a percutaneous midaxillary line. The needle is passed several times until the biliary tree is opacified. In the second step, a separate puncture is performed into a peripheral right posterior duct. After placement of a dilator-sheath assembly set (Neff Percutaneous Access Set, Cook), the occluded biliary duct is traversed with a hydrophilic guidewire, and a 10-French biliary drainage catheter (Boston Scientific, Natick, Massachusetts) is inserted in a standard fashion over a stiff wire. All patients are admitted overnight to monitor for sepsis and hemobilia.

In patients with a newly inserted biliary tube, IBMR should not be performed for at least 1 to 2 weeks to allow for proper biliary decompression. Due to trauma that can occur to the hepatobiliary system during the procedure, patients may experience hemobilia or transient cholangitis, which may potentially complicate an IBMR procedure. In addition, a biliary tree that has been obstructed for a prolonged period may have a dramatically different appearance and tortuosity after a short period of decompression. Finally, in situations in which patients are malnourished or infected from prolonged obstruction, this delay will allow patients to recover before IBMR.

Intrabiliary MR imaging

Candidates for IBMR should be able to tolerate an MR imaging examination of 1 hour. In addition to standard contraindications for MR imaging, additional exclusion criteria for IBMR include patients with metallic stents in the biliary tree, surgical clips in the porta hepatis, or vascular stents or embolization coils in the hepatic artery. Because IBMR is an off label use of an FDA-approved product, institutional review board–approved consents were obtained on all patients enrolled in the pilot trial.

The intravascular MR imaging wire (Surgivision, Frederick, Maryland) has been previously described for high-resolution vessel wall imaging [6,18]. The wire, 75 cm long with a diameter of 0.030 in, is a loopless antenna consisting of a soft conducting wire that has an inner conductor from a 50-Ω, 0.6-mm coaxial cable with a polyester jacket (Pico-Coax, Axon Cable, Norwood, Massachusetts). The inner and outer conductors of the coaxial cable are made of silver-plated copper alloy with a fluoroethylene polymer as the dielectric. The wire has a soft floppy tip and a flexible shaft that is composed of nitinol. Due to this design, the wire can be safely advanced and visualized under fluoroscopy into any vascular or nonvascular lumen with minimal friction, especially when introduced through standard catheters or biliary tubes (Fig. 1A–C). The proximal end of the coaxial cable is connected through a matching tuning-decoupling circuit to the MR scanner. In the United States, intravascular MR imaging coils are FDA-approved devices for internal imaging of aorta and surrounding area. Use of the Surgi-Vision intravascular wire for IBMR is an off-label use of this FDA approved product.

The placement of the intravascular MR imaging wire does not require significant expertise, but the operator should understand the basic concepts and management of biliary tubes and the intravascular MR receiver coils. Before performing IBMR, all patients should receive a broad-spectrum antibiotic. The authors prefer to not use any sedation for placing the wire because patients are often not monitored on a continuous basis in the MR imaging suite. A tube cholangiogram is initially performed to confirm proper location of the biliary tube and, in cases in which two biliary tubes are present, to determine which tube will

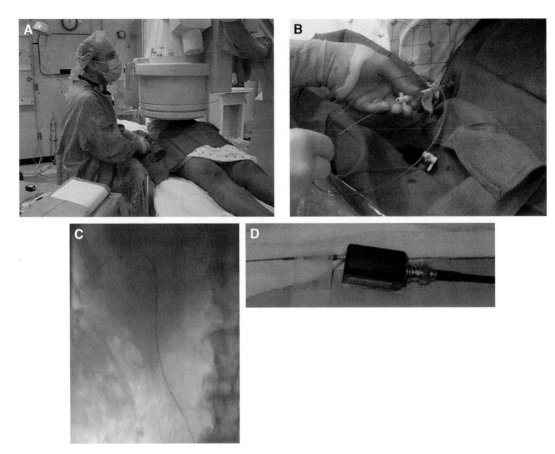

Fig. 1. (*A*) Interventional radiologist advancing an intravascular MR imaging wire under fluoroscopy into a biliary tube. (*B*) The Intravascular MR Coil (Surgivision, Frederick, Maryland) is 75 cm long with a soft, floppy platinum tip and a flexible nitinol shaft. Note the relative flexibility of the wire as it is being introduced directly into the biliary tube. (*C*) The intravascular MR imaging wire being introduced under fluoroscopy directly into a biliary tube. Note the clear visibility of the platinum wire tip, which is positioned in the duodenum. The biliary tube is made of silicon and therefore translucent under fluoroscopy. (*D*) Interface adapter that connects the intravascular MR imaging wire to the MR scanner. The proximal end of the coaxial cable is connected through a matching tuning-decoupling circuit to the MR scanner.

serve as the best access site for imaging the biliary tree of interest. The intravascular MR imaging wire should be gently advanced under direct fluoroscopic imaging to avoid exiting any side holes and allowing the wire to properly egress out the end hole of the biliary tube, which is within the duodenum (see Fig. 1A–C). By advancing the distal tip of the wire well into the duodenum, the entire imaging length of the intravascular wire should now be in proper place to image the entire biliary tract. Final positioning should have the wire in a relatively straight course, with the distal tip outside the biliary tube in the duodenum (see Fig. 1C). Because most biliary tubes do not have metallic braiding, the intravascular MR imaging wire may be placed directly into most biliary tubes.

In situations in which a braided tube is present, the tube can readily be changed for a nonbraided biliary catheter (Boston Scientific) by an interventional radiologist. In addition, because the biliary tube is placed through a peripheral duct, the entire course of the biliary tube is available for high-resolution imaging (Fig. 2). After the wire is properly positioned, it should be secured with sterile tape or a Tuohy-Borst adapter to prevent migration and then connected to the interface adapter (see Fig. 1D). This adapter creates a matching tuning-decoupling circuit that allows the intravascular MR imaging wire to connect to the scanner by way of a coaxial cable. After placement of the wire, patients are transferred to the MR suite for further imaging.

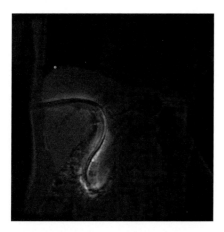

Fig. 2. Breath-hold coronal fast spoiled gradient sequence with a 40-cm field of view is created for a scout image. Note the increased signal through the entire biliary tube from the intravascular MR imaging wire.

All IBMR examinations at the authors' institution are performed on a 1.5-T MR imaging system (CV/i, General Electric, Waukesha, Wisconsin). Using the body coil, an initial breath-held fast multiplanar spoiled gradient sequence (TR [repetition time], 10 milliseconds; TE [time to echo], 1.2 milliseconds) with a 40-cm field of view is created for a scout image (see Fig. 2). This scout image serves as the source for planning all high-resolution planes that will be needed for the rest of the study. For the remaining MR sequences, the IBMR coil serves as one channel of a phased array, with two additional anterior surface coils and one posterior surface coil forming the phased array. Axial T2 fast spin echo (TR, 3000 milliseconds; TE, 105 milliseconds; echo train length, 16) and single-shot fast spin echo (TR, infinite; TE, 90 milliseconds) (Fig. 3A) images are acquired. Axial and coronal T1-weighted two-dimensional fast multiplanar spoiled gradient sequence (TR, 100 milliseconds; TE, 2.8 milliseconds; flip angle, 70°) and three-dimensional fast spoiled gradient breath-hold sequence (TR, 4.1 milliseconds; TE, 1.6 milliseconds; flip angle, 15°) images were acquired before and 20 and 70 seconds after 0.1 mmol/kg intravenous Gadodiamide administration (see Fig. 3B, C). Often, tailored direct-axial imaging of the intravascular MR coils (two-dimensional fast multiplanar spoiled gradient sequence; TR, 100 milliseconds; TE, 2.8 milliseconds; flip angle, 70°) is performed to obtain a dedicated high-resolution imaging of the bile ducts of interest. Sequences are prescribed so that

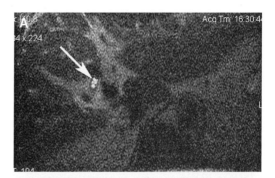

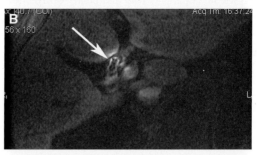

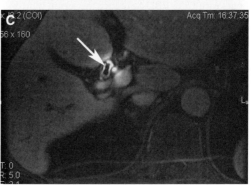

Fig. 3. Axial IBMR performed through the same area of the common bile duct with various sequences. White arrows point to common bile duct. (A) Axial T2-weighted fast spin echo sequence (TR, 3000 milliseconds; TE, 105 milliseconds; echo train length, 16) shows increased signal from fluid in the common bile duct. Poor visualization of the adjacent liver is noted. (B) Axial fast spoiled gradient breath-hold sequence (TR, 4.1 milliseconds; TE, 1.6 milliseconds; flip angle, 15°) before contrast and (C) 70 seconds after 0.1 mmol/kg intravenous Gadodiamide administration. Note the improved visualization of the adjacent liver and pertinent vascular structures with administration of contrast. Note the biliary wall is well defined with intact fat planes between the bile ducts and other structures in the porta hepatis (arrow).

the in-plane resolution is approximately 400 to 500 μm (field of view, 19–20 cm; 512 frequency imaging matrix, 256 phase encodes interpolated to 512 pixels).

When the IBMR examination is finished, the intravascular MR imaging wire may be removed without the need for fluoroscopy and patients may be immediately discharged. The patient should be instructed to contact a physician if there is development of any fevers/chills over the next 24-hour period.

Clinical experience with intrabiliary MR imaging

From 2002 to 2004, the authors performed IBMR in 12 patients who had biliary obstruction of unknown etiology. IBMR was conducted as a single-center, prospective clinical trial at Johns Hopkins Medical Institutes and funded by the Cardiovascular and Interventional Radiology Research and Education Fund. The following guidelines were used to enroll patients for the trial: (1) patients had biliary obstruction/dilatation from an unknown etiology as diagnosed by standard axial imaging (contrast-enhanced CT or MR imaging); (2) biliary decompression was performed on patients with PTC/PBD to reduce the serum bilirubin concentration below 2 mg/dL and to control cholangitis; and (3) patients were surgical candidates for resection and biliary reconstruction.

There were two aims for this trial. First, the authors wanted to optimize MR imaging parameters to develop consistent imaging protocols that are tailored for patients who have biliary obstruction. Next, based on experience [8], the authors wanted to determine the accuracy of IBMR to detect tumor extension by correlation with standard axial imaging, cholangiograms, and biliary biopsies. The following results describe the authors' preliminary experience and results of IBMR.

In the authors' pilot trial, all patients tolerated placement of the intravascular MR imaging wire under fluoroscopy without any difficulty. There were no episodes of cholangitis or difficulty with biliary tubes. One of 15 patients could not tolerate the MR imaging examination due to claustrophobia. The average age of the patients was 60 years (±9.0); 60% were men. All patients presented with biliary obstruction of unknown etiology and were assessed with IBMR without a diagnosis or review of other imaging studies. Because the authors' institute is a referral center, most of their patients had been screened for surgery in previous hospitals and had extensive imaging before IBMR procedures. Therefore, all patients had adjuvant axial contrast-enhanced CT/MR imaging, cholangiography, and biliary biopsies for comparison with IBMR procedures.

Optimal MR imaging parameters

All MR imaging examinations were performed in less than 1 hour. Diaphragmatic motion was a limiting factor in decreasing the field of view. The average in-plane resolution of the biliary tree that was achieved was 740 ± 20 μm $\times 1150 \pm 20$ μm, which was obtained using an average field of view of 18 cm $\times$ 18 cm (range, 15–24 cm) and an average acquisition matrix of 256 $\times$ 160. When the displayed matrix size was increased to 512 $\times$ 512 (using zero-fill interpolation processing), the in-plane resolution decreased to 350 ± 50 μm $\times$ 356 ± 48 μm. T2-weighted sequences, although diagnostic, were more often susceptible to respiratory motion artifact than other sequences. T1-weighted imaging with gadolinium (three-dimensional fast spoiled gradient sequence) was superior in quality in depicting adjacent liver parenchyma and displaying the biliary wall (see Fig. 3A–C). For the common bile duct, the optimal plane of imaging was standard axial sections through the liver. In patients who did not have malignancies, biliary wall enhancement was noted and clear definition of biliary wall boundaries could be seen that allowed distinction of adjacent fat planes and vasculature (see Fig. 3C; Fig. 4A). For intrahepatic ducts, coronal or direct axial imaging of the intravascular MR imaging coil provided better depiction of biliary lumen and adjacent structures, which allowed for easier identification of biliary tumors (see Fig. 4A–C).

Formal signal intensity analysis was also performed in these patients by creating a region of interest in the common bile duct with the IBMR coil image alone and with the three surface coils active (least squares method) on the contrast-enhanced sequence. This analysis showed that in the common bile duct, the average contrast-to-noise ratio of the IBMR coil, the three surface coils, and the combined image was 110 ± 63, 12.4 ± 7.6, and 109.7 ± 67, respectively, resulting in a tenfold increase in signal in the common bile duct by using the IBMR technique ($P < .0001$).

Accuracy of intrabiliary MR imaging to detect tumor extension

In 12 of the 15 patients, final pathology was available to determine the clinical utility of IBMR. Specifically, the accuracy of this technique was compared with axial contrast-enhanced CT/MR imaging, tube cholangiograms, and surgical pathology (Table 1). All modalities were interpreted with regard to etiology of obstruction, level of

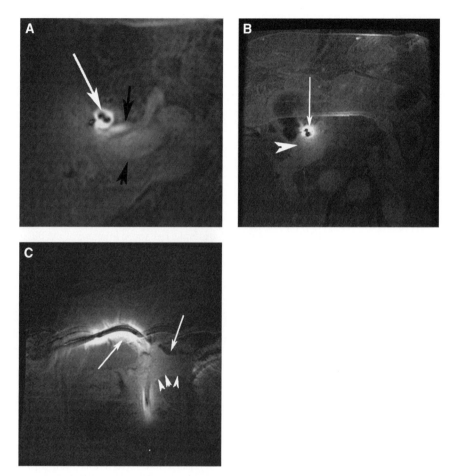

Fig. 4. Axial (*A*, *B*) and coronal (*C*) IBMR in a patient after administration of Gadodiamide. (*A*) The biliary wall is somewhat intact in common bile duct (*white arrow*) just below the tumor. Some of the fat planes are intact. Short dark arrow indicates the portal vein and the long dark arrow indicates the hepatic artery. (*B*) Note at the level of the tumor, there is loss of all fat planes due to tumor (*arrowhead*) encasing the bile duct (*long arrow*). (*C*) On coronal view, soft tissue tumor extends to the biliary bifurcation and extends to the left biliary duct (*arrowheads*). Right and left biliary ducts are also seen (*long arrows*).

obstruction, and degree of tumor visualization. This analysis demonstrated that IBMR had a higher sensitivity and positive predictive value compared with CT and higher specificity than cholangiograms (see Table 1). Overall, the clear advantage of this technique to identify tumor infiltration into the liver and the biliary wall allowed for higher accuracy in detecting biliary malignancies.

Limitations and human biohazards

Due to the infancy of this technique, several limitations were encountered during this pilot trial. Although the field of view was reduced from standard imaging, respiratory motion caused significant artifacts that limited the diagnostic quality of some studies. Attempts to correct this problem with respiratory bellows and faster MR imaging acquisitions helped to reduce some of the artifacts, but the problem persisted. Potential cardiac MR imaging techniques used to minimize respiratory and motion artifacts may alleviate problems with diaphragmatic motion and are currently under investigation [19,20]. Another limitation of this technique is that the high-resolution imaging plane is limited to the region of the active portion of the wire. Therefore, the reader should be cautioned that IBMR should be reserved for

Table 1

Comparison of intrabiliary MR imaging technique with contrast-enhanced CT/MR imaging and percutaneous cholangiograms in 12 patients

	IBMR	CT/MR imaging	Cholangiogram
Sensitivity	100.0%	57.0%	100.0%
Specificity	80.0%	100.0%	20.0%
Positive predictive value	87.5%	60.8%	56.5%
Negative predictive value	100.0%	42.9%	100.0%
P	.023*	.15	.86

χ^2 analysis was performed with each modality utilizing surgical pathology as the "gold standard."
* Statistical significance.

patients who require a dedicated, localized examination of the biliary tree. Because IBMR improves signal only in the biliary system that is intubated, it will not provide high-resolution imaging of the entire liver. Therefore, patients should have standard imaging of the liver in addition to IBMR to fully assess the liver and surrounding organs.

Finally, IBMR does not entail substantial risk. The most important risk of this protocol is local tissue heating due to the MR imaging catheter coil. Current research under way at the authors' institution has shown the safety of interventional MR imaging devices for human applications [21,22]. The probes have been safely used in various lumens, including transesophageal intubation for aortic imaging and transvenous insertion for arterial wall imaging in human subjects [7,18]. No hazards or risks to the patients have been encountered. To minimize the potential risk of local tissue heating during the examination, the length of the overall IBMR procedure was kept to less than 60 minutes to minimize overall radiofrequency power deposition. In addition, careful selection of MR imaging sequences and parameters were made to use low radiofrequency intensive sequences. Finally, the coil itself was placed within a biliary drainage tube so that it did not directly contact the bile duct walls. Given the experience with transesophageal MR imaging and transvenous MR imaging of the arteries and the extensive animal testing already performed [7,18,22], the authors believe that the risk of this procedure is minimal.

Summary

The goal of this research is to illustrate the potential role of interventional MR imaging in a clinical setting. As shown by this study, IBMR is feasible, is well tolerated, and positively affects patient management. IBMR allowed for significantly decreased field of view and high in-plane resolution and provided contrast between the biliary lumen and adjacent structures with high diagnostic accuracy. This technique enabled clinicians not only to improve imaging of the biliary tree but also to make a more accurate diagnosis. Based on this pilot work, there are several potential avenues of further expansion for IBMR. For example, enhanced imaging of the biliary tree may allow for monitoring of new biliary treatment regimens such as photodynamic therapy or molecular targeting [23,24]. In addition, this technique may also foster development of innovative new percutaneous procedures [25] that may eventually treat some biliary disorders under MR imaging guidance.

References

[1] Moon SG, Han JK, Kim AY, et al. Biliary obstruction in metastatic disease: thin-section helical CT findings. Abdom Imaging 2003;28(1):45–52.

[2] Manfredi R, Brizi MG, Masselli G, et al. [Malignant biliary hilar stenosis: MR cholangiography compared with direct cholangiography.] Radiol Med (Torino) 2001;102(1–2):48–54 [in Italian].

[3] Ferrari AP Jr, Lichtenstein DR, Slivka A, et al. Brush cytology during ERCP for the diagnosis of biliary and pancreatic malignancies. Gastrointest Endosc 1994;40(2 Pt 1):140–5.

[4] Savader SJ, Prescott CA, Lund GB, et al. Intraductal biliary biopsy: comparison of three techniques. J Vasc Interv Radiol 1996;7(5):743–50.

[5] Atalar E, Bottomley PA, Ocali O, et al. High resolution intravascular MRI and MRS by using a catheter receiver coil. Magn Reson Med 1996;36(4):596–605.

[6] Ocali O, Atalar E. Intravascular magnetic resonance imaging using a loopless catheter antenna. Magn Reson Med 1997;37(1):112–8.

[7] Shunk KA, Lima JA, Heldman AW, et al. Transesophageal magnetic resonance imaging. Magn Reson Med 1999;41(4):722–6.

[8] Arepally A, Georgiades C, Hofmann LV, et al. Hilar cholangiocarcinoma: staging with intrabiliary MRI. AJR Am J Roentgenol 2004;183(4):1071–4.

[9] Klempnauer J, Ridder GJ, von Wasielewski R, et al. Resectional surgery of hilar cholangiocarcinoma: a multivariate analysis of prognostic factors. J Clin Oncol 1997;15(3):947–54.

[10] Kondo S, Hirano S, Ambo Y, et al. Forty consecutive resections of hilar cholangiocarcinoma with no postoperative mortality and no positive ductal margins: results of a prospective study. Ann Surg 2004; 240(1):95–101.

[11] Bismuth H, Corlette MB. Intrahepatic cholangioenteric anastomosis in carcinoma of the hilus of the liver. Surg Gynecol Obstet 1975;140(2): 170–8.

[12] Tillich M, Mischinger HJ, Preisegger KH, et al. Multiphasic helical CT in diagnosis and staging of hilar cholangiocarcinoma. AJR Am J Roentgenol 1998; 171(3):651–8.

[13] Choi BI, Han JK, Shin YM, et al. Peripheral cholangiocarcinoma: comparison of MRI with CT. Abdom Imaging 1995;20(4):357–60.

[14] Lee SS, Kim MH, Lee SK, et al. MR cholangiography versus cholangioscopy for evaluation of longitudinal extension of hilar cholangiocarcinoma. Gastrointest Endosc 2002;56(1):25–32.

[15] Courbiere M, Pilleul F, Henry L, et al. Value of magnetic resonance cholangiography in benign and malignant biliary stenosis: comparative study with direct cholangiography. J Comput Assist Tomogr 2003;27(3):315–20.

[16] Otto G, Romaneehsen B, Bittinger F, et al. Preoperative imaging of hilar cholangiocarcinoma: surgical evaluation of standard practises. Z Gastroenterol 2004;42(1):9–14.

[17] Jarnagin WR, Fong Y, DeMatteo RP, et al. Staging, resectability, and outcome in 225 patients with hilar cholangiocarcinoma. Ann Surg 2001;234(4):507–17 [discussion: 517–9].

[18] Hofmann LV, Liddell RP, Arepally A, et al. In vivo intravascular MR imaging: transvenous technique for arterial wall imaging. J Vasc Interv Radiol 2003;14(10):1317–27.

[19] Stuber M, Botnar RM, Danias PG, et al. Breathhold three-dimensional coronary magnetic resonance angiography using real-time navigator technology. J Cardiovasc Magn Reson 1999;1(3):233–8.

[20] McConnell MV, Khasgiwala VC, Savord BJ, et al. Comparison of respiratory suppression methods and navigator locations for MR coronary angiography. AJR Am J Roentgenol 1997;168(5):1369–75.

[21] Yeung CJ, Susil RC, Atalar E. RF heating due to conductive wires during MRI depends on the phase distribution of the transmit field. Magn Reson Med 2002;48(6):1096–8.

[22] Yeung CJ, Susil RC, Atalar E. RF safety of wires in interventional MRI: using a safety index. Magn Reson Med 2002;47(1):187–93.

[23] Sirica AE. Cholangiocarcinoma: molecular targeting strategies for chemoprevention and therapy. Hepatology 2005;41(1):5–15.

[24] Nanashima A, Yamaguchi H, Shibasaki S, et al. Adjuvant photodynamic therapy for bile duct carcinoma after surgery: a preliminary study. J Gastroenterol 2004;39(11):1095–101.

[25] Abu-Hamda EM, Baron TH. Endoscopic management of cholangiocarcinoma. Semin Liver Dis 2004;24(2):165–75.

ELSEVIER
SAUNDERS

Magn Reson Imaging Clin N Am
13 (2005) 491–504

MAGNETIC
RESONANCE
IMAGING CLINICS
of North America

MR-Guided Interventions for Prostate Cancer

Ergin Atalar, PhD[a,b,]*, Cynthia Ménard, MD[c]

[a]*Departments of Radiology, BME, and ECE, The Johns Hopkins University, 720 Rutland Avenue,
Traylor 330, Baltimore, MD 21205, USA*
[b]*Electrical and Electronics Engineering Department, Bilkent University, Ankara 06800, Turkey*
[c]*Princess Margaret Hospital, University Health Network, University of Toronto, 5th Floor,
610 University Avenue, Toronto, Ontario, M5G 2M9, Canada*

With an estimated annual incidence of 230,000 cases in 2004, prostate cancer is the most common noncutaneous cancer in men in the United States [1]. Despite an impressive scope of research efforts, difficult challenges persist in various aspects of prostate cancer care, including diagnosis, prognostication, and treatment.

First and foremost is a pressing need to appropriately tailor therapeutic interventions to the spatial extent and biologic aggressiveness of disease for individual patients. Individualized therapy for localized disease could significantly reduce the treatment-related morbidity incurred by this population of patients but requires the development of better measures to delineate and characterize disease. At present, these measures are limited to nonspecific prostate-specific antigen (PSA) serum levels [2], histopathologic estimates of tumor burden, and Gleason grading, which is subject to random biopsy sampling error [3–5] and insensitive digital rectal examinations that are poorly reproducible among observers [6].

The authors believe that in the near future, imaging will bridge the gap between characterization of disease and individualized therapy. An ability to visualize the complete extent and biologic profile of prostate cancer with regard to

prostatic anatomy may counter biopsy sampling error, enable appropriate patient selection for local therapy, guide local therapy to the disease rather than to the entire prostate gland, and provide a noninvasive means of monitoring progression or response to therapy.

Here, the authors review the studies that are currently investigating the potential role of MR imaging in guiding needle-based prostate interventions. This review omits studies that use MR images for guidance of external beam radiotherapy [7] and, instead, focuses primarily on interventional procedures that are conducted in the MR imaging scanner room. The article starts with a brief overview of the role of diagnostic MR imaging in prostate cancer.

MR imaging for prostate cancer

It is unfortunate that there is no single imaging method that embodies all of the optimal characteristics for the integration of diagnostic and interventional procedures for prostate cancer. CT permits accurate spatial visualization of interventional devices (Fig. 1A) but does not provide real-time feedback or adequate soft tissue delineation. Transrectal ultrasound (TRUS) is the current "gold standard" for guiding prostate interventions due to its ease of use and real-time image feedback. Soft tissue delineation is better with TRUS than with CT, but most tumors are not visible under ultrasound, and biologic profiling is currently limited [8]. In addition, accurate visualization of interventional needles remains challenging (see Fig. 1B). The interventional

This work was supported in part by the National Science Foundation grant NSF ERC9731478, the US Army grant PC10029, and the National Institutes of Health grants R01 HL 57483 and R01 HL 61672.

* Corresponding author. Departments of Radiology, BME, and ECE, Johns Hopkins University, 720 Rutland Avenue, Traylor 330, Baltimore, MD 21205.

E-mail address: eatalar@jhu.edu (E. Atalar).

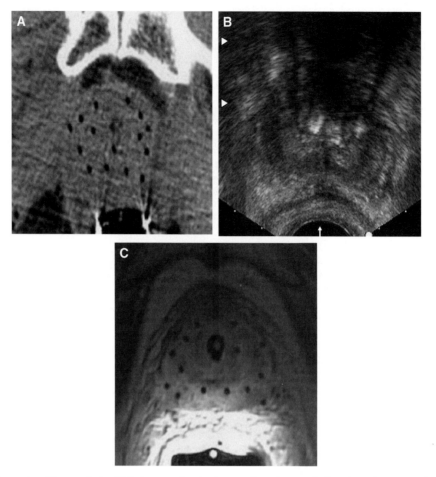

Fig. 1. Interventional images during high dose rate brachytherapy show the superiority of MR imaging in depicting the prostate anatomy and the interventional catheters. (*A*) CT scan image. (*B*) Transrectal ultrasound image. (*C*) MR image.

needles and the prostate anatomy are clearly visible in MR images (see Fig. 1C). From this perspective, MR imaging is well suited for guidance of interventional procedures. The principal limitations to its routine use include a lack of real-time feedback and a complex and technically challenging environment.

A number of anatomic structures can be clearly delineated on MR imaging, including the distal prostatic urethra (up to the point of insertion in the central gland), the central zone, the peripheral zone, the prostatic capsule, the levator ani, and the rectal mucosa [9]. On contrast-enhanced MR images, the neurovascular bundles can also be identified (Fig. 2) [10]. Diagnostic MR imaging, however, has the potential to provide more than high image resolution of the prostate

anatomy. Endorectal coil MR imaging of the prostate gland has demonstrated value for staging and prognostication in patients with localized disease [11–16]. When T2-weighted anatomic images, which are sensitive but not specific for malignancy, are combined with biologic imaging techniques such as MR spectroscopic imaging [17–20] and dynamic contrast-enhanced (DCE) MR imaging [8], MR imaging may be able to accurately identify predominant subsites of tumor burden.

DCE MR imaging is a promising tool for visualizing the vascular physiology of solid tumors. With the advent of modern multislice imaging techniques and data analysis tools, imaging the entire prostate gland with high spatial and temporal resolution using DCE MR imaging is

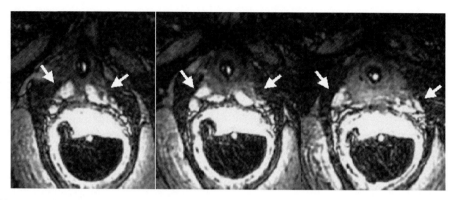

Fig. 2. Neurovascular bundle imaging. The neurovascular bundle (*arrows*) along the prostate gland can be visualized post contrast three-dimensional TrueFISP images. Each panel represents contiguous axial slices at the prostate apex. (*From* Citrin D, Ning H, Guion P, et al. Inverse treatment planning based on MRI for high dose rate prostate brachytherapy. Int J Radiat Oncol Biol Phys 2005;61(4):1272; with permission.)

feasible. In a recent study [8], the sensitivity and specifity of DCE MR imaging for localizing malignancy in the peripheral zone were estimated to be 87% and 74%, respectively, based on a subjective coregistration to TRUS-guided biopsies. This level of accuracy is not maintained in the central gland (sensitivity 96%, specificity 46%) because coexisting benign prostatic hyperplasia is also characterized by high vascularity.

Kurhanewicz and colleagues [17] proposed a three-dimensional MR spectroscopic imaging technique for the detection of prostate cancer. This promising method compares the ratios of choline and creatine to citrate peak levels as a marker of malignancy in the peripheral zone. One of the main limitations of this MR spectroscopic imaging technique is the relatively long data acquisition time and the low signal-to-noise ratio inherent to spectroscopy. The use of large voxels in the imaging protocol partially solves this problem but introducs partial volume effects whereby small lesions may become invisible.

In addition to the techniques of T2-weighted MR imaging, DCE MR imaging, and MR spectroscopic imaging, there are a number of complementary techniques under investigation to improve the diagnostic accuracy of MR imaging. For example, tissue hypoxia, a known biomarker associated with prostate cancer, can be interrogated using blood oxygen level–dependent imaging techniques [21,22]. Diffusion maps of the prostate gland can also be generated with MR imaging, thus providing noninvasive information related to interstitial fluid pressure changes in normal and malignant prostate tissue [23,24].

Needle core biopsy

Currently, prostate biopsy is conducted under TRUS guidance. Although a positive biopsy result is a clear indication of cancer, a negative biopsy result is often indefinite and problematic because it is known that the sextant biopsy procedure has a relatively low sensitivity and high sampling error [25]. To address this problem, an 8- to 10-biopsy regimen, depending on prostate size, has been proposed [26], with sensitivity increasing up to 80%. Repeat sextant biopsy is another approach, which further increases the sensitivity of this approach [27]. Image-guided biopsy may be the best approach to this problem, but ultrasound can be blind to 40% of lesions, which are isoechoic [28].

MR-guided biopsy may have an immediate impact by improving the sensitivity of needle core biopsies to detect prostate cancer, specifically for those 20% of patients who have false-negative biopsy results from sampling error when performed under TRUS guidance [29]. By combining tissue biopsy with MR imaging (ie, to directly biopsy tissue regions with a suspicious MR imaging appearance), the high sensitivity of MR imaging [30] may be obtained while gaining the specificity of tissue biopsy.

In addition, MR imaging guidance of needle biopsies is a critical step in the histopathologic validation of emerging MR imaging techniques for prostate cancer delineation and characterization. These new imaging techniques must be validated against gold standard measures to establish their accuracy, and in this case, the gold standard is prostate biopsy and histopathology. Notable intraprostatic [31] and intratumoral [32] biologic heterogeneity mandates millimeter colocalization accuracy between tissue samples and their corresponding image pixels. When prostate MR imaging and tissue acquisition procedures are performed in different settings and at different times, however, spatial coregistration is fraught with error.

Stereotactic needle placement under MR imaging guidance enables two critical steps in the coregistration of tissue and MR imaging data. First, it directly guides biopsies to sites of suspected tumor on MR imaging, and second, it permits volumetric verification and documentation of the actual biopsy location with regard to MR imaging data.

Investigators at Harvard University were the first to report MR-guided prostate biopsies, which were performed in patients with suspicion of prostate cancer who were not candidates for the standard TRUS-guided technique because of a previous proctocolectomy [33,34]. Using an open-configuration 0.5-T MR imaging scanner and a pelvic coil, transperineal needle core biopsies were performed with patients in the dorsal lithotomy position. Sites deemed suspicious for cancer on previously acquired diagnostic MR imaging were subjectively correlated to corresponding sites on the interventional MR imaging images and specifically targeted through a stereotactically registered perineal template (Fig. 3). A nonconventional transgluteal approach has also been reported using an open low-field MR

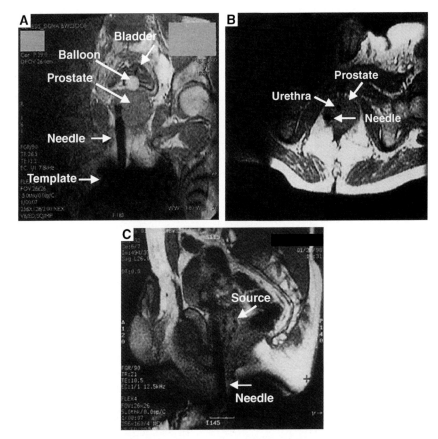

Fig. 3. Images obtained during MR-guided diagnosis and treatment of prostate cancer in a 62-year-old man. (*A*) Coronal view of the prostate gland and bladder. The tip of the biopsy needle has been placed through the perineum and into the lesion, located in the right midportion of the gland. The template was used for accurate placement of the needle. (*B*) Axial view of the prostate gland with the tip of the biopsy needle in the right midportion of the gland. (*C*) Real-time intraoperative catheter placement in the sagittal plane during MR-guided prostate brachytherapy. The black spots are previously deposited radioactive sources posterior to the needle. (*From* D'Amico AV, Cormack RA, Tempany CM. MRI-guided diagnosis and treatment of prostate cancer. N Engl J Med 2001;344(10):776; with permission.)

imaging scanner in patients with uncertain or suspicious prostate lesions on diagnostic MR imaging [35]. Diagnostic images were similarly subjectively correlated to interventional MR images to define biopsy target sites. Using T1-weighted sequences, 25 biopsy procedures were performed successfully with MR guidance in all cases without any side effects or complications. Alternatively, diagnostic MR images have been rigidly coregistered to interventional ultrasound images for guidance [36].

To circumvent the need for and the error associated with deformable or rigid registration of previously acquired diagnostic MR images, transperineal biopsies have been performed under direct MR imaging guidance in a cylindric 1.5-T scanner [37]. To address the challenge of accessing the perineum under the geometric constraint of a 60-cm diameter bore, patients were positioned in the left lateral decubitus position (Fig. 4). Biopsies were again performed through a stereotactically registered perineal template that in this case was affixed perpendicularly to a rigid endorectal coil,

thereby increasing signal-to-noise ratio and image quality. The mean biopsy-needle targeting accuracy of the stereotactic system was 2.1 mm.

Finally, two competing devices for transrectal prostate biopsy in a cylindric 1.5-T scanner have recently been developed [38,39] and clinically tested in patients with prostate cancer [39,40]. The main advantage of the transrectal approach is a shorter needle path length, which translates to less tissue trauma and patient discomfort. For access, patients are positioned prone on the MR imaging table.

The first MR-guided transrectal biopsy system was developed at Charité, Humboldt-Universität zu Berlin in cooperation with MRI Devices/Daum (Schwerin, Germany). This device is made of polyoxymethylene and consists of a base plate, an adjustable arm, and a needle guide filled with contrast material gel that can be visualized on MR imaging. After the patient is positioned, the needle guide is inserted into the rectum and connected to the arm of the biopsy device (Fig. 5). The arm enables the needle guide to be rotated, translated

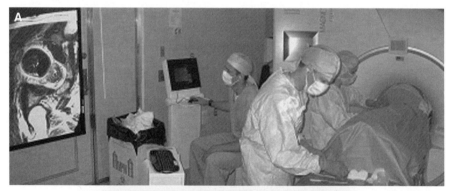

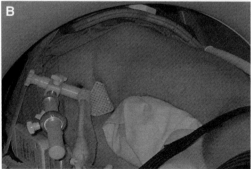

Fig. 4. Setup for transperineal biopsy in a conventional 1.5-T MR imaging scanner. (*A*) Prostate images are displayed within the scanner room using stereotactic targeting software. (*B*) The patient is positioned in the left lateral decubitus position. An endorectal coil is affixed perpendicular to the perineal template. (*From* Menard C, Susil RC, Choyke P, et al. MRI-guided HDR prostate brachytherapy in standard 1.5T scanner. Int J Radiat Oncol Biol Phys 2004;59(5):1417; with permission.)

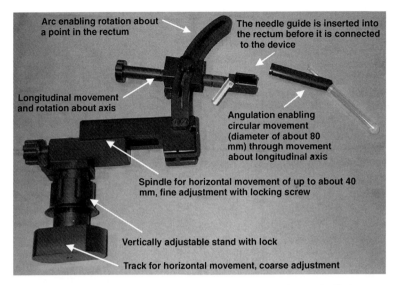

Fig. 5. The endorectal biopsy system developed at Charité, Humboldt-Universität zu Berlin in cooperation with MRI Devices/Daum. Passive markers are imaged to register the device with respect to the prostate. (*From* Beyersdorff D, Winkel A, Hamm B, et al. MR imaging-guided prostate biopsy with a closed MR unit at 1.5 T: initial results. Radiology 2005;234(2):577; with permission.)

forward and backward, and adjusted in height. In addition, the insertion angle can be changed by rotating the needle guide about a point inside the rectum.

In the initial study, biopsies were obtained from suspicious areas of the prostate (Fig. 6) in 12 patients by means of an MR imaging–compatible automatic (n = 5) or semiautomatic (n = 7) 16-gauge core needle biopsy device (Double-Shoot Biopsy Gun or Semi-Automatic Biopsy Gun; MRI Devices/Daum). The authors reported that

of the 16 biopsy specimens from areas that were highly suspicious for prostate cancer at prebiopsy MR imaging, 8 were positive and 8 were negative. Of the 24 biopsy specimens from moderately suspicious areas, 4 showed prostate cancer and 20 showed no prostate cancer. Of the 57 specimens from nonsuspicious areas, 2 showed prostate cancer and 55 did not.

It is important to note that the investigators did not use DCE MR imaging or MR spectroscopic imaging to identify the suspected tumor

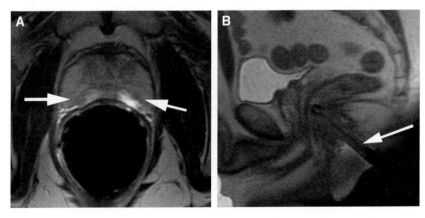

Fig. 6. (*A*) Axial T2-weighted diagnostic MR image of the prostate showing suspicious lesions (*arrows*). (*B*) Sagittal interventional image of the endorectal biopsy procedure. The arrow shows the location of the biopsy device. (*From* Beyersdorff D, Winkel A, Hamm B, et al. MR imaging-guided prostate biopsy with a closed MR unit at 1.5 T: initial results. Radiology 2005;234(2):579; with permission.)

locations; however, they demonstrated a very strong correlation between MR imaging findings and biopsy results. These results are very encouraging for the future widespread use of MR-guided biopsy procedures.

The other transrectal biopsy device, the "access to prostate tissue under MR imaging guidance" (APT MR imaging) system (Fig. 7) [38,40], consists of a 23-mm diameter hollow endorectal sheath, placed at the beginning of the procedure, that remains immobile throughout the intervention. The sheath includes an integrated 20-mm diameter single-turn imaging coil surrounding an anterior window that allows for needle access to the prostate. An 18-mm diameter cylindric needle guide fits inside the stationary rectal sheath and contains three MR tracking microcoils (allowing for device registration). Needle channels at 20° and 30° of angulation permit transrectal needle access to the prostate gland. The cylindric needle guide is mounted on a positioning stage containing the mechanism that converts the rotation of two flexible control rods—each extending to the edge of the scanner bore—into the rotation and translation of the needle guide. Finally, the positioning stage is attached to an immobilization arm mounted on a linear rail.

Four MR-guided prostate biopsy procedures have been reported to date with the APT MR imaging system for the histomolecular validation of DCE MR imaging [41]. Biopsy locations were selected throughout the peripheral zone of the prostate using T2-weighted fast spin-echo images and DCE MR images. Subsequently, after inserting the biopsy needle but before collecting the tissue core biopsy, T1-weighted fast spin-echo images were acquired to confirm biopsy needle placement accuracy. Fifteen tissue biopsies were collected; the mean biopsy needle placement accuracy was 1.8 mm (maximum error, 4.0 mm) [41]. All biopsy cores were suitable for histologic evaluation and for genomic and proteomic microarray profiling. These data demonstrate the feasibility and value of stereotactic biopsies under MR imaging guidance and verification to provide a platform for rigorous histopathologic and biologic validation of MR imaging techniques (Fig. 8).

The APT MR imaging system has also been adapted to a 3-T MR imaging scanner and tested in six patients to date [41]. Because higher field strength translates to higher MR signal, the authors expect an improvement in the resolution of diagnostic images.

In summary, five different techniques of MR-guided prostate biopsy have been reported in the clinical literature. Given the need and rationale for needle guidance to be based on diagnostic-quality MR images, the authors favor a stereotactic approach without real-time image guidance within a diagnostic scanner. One of the limitations to a broader application of the latter cylindric scanner techniques relates to the instability and discomfort associated with the left lateral decubitus and prone positions. Although spatially accurate and robust, stereotactic guidance systems mandate an immobile prostate gland. A number of studies have shown that prostate motion is greatly reduced when patients are positioned supine, stemming from greater patient comfort and reduced respiratory motion [42–44]. Supine immobilization and perineal access in the cylindric

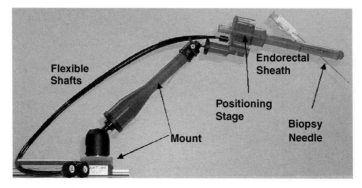

Fig. 7. The APT MR imaging system developed at the Johns Hopkins University. A stationary sheet minimizes the motion of the prostate during rotation and translation of the needle guide. The position of the needle guide is determined by active tracking coils.

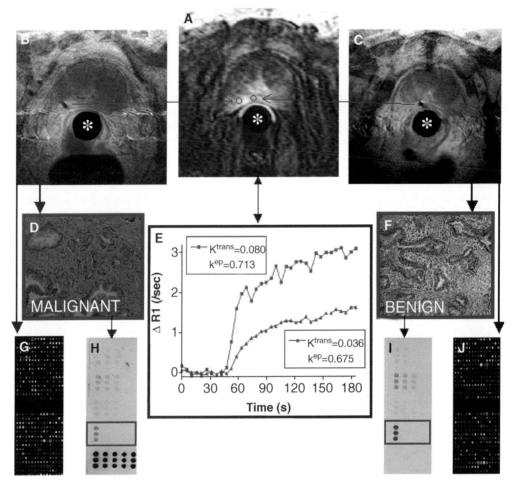

Fig. 8. Case example demonstrating the feasibility and integration of prostate interventional MR imaging for the correlation of molecular biology and DCE MR imaging. The stationary interventional endorectal coil (*) is used for diagnostic and interventional MR imaging. (*A*) DCE MR imaging at 120 seconds shows a small area of increased signal intensity in the left peripheral zone of the prostate. Regions of interest (ROIs; *red and blue*) corresponding to the subsequent needle biopsy voids (*B, C*) are defined for image analysis. (*E*) Time-intensity curves (corrected for T1 heterogeneity) from each ROI are fit to a general kinetic model convolution integral using an arterial input function measured from the external iliac artery. The transfer constant K^{trans} (corresponding to the magnitude of the enhancement curve, unit minute^{-1}) and the rate constant k^{ep} (describing the rate of clearance, unit minute^{-1}) are thought to reflect differences in the perfusion and microvascular permeability underlying each ROI, respectively. Hematoxylin-eosin staining shows adenocarcinoma (*D*) corresponding in this case to higher K^{trans} and k^{ep} than benign tissue (*F*). cDNA microarray (*G, J*) and reverse-phase protein array (*H, I*; array probed with STAT3 antibody) analysis can be performed on the biopsy cores. (*From* Menard C, Susil RC, Choyke P, et al. An interventional magnetic resonance imaging technique for the molecular characterization of intraprostatic dynamic contrast enhancement. Mol Imaging 2005;4(1):63–6; with permission.)

scanner is only be possible with custom-designed interventional MR imaging tables, which is the subject of ongoing work. Finally, larger studies are required to confirm the clinical value and role of MR-guided biopsy in patients with prostate cancer.

Brachytherapy

Permanent implant

For patients with localized prostate cancer at low risk for extraprostatic extension, permanent-seed brachytherapy is an accepted and effective minimally invasive treatment strategy. Radioactive seeds are conventionally placed and left throughout the prostate gland under ultrasound guidance using a transperineal template. One important performance measure of the procedure is the proportion of the prostate gland receiving the minimum desired dose. Treatment-related toxicity is associated with radiation dose delivered to the surrounding normal organs, including the urethra, bladder wall, rectal wall, penile bulb, and neurovascular bundles.

In an effort to avoid toxicity with permanent-seed brachytherapy, investigators at Harvard University translated the conventional transperineal ultrasound technique to an open MR imaging scanner architecture [45]. Even at low field strength, the peripheral zone of the prostate gland (where most cancers are known to reside) could be distinguished from the central gland, thus permitting partial prostatic irradiation whereby permanent seeds were placed in the peripheral zone only, thereby reducing the radiation dose to the urethra and bladder wall (Fig. 9). Five-year results confirmed the equivalence of this approach to radical prostatectomy in biochemical disease-free survival [46].

Ultrasound or low-field interventional MR images, however, cannot accurately identify prostatic subsites of tumor burden that may benefit from targeted radiation dose escalation. For this reason, a number of investigators have attempted to coregister previously acquired diagnostic MR images to interventional images using techniques ranging from subjective interpretation to finite element–based deformable registration [47–52]. Permanent-seed brachytherapy performed directly in a high-field diagnostic scanner would circumvent this step and potentially reduce the error introduced by coregistration. This methodology is currently being investigated in the Netherlands, where the technical feasibility of a novel single-needle technique has been proposed [53].

Temporary implant

Patients with intermediate- or high-risk prostate cancer have a higher intraprostatic burden of disease. A number of prospective randomized studies have confirmed that such patients may benefit from escalation of radiation dose [54–56]. By virtue of the "inverse square" law, brachytherapy "radiation boosts" result in a much steeper dose gradient and, hence, can achieve better sparing of adjacent normal structures compared with external beam radiotherapy. Such a highly desirable quality can paradoxically lead to important errors; therefore, the technique demands a high level of accuracy and precision and mandates optimal image guidance.

High dose rate temporary implants offer several advantages over permanent-seed implants. Dosimetric calculations are performed immediately following the catheter placement procedure, which permits the treatment plan to be based on the actual geometry of the implant relative to the anatomy. The treatment is immediately delivered with an afterloading technique, and problems with organ motion, setup error, and postimplant edema are circumvented. A single high-intensity ^{192}Ir source can be placed at any position for any length of time within each needle. These two variables (dwell position and dwell time) can be optimized using computer programs designed to achieve dose distribution that conforms to the target volume, while limiting dose to normal structures at risk of radiation injury.

Investigators at the University of California–San Francisco have manually aligned previous diagnostic MR imaging/MR spectroscopic imaging datasets to "treatment planning" CT or MR images acquired after brachytherapy catheters were inserted into the prostate gland under ultrasound guidance [57]. Based on the diagnostic images, subprostatic sites suspicious for tumor burden that were specifically targeted for further dose escalation were defined. It was found that the dose could be safely escalated to these sites without overdosing the urethra or the rectum.

To circumvent the error associated with coregistration of previously acquired diagnostic images, a technique for transperineal placement of brachytherapy catheters in a 1.5-T scanner was developed [37]. This technique is identical to the biopsy technique described previously, whereby patients are placed under general anesthesia in the left lateral decubitus position on the MR imaging table. This approach permits diagnostic images to be acquired first, followed immediately by the placement of brachytherapy catheters throughout the prostate gland. After the catheters are in place, a final diagnostic-quality T2-weighted image set can be acquired and directly used to plan and optimize radiation delivery [58]. The authors have used this approach to demonstrate a unique ability to limit radiation dose to the neurovascular bundle—a structure critical to sexual function—which is immediately adjacent to the prostate gland and best visualized on MR imaging [10].

A   B   C

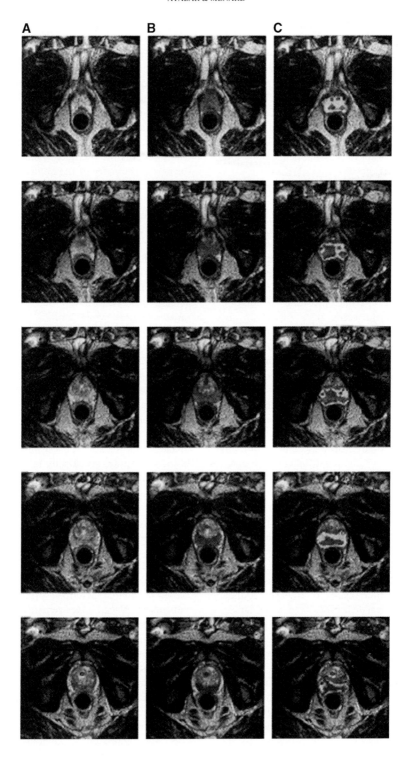

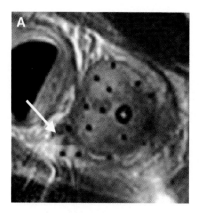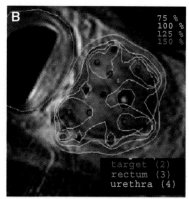

Fig. 10. High dose rate brachytherapy in a 1.5-T scanner. (*A*) Fourteen brachytherapy catheters (signal voids) were placed throughout the prostate gland and at sites of visualized extracapsular extension (*arrow*). (*B*) Radiation was delivered according to a dosimetry plan whereby the target volume including the prostate gland and extracapsular sites of disease extension (*purple line*) is encompassed by 100% of the prescription dose (*outer yellow outline*). The urethral dose (*orange outline*) is kept below 125% of the prescription dose, and the rectal mucosa (*white outline*) is kept below 75% of the prescription dose. (*From* Menard C, Susil RC, Choyke P, et al. MRI-guided HDR prostate brachytherapy in standard 1.5T scanner. Int Radiat Oncol Biol Phys 2004;59(5):1420; with permission.)

This procedure may also offer a therapeutic advantage for those patients who have extracapsular extension of disease visualized on MR images, whereby extracapsular disease may be included in the radiation target volume (Fig. 10).

Thermal therapy

The role of thermal therapies for patients with prostate cancer remains investigational at this time. Beyond anatomic guidance, there is a strong rationale for integrating thermal treatment, specifically heat therapy, in the MR imaging environment where temperature can be monitored noninvasively during the procedure [59]. This treatment has been demonstrated by Chen and colleagues [60], whereby patients who had locally recurrent prostate carcinoma received percutaneous interstitial microwave thermoablation continually guided with MR imaging. Four MR imaging–compatible microwave applicators were placed in the four quadrants of the prostate gland under ultrasound guidance. Patients were transferred to MR imaging, where treatment was delivered while phase images were obtained with a rapid gradient-echo technique to derive tissue temperature change on the basis of proton-resonance frequency shift (Fig. 11).

Prostate treatments with high-intensity focused ultrasound under MR imaging guidance with a transurethral [61,62] or transrectal [63] approach have been reported in the literature only at the preclinical stage to date.

Summary

MR imaging is currently the most effective diagnostic imaging tool for visualizing the anatomy and pathology of the prostate gland. Currently, the practicality and cost effectiveness of transrectal ultrasound dominates image guidance for needle-based prostate interventions. Challenges to the integration of diagnostic and interventional MR imaging have included the lack of real-time feedback, the complexity of the imaging technique, and limited access to the perineum within the geometric constraints of the MR imaging scanner.

Fig. 9. MR-guided permanent seed brachytherapy in an open MR imaging scanner. (*A*) Series of axial T2-weighted MR images used to identify the clinical target volume, the anterior rectal wall, and the prostatic urethra. (*B*) Series showing segmentation of the prostate peripheral zone, the anterior rectal wall, and the prostatic urethra. (*C*) Series after total dose received based on final [125]iodine source positions. Red, ≥ 240 Gy; yellow, ≥ 160 and < 240 Gy; blue, ≥ 100 and < 160 Gy; no color, < 100 Gy. (*From* D'Amico AV, Cormack R, Tempany CM, et al. Real-time magnetic resonance image-guided interstitial brachytherapy in the treatment of select patients with clinically localized prostate cancer. Int J Radiat Oncol Biol Phys 1998;42(3):513; with permission.)

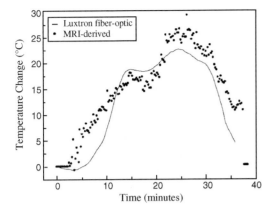

Fig. 11. Graph demonstrates the temperature measurements (Luxtron fiber-optic) and proton-resonance frequency shift temperature estimates (MR imaging–derived) as a function of elapsed time (in minutes) during the prostate ablation process. Active heating began at 2 minutes and was terminated at 38 minutes. (*From* Chen JC, Moriarty JA, Derbyshire JA, et al. Prostate cancer: MR imaging and thermometry during microwave thermal ablation-initial experience. Radiology 2000;214(1):295; with permission.)

Two basic strategies have been explored and clinically demonstrated in the literature: (1) coregistration of previously acquired diagnostic MR imaging to interventional TRUS or open scanner MR images, and (2) stereotactic needle interventions within conventional diagnostic scanners using careful patient positioning or the aid of simple manipulators.

Currently, researchers are developing techniques that render MR imaging the method of choice for the direct guidance of many procedures. This article focuses on needle-based interventions for prostate cancer, including biopsy, brachytherapy, and thermal therapy. With rapid progress in biologic imaging of the prostate gland, the authors believe that MR imaging guidance will play an increasing role in the diagnosis and treatment of prostate cancer.

References

[1] Jemal A, Tiwari RC, Murray T, et al. Cancer statistics, 2004. CA Cancer J Clin 2004;54(1):8–29.

[2] So A, Goldenberg L, Gleave ME. Prostate specific antigen: an updated review. Can J Urol 2003;10(6): 2040–50.

[3] Bostwick DG. Gleason grading of prostatic needle biopsies. Correlation with grade in 316 matched prostatectomies. Am J Surg Pathol 1994;18(8): 796–803.

[4] Humphrey PA. Gleason grading and prognostic factors in carcinoma of the prostate. Mod Pathol 2004; 17(3):292–306.

[5] D'Amico AV, Renshaw AA, Cote K, et al. Impact of the percentage of positive prostate cores on prostate cancer-specific mortality for patients with low or favorable intermediate-risk disease. J Clin Oncol 2004;22(18):3726–32.

[6] Obek C, Louis P, Civantos F, et al. Comparison of digital rectal examination and biopsy results with the radical prostatectomy specimen. J Urol 1999; 161(2):494–8 [discussion: 498–9].

[7] Debois M, Oyen R, Maes F, et al. The contribution of magnetic resonance imaging to the three-dimensional treatment planning of localized prostate cancer. Int J Radiat Oncol Biol Phys 1999; 45(4):857–65.

[8] Ito H, Kamoi K, Yokoyama K, et al. Visualization of prostate cancer using dynamic contrast-enhanced MRI: comparison with transrectal power Doppler ultrasound. Br J Radiol 2003;76(909):617–24.

[9] Mayr NA, Menard C, Molloy AR, et al. Computed tomography and magnetic resonance imaging of the prostate, uterus, and cervix. In: Chao CKS, editor. Practical essentials of intensity modulated radiation therapy. Philadelphia: Lippincott Williams & Wilkins; 2004. p. 47–61.

[10] Citrin D, Ning H, Guion P, et al. Inverse treatment planning based on MRI for HDR prostate brachytherapy. Int J Radiat Oncol Biol Phys 2005;61(4): 1267–75.

[11] Cheng GC, Chen MH, Whittington R, et al. Clinical utility of endorectal MRI in determining PSA outcome for patients with biopsy Gleason score 7, PSA < or = 10, and clinically localized prostate cancer. Int J Radiat Oncol Biol Phys 2003;55(1): 64–70.

[12] D'Amico AV, Whittington R, Malkowicz SB, et al. Combined modality staging of prostate carcinoma and its utility in predicting pathologic stage and postoperative prostate specific antigen failure. Urology 1997;49(Suppl 3A):23–30.

[13] D'Amico AV, Schnall M, Whittington R, et al. Endorectal coil magnetic resonance imaging identifies locally advanced prostate cancer in select patients with clinically localized disease. Urology 1998;51(3):449–54.

[14] D'Amico AV, Whittington R, Malkowicz SB, et al. Combination of the preoperative PSA level, biopsy Gleason score, percentage of positive biopsies, and MRI T-stage to predict early PSA failure in men with clinically localized prostate cancer. Urology 2000;55(4):572–7.

[15] Nguyen PL, Whittington R, Koo S, et al. Quantifying the impact of seminal vesicle invasion identified using endorectal magnetic resonance imaging on PSA outcome after radiation therapy for patients with clinically localized prostate cancer. Int J Radiat Oncol Biol Phys 2004;59(2):400–5.

[16] Poulakis V, Witzsch U, De Vries R, et al. Preoperative neural network using combined magnetic resonance imaging variables, prostate specific antigen and Gleason score to predict prostate cancer stage. J Urol 2004;172(4 Pt 1):1306–10.

[17] Kurhanewicz J, Vigneron DB, Hricak H, et al. Three-dimensional H-1 MR spectroscopic imaging of the in situ human prostate with high (0.24–0.1-cm^3) spatial resolution. Radiology 1996;198(3):795–805.

[18] Hasumi M, Suzuki K, Taketomi A, et al. The combination of multi-voxel MR spectroscopy with MR imaging improve the diagnostic accuracy for localization of prostate cancer. Anticancer Res 2003;23(5b):4223–7.

[19] Scheidler J, Hricak H, Vigneron DB, et al. Prostate cancer: localization with three-dimensional proton MR spectroscopic imaging—clinicopathologic study. Radiology 1999;213(2):473–80.

[20] Coakley FV, Kurhanewicz J, Lu Y, et al. Prostate cancer tumor volume: measurement with endorectal MR and MR spectroscopic imaging. Radiology 2002;223(1):91–7.

[21] Carnell D, Smith R, Taylor J, et al. Evaluation of hypoxia within human prostate carcinoma using quantified BOLD MRI and pimonidazole immunohistochemical mapping. Br J Cancer 2003;88:S12.

[22] Jiang L, Zhao DW, Constantinescu A, et al. Comparison of BOLD contrast and Gd-DTPA dynamic contrast-enhanced imaging in rat prostate tumor. Magn Reson Med 2004;51(5):953–60.

[23] Issa B. In vivo measurement of the apparent diffusion coefficient in normal and malignant prostatic tissues using echo-planar imaging. J Magn Reson Imaging 2002;16(2):196–200.

[24] Chan I, Wells W, Mulkern RV, et al. Detection of prostate cancer by integration of line-scan diffusion, T2-mapping and T2-weighted magnetic resonance imaging; a multichannel statistical classifier. Med Phys 2003;30(9):2390–8.

[25] Kantoff P, Carroll PR, D'Amico AV. Prostate cancer: principles and practice. Philadelphia: Lippincott Williams & Wilkins; 2002.

[26] Norberg M, Egevad L, Holmberg L, et al. The sextant protocol for ultrasound-guided core biopsies of the prostate underestimates the presence of cancer. Urology 1997;50(4):562–6.

[27] Levine MA, Ittman M, Melamed J, et al. Two consecutive sets of transrectal ultrasound guided sextant biopsies of the prostate for the detection of prostate cancer. J Urol 1998;159(2):471–5 [discussion: 475–6].

[28] Shinohara K, Wheeler TM, Scardino PT. The appearance of prostate cancer on transrectal ultrasonography: correlation of imaging and pathological examinations. J Urol 1989;142(1):76–82.

[29] Rabbani F, Stroumbakis N, Kava BR, et al. Incidence and clinical significance of false-negative sextant prostate biopsies. J Urol 1998;159(4):1247–50.

[30] Beyersdorff D, Taupitz M, Winkelmann B, et al. Patients with a history of elevated prostate-specific antigen levels and negative transrectal US-guided quadrant or sextant biopsy results: value of MR imaging. Radiology 2002;224(3):701–6.

[31] Aihara M, Wheeler TM, Ohori M, et al. Heterogeneity of prostate cancer in radical prostatectomy specimens. Urology 1994;43(1):60–6 [discussion: 66–7].

[32] Evans SM, Hahn SM, Magarelli DP, et al. Hypoxic heterogeneity in human tumors—EF5 binding, vasculature, necrosis, and proliferation. Am J Clin Oncol Cancer Clin Trials 2001;24(5):467–72.

[33] D'Amico AV, Tempany CM, Cormack R, et al. Transperineal magnetic resonance image guided prostate biopsy. J Urol 2000;164(2):385–7.

[34] D'Amico AV, Cormack RA, Tempany CM. MRI-guided diagnosis and treatment of prostate cancer. N Engl J Med 2001;344(10):776–7.

[35] Zangos S, Eichler K, Engelmann K, et al. MR-guided transgluteal biopsies with an open low-field system in patients with clinically suspected prostate cancer: technique and preliminary results. Eur Radiol 2005;15(1):174–82.

[36] Kaplan I, Oldenburg NE, Meskell P, et al. Real time MRI-ultrasound image guided stereotactic prostate biopsy. Magn Reson Imaging 2002;20(3):295–9.

[37] Susil RC, Camphausen K, Choyke P, et al. System for prostate brachytherapy and biopsy in a standard 1.5 T MRI scanner. Magn Reson Med 2004;52(3):683–7.

[38] Susil RC, Krieger A, Derbyshire JA, et al. System for MR image-guided prostate interventions: canine study. Radiology 2003;228(3):886–94.

[39] Beyersdorff D, Winkel A, Hamm B, et al. MR imaging-guided prostate biopsy with a closed MR unit at 1.5 T: initial results. Radiology 2005;234:576–81.

[40] Krieger A, Susil RC, Menard C, et al. Design of a novel MRI compatible manipulator for image guided prostate interventions. IEEE Trans Biomed Eng 2005;I52(2):306–13.

[41] Menard C, Susil RC, Choyke P, et al. An interventional magnetic resonance imaging technique for the molecular characterization of intraprostatic dynamic contrast enhancement. Mol Imaging 2005;4(1):63–6.

[42] Mah D, Freedman G, Milestone B, et al. Measurement of intrafractional prostate motion using magnetic resonance imaging. Int J Radiat Oncol Biol Phys 2002;54(2):568–75.

[43] Kitamura K, Shirato H, Seppenwoolde Y, et al. Three-dimensional intrafractional movement of prostate measured during real-time tumor-tracking radiotherapy in supine and prone treatment positions. Int J Radiat Oncol Biol Phys 2002;53(5):1117–23.

[44] Bayley AJ, Catton CN, Haycocks T, et al. A randomized trial of supine vs. prone positioning in patients undergoing escalated dose conformal

radiotherapy for prostate cancer. Radiother Oncol 2004;70(1):37–44.

[45] D'Amico AV, Cormack R, Tempany CM, et al. Real-time magnetic resonance image-guided interstitial brachytherapy in the treatment of select patients with clinically localized prostate cancer. Int J Radiat Oncol Biol Phys 1998;42(3):507–15.

[46] D'Amico AV, Tempany CM, Schultz D, et al. Comparing PSA outcome after radical prostatectomy or magnetic resonance imaging-guided partial prostatic irradiation in select patients with clinically localized adenocarcinoma of the prostate. Urology 2003; 62(6):1063–7.

[47] Reynier C, Troccaz J, Fourneret P, et al. MRI/TRUS data fusion for prostate brachytherapy. Preliminary results. Med Phys 2004;31(6):1568–75.

[48] Bharatha A, Hirose M, Hata N, et al. Evaluation of three-dimensional finite element-based deformable registration of pre- and intraoperative prostate imaging. Med Phys 2001;28(12):2551–60.

[49] Mizowaki T, Cohen GN, Fung AY, et al. Towards integrating functional imaging in the treatment of prostate cancer with radiation: the registration of the MR spectroscopy imaging to ultrasound/CT images and its implementation in treatment planning. Int J Radiat Oncol Biol Phys 2002;54(5): 1558–64.

[50] Clarke DH, Banks SJ, Wiederhorn AR, et al. The role of endorectal coil MRI in patient selection and treatment planning for prostate seed implants. Int J Radiat Oncol Biol Phys 2002;52(4): 903–10.

[51] Wu X, Dibiase SJ, Gullapalli R, et al. Deformable image registration for the use of magnetic resonance spectroscopy in prostate treatment planning. Int J Radiat Oncol Biol Phys 2004;58(5):1577–83.

[52] DiBiase SJ, Hosseinzadeh K, Gullapalli RP, et al. Magnetic resonance spectroscopic imaging-guided brachytherapy for localized prostate cancer. Int J Radiat Oncol Biol Phys 2002;52(2):429–38.

[53] Van Gellekom MP, Moerland MA, Battermann JJ, et al. MRI-guided prostate brachytherapy with single needle method—a planning study. Radiother Oncol 2004;71(3):327–32.

[54] Pollack A, Zagars GK, Smith LG, et al. Preliminary results of a randomized radiotherapy dose-escala-tion study comparing 70 Gy with 78 Gy for prostate cancer. J Clin Oncol 2000;18(23):3904–11.

[55] Zeitman A, DeSilvio M, Slater JD, et al. A randomized trial comparing conventional dose (70.2GyE) and high-dose (79.2GyE) conformal radiation in early stage adenocarcinoma of the prostate: results of an interim analysis of PROG 95–09. In: Cox J, editor. ASTRO 2004. Atlanta (GA): Elsevier; 2004. p. S131–2.

[56] Sathya J, Davis I, Julian J, et al. A randomized trial comparing a conbination of iridium implant and external beam radiation to external beam radiation alone for patients with locally advanced prostate cancer. In: Cox J, editor. ASTRO 2004. Atlanta (GA): Elsevier; 2004. p. S448.

[57] Pouliot J, Kim Y, Lessard E, et al. Inverse planning for HDR prostate brachytherapy used to boost dominant intraprostatic lesions defined by magnetic resonance spectroscopy imaging. Int J Radiat Oncol Biol Phys 2004;59(4):1196–207.

[58] Menard C, Susil RC, Choyke P, et al. MRI-guided HDR prostate brachytherapy in standard 1.5T scanner. Int J Radiat Oncol Biol Phys 2004;59(5). 1414–23.

[59] Peters RD, Chan E, Trachtenberg J, et al. Magnetic resonance thermometry for predicting thermal damage: an application of interstitial laser coagulation in an in vivo canine prostate model. Magn Reson Med 2000;44(6):873–83.

[60] Chen JC, Moriarty JA, Derbyshire JA, et al. Prostate cancer: MR imaging and thermometry during microwave thermal ablation-initial experience. Radiology 2000;214(1):290–7.

[61] Diederich CJ, Stafford RJ, Nau WH, et al. Transurethral ultrasound applicators with directional heating patterns for prostate thermal therapy: in vivo evaluation using magnetic resonance thermometry. Med Phys 2004;31(2):405–13.

[62] Ross AB, Diederich CJ, Nau WH, et al. Highly directional transurethral ultrasound applicators with rotational control for MRI-guided prostatic thermal therapy. Phys Med Biol 2004;49(2):189–204.

[63] Sokka SD, Hynynen KH. The feasibility of MRI-guided whole prostate ablation with a linear aperiodic intracavitary ultrasound phased array. Phys Med Biol 2000;45(11):3373–83.

ELSEVIER
SAUNDERS

Magn Reson Imaging Clin N Am
13 (2005) 505–517

**MAGNETIC
RESONANCE
IMAGING CLINICS**
of North America

MR-Guided Interventions of the Breast

Maurice A.A.J. van den Bosch, MD, PhD[a], Bruce L. Daniel, MD[b],*

[a]Department of Radiology, University Medical Center Utrecht,
Heidelberglaan 100, 3584CX Utrecht, The Netherlands
[b]Department of Radiology, Stanford University Medical Center,
Room H1307, 300 Pasteur Drive, Stanford, CA 94305-5105, USA

MR imaging of the breast has become a well-established method for detecting invasive breast carcinoma. It is a more sensitive method than conventional mammography and ultrasound for detection of invasive tumors, with a sensitivity approaching 100% [1–4]. The specificity of MR imaging of the breast, however, is limited, ranging from 40% to 95% depending on patient selection and imaging techniques used [5–7]. To standardize reporting of breast MR images, the American College of Radiology breast imaging reporting and data system–MR imaging (BI-RADS-MRI-lexicon was developed [8]. Currently, well-accepted indications for MR imaging of the breast include analysis of questionable breast lesions detected with conventional imaging modalities, screening high-risk patients, follow-up after breast-conserving therapy or silicon implant, and preoperative staging of patients before breast-conserving therapy. In these patients, MR imaging has proved to reveal therapeutically relevant multicentric or contralateral disease in up to 15% of patients [9–12].

Because of its high sensitivity, MR imaging of the breast may reveal suspicious breast lesions that are clinically and mammographically occult. In these cases, MR-guided tissue sampling is necessary to make a diagnosis [12]. Furthermore, even when an MR-detected breast lesion can be presumptively identified by corroborating physical examination, mammography, or sonography, MR-guided tissue sampling may be preferred because it may be impossible to prove that the purported palpable, sonographic, or mammographic lesion is the same as the suspicious MR imaging lesion [13]. Several techniques have been developed during recent years to allow MR-guided preoperative localization and percutaneous biopsy of suspicious breast lesions. The capability to localize and perform biopsies on breast lesions using MR imaging guidance has to be considered a crucial part of each state-of-the-art breast MR imaging program. In the following two sections, the current techniques used for MR-guided preoperative localization and percutaneous biopsy are discussed.

MR-guided needle localization

The primary method for sampling MR-detected lesions remains preoperative MR-guided needle localization and hookwire placement, followed by surgical biopsy [12]. Although "second-look" sonography is frequently attempted to identify suspicious lesions found on MR imaging, not all MR-detected tumors are sonographically visible. Even when a sonographic abnormality is detected, it can be difficult to be sure that it corresponds to the MR imaging lesion because the breast is imaged supine during sonography and prone during MR imaging. In the early 1990s, MR-compatible needle and hookwire sets using low-susceptibility alloys were developed. Several techniques were reported that allowed localization in supine patient position, including a freehand technique similar to localization of lesions under CT or ultrasound guidance and stereotactic localization by means of a surface coil with an integrated perforated plate [14]. The main

* Corresponding author.
E-mail address: bdaniel@stanford.edu (B.L. Daniel).

1064-9689/05/$ - see front matter © 2005 Elsevier Inc. All rights reserved.
doi:10.1016/j.mric.2005.04.003

disadvantages of these supine patient methods are respiratory motion artifacts and direction of needle insertion toward the chest wall.

The development of prone-position breast coils that have open access to the breast improved MR-guided needle placement techniques by eliminating respiratory motion, by allowing needle trajectories that parallel the chest wall, and by positioning the breast for biopsy in the same (or nearly the same) position in which diagnostic breast MR imaging is performed (Fig. 1A). Currently, localization with the patient in the prone position is considered more adequate and feasible and has been the subject of the more recent studies [12,15–17]. In general, two successful MR-guided needle localization techniques with the patient in the prone position have been described: the stereotactic technique, with the patient in the prone or lateral decubitus position in a closed magnet; and the freehand technique, with the patient in the prone position in an open MR imaging unit.

In sterotactic MR-guided needle localization methods, breast fixation is maintained by breast compression between two perforated plates (grids), allowing needle insertion through the holes (see Fig. 1B). The first report on MR-guided localization using a grid was published by Heywang-Köbrunner and colleagues [18] in 1994. The patient lies prone on the compression device, with the breast compressed between the two plates. The position is maintained throughout the procedure. Medial and lateral access is possible with this system. Other reported grid techniques, based on the same principle, also use perforated compression plates but only allow needle insertion on the lateral side of each breast [12,17,19]. The most recent study by Morris and colleagues [17] reported on the results of this technique in 69 patients with 101 breast lesions (Fig. 2). They concluded that MR-guided needle localization using a grid could be performed quickly and safely and that 31% of the localized lesions proved to be malignant. These results are in concordance with those of previous studies on mammographic or ultrasound-guided needle localization, which reported breast cancers to be present in 12% to 55% of the cases [20]. There are some limitations of MR-guided needle localization using breast compression devices. First, breasts can only be approached from the lateral side, necessitating longer tissue needle penetration and difficult wire trajectory to lesions located medially in the breast. Second, by using a grid, several parts of the breast are difficult to access, especially posterior localized lesions near the chest wall and the axillary tail. In addition, lesions localized in the retroareolar region are difficult to target because the anterior part of the breast may not be adequately stabilized between two sagittal compression plates. Third, the prearrangement of holes within the grid limits access to areas that are located between the holes, which may be of special importance when localizing small lesions. Fourth, it has been reported that strong breast compression might interfere with lesion enhancement [21].

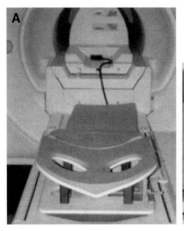
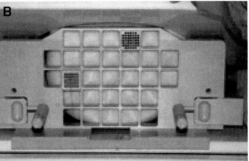

Fig. 1. Breast MR imaging grid localization system. (*A*) Bilateral open prone breast coil (Biopsy-System No. NMR NI 160; MRI Devices, Waukesha, Wisconsin) with lateral positioned grid system that allows immobilization, localization, and biopsy. (*B*) Close-up image of the grid plate. Note needle guides and wires. (Courtesy of Elizabeth Morris, MD, New York, New York.)

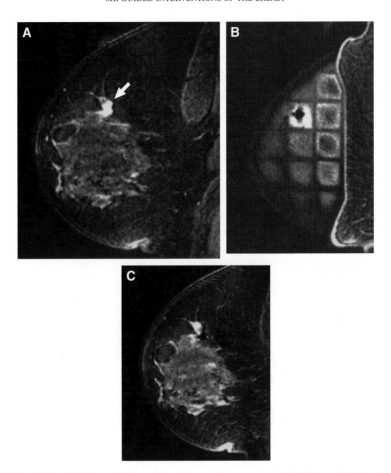

Fig. 2. MR-guided needle localization with the grid technique of a mammographically occult lesion in the right breast. (*A*) Contrast-enhanced sagittal fat-suppressed three-dimensional T1-weighted MR image shows irregular, speculated mass (*arrow*) in the right upper outer quadrant. Sequential sagittal MR images depict the lesion in relation to the grid. (*B*) The radiologist places the needle in the needle guide hole of the grid estimated to be closest to the lesion. (*C*) Needle artifact is shown at the level of the grid and through the lesion. (Courtesy of Elizabeth Morris, MD, New York, New York.)

The second technique (needle localization of suspicious breast lesions using a freehand technique) addresses some of these problems [13]. The authors reported the results of freehanded MR-guided needle localization in 14 patients prone positioned on an open-platform breast coil in a vertically open 0.5-T imager (Signa-SP, General Electric Medical Systems, Milwaukee, Wisconsin) (Fig. 3) [13]. In this procedure, the needle is advanced in small increments toward the target, alternating with rapid imaging of the progress of needle insertion on a stack of approximately 5 to 7 adjacent image slices. This technique has primarily been reported using open magnets that allow direct monitoring of the procedure [21]; however, it can be performed using conventional cylindric magnets by shuttling the patient in and out of the

bore for each set of images. With this technique, fast and accurate localization within 9 mm from the target lesion was possible. Between 1997 and 2004, the authors performed 304 needle localizations in 220 patients and found that 34% of the lesions were malignant, which is comparable to the results of studies reporting on the grid technique (Fig. 4) [17].

The main advantage of the freehand technique compared with the grid technique is the freely chosen needle insertion angle, enabling localization of lesions throughout the breast, from lesions near the chest wall to those superficially located near the nipple. The freehand technique facilitates a circumareolar needle insertion, which some surgeons prefer to preserve breast cosmesis (see Fig. 4). It allows needle trajectories that parallel

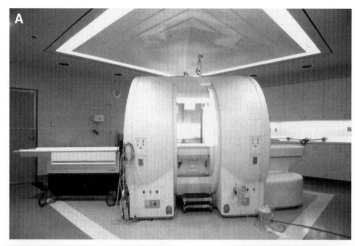

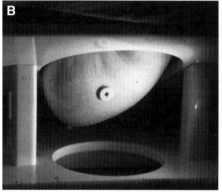

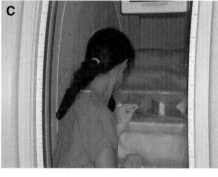

Fig. 3. (*A*) The open 0.5-T MR imager (Signa-SP; General Electric Medical Systems, Milwaukee, Wisconsin). With the use of an open platform-type phased-array breast coil (MRI Devices, Waukesha, Wisconsin), interventional procedures can be performed. (*B*) The open architecture of the coil provides unrestricted access to the lateral breast and limited access to the superior, inferior, anterior, and medial breast. (*C*) In the open magnet, the radiologist has direct access to the breast for needle placement without removing the patient from the scanner.

the surface of silicon implants, thereby minimizing the risk of incidental puncture. Even medial, cranial, and caudal approaches have been performed. Another advantage of the freehand method is that the configuration of the uncompressed breast during the procedure is the same as the configuration of the breast during the preprocedural diagnostic MR imaging, facilitating proper identification of the target lesion in the beginning of the needle localization by using non–contrast-enhanced T1-weighted images of the breast architecture as a map [13,21]. This identification is important because after contrast injection, the target lesions will be visualized only for a limited period (approximately 5 to 15 minutes). To make best use of this time, all steps, including preliminary imaging, skin site preparation, and any necessary anesthesia and initial needle placement

toward the lesion are performed before contrast injection. A potential limitation of the freehand technique is possible motion of the target lesion in the noncompressed breast, especially in patients with dense breast tissue. In the authors' experience, however, substantial breast motion does not occur because the weight of the patient's prone body fixes the chest wall to the coil platform. When less critical breast motion occurs, the rapid interactive imaging approach allows redirecting of the needle to the target despite motion.

Devices and pulse sequences

For MR-guided localization or biopsy, equipment that is fully MR-compatible should be used. MR-compatible needles and hookwires of different shapes, sizes, and lengths are now

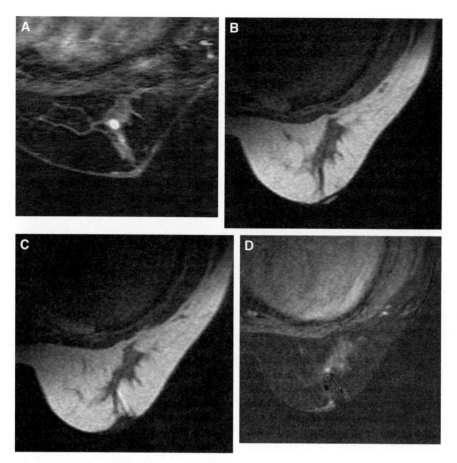

Fig. 4. Freehanded MR-guided needle localization and hookwire placement. (*A*) Contrast-enhanced T1-weighted axial image, reformatted from a high-resolution three-dimensional water-selective spoiled gradient-echo image with a magnetization transfer contrast pulse, revealed a mammographically occult, rapidly enhancing indeterminant lesion in the central right breast. (*B*) Initial precontrast T1-weighted image reveals a fiducial marker (*arrow*) on the skin at the corresponding slice location. (*C*) The needle is inserted to the suspicious area using the breast architecture on T1-weighted images as an initial guide to placement. (*D*) Finally, contrast-enhanced water-specific three-point Dixon gradient-echo sequence image confirms that the suspicious enhancing target is located at the tip of the needle.

commercially available (E-Z-EM, Westbury, New York; Daum Medical USA, Chicago, Illinois; Cook, Bloomington, Indiana). Several MR-compatible stereotaxy devices have become commercially available. Heywang-Köbrunner and colleagues [18] built one in collaboration with Siemens Medical Solutions (Erlangen, Germany) in which the stereotactic device was integrated in a dedicated phased-array breast coil. More recently, systems consisting of a phased-array breast coil and a removable stereotactic device have been developed and are commercially available (Biopsy-System No. NMR NI 160, MRI Devices, Waukesha, Wisconsin; Noras, Würzburg, Germany), allowing MR-guided interventions and diagnostic MR imaging of the breast [17].

For lesion detection and localization, contrast-enhanced studies that combine high spatial and temporal resolution are generally performed. Usually, three-dimensional gradient-echo sequences are used with and without subtraction or with fat suppression. A gadolinium diethylenetriamine pentaacetic acid dose of 0.1 mmol/kg is used for contrast-enhanced images [16]. New techniques have improved MR images; fast imaging of a reduced number of slices is sufficient. Pulse sequence parameters can be adjusted to increase or decrease the conspicuity of needle artifacts [22,23]. Standard two-dimensional slice-selective sequences enable rapid imaging of just a few slices through the region of the breast with the suspected target and can be faster than whole-breast three-dimensional

sequences. Radiofrequency (RF)-refocused sequences, such as high-bandwidth T1-weighted
fast-spin-echo with short-echo train length can
minimize needle artifact size. Water-specific imaging can increase the conspicuity of target lesions by
eliminating competing bright fat signals on T1-
weighted images. Fat suppression is generally
preferred over subtraction techniques because
even small amounts of motion due to needle
manipulations can cause subtraction artifacts.
Three-point Dixon imaging can provide high-
quality water-specific images even at low field or
on open MR imaging systems [13] in which poor
shim and limited spectral separation of fat and
water results in poor fat suppression using conventional fat saturation pulses.

MR-guided biopsy

MR-guided fine-needle aspiration and large-
gauge core needle biopsy can provide a cytologic
or pathologic diagnosis without surgery. Fine-
needle aspiration provides only cytology and
cannot distinguish in situ and invasive cancer.
Several MR-compatible needles are available and,
attached to a syringe, these needles can be used for
fine-needle aspiration under MR imaging guidance [24]. Fine-needle aspiration requires a high
level of quality assurance of cytology, and acquisition of insufficient material is a well-known
problem. As a consequence, fine-needle aspiration
has only rarely been performed under MR imaging guidance. On the other hand, large-gauge core
needle biopsy has proved to be an accurate and
reliable alternative to surgical excision biopsy.
MR-compatible core needle biopsy needles ranging from 18 to 14 gauge have become available (E-
Z-EM; Cook; MRI Devices/Daum, Waukesha,
Wisconsin) [25–27]. Accurate biopsy requires
sampling from within the target lesion, unlike
needle localization, which merely requires close
proximity to the target [28]. Thus, meticulous,
accurate technique is crucial. MR imaging pulse
sequences must be chosen that can provide "post-
fire" images of the needle within the target to
prove sampling accuracy (Fig. 5).

MR-compatible needles used for biopsy have
two major disadvantages. First, depending on the
diameter, needle artifacts can obscure small target
lesions, making core biopsy of small lesions (<1
cm) difficult. Second, current MR-compatible
needles are not as sharp as regular steel needles
and yield smaller samples compared with conventional steel needles of similar design, thereby

limiting the amount of tissue available to the
pathologist. Small sample volumes are a potential
problem because they provide less accurate pathologic diagnoses. Performing the biopsy in an
open MR imaging scanner can facilitate removal
of multiple samples, provided that satisfactory
image quality is available [29,30]. Different groups
have reported on repeated tissue sampling facilitated by coaxial systems or substitute needles
in combination with a conventional automatic
biopsy gun; however, coaxial systems may further
increase the size of the needle system and associated artifacts. The conventional automatic biopsy
gun can only be used outside the magnet, which
has the disadvantage that possible lesion shift
caused by biopsy gun needle insertion or bleeding
cannot be detected. Because images cannot be
obtained that show the actual biopsy device in the
target lesion, it may be difficult to prove that the
target did not move transiently out of the way
during biopsy.

More recently, MR-compatible vacuum-assisted breast biopsy devices have been developed
(ATEC Breast Biopsy System, Suros Surgical
Systems, Indianapolis, Indiana; Vacora, Bard
Biopsy Systems, Tempe, Arizona) [31–33]. With
these methods, a sharp trocar, placed inside an
introducer sheath, is inserted after skin incision
and advanced toward the lesion. After appropriate positioning is confirmed on MR imaging, the
trocar is replaced by the biopsy device, which is
fully inserted through the introducer sheath into
the target lesion to obtain tissue specimens. A
recent study by Liberman and colleagues [31]
reported a technically successful MR-guided
vacuum-assisted core biopsy in 19 of 20 (95%)
women using the Suros Surgical Systems device.
Biopsies were performed on 27 MR-detected
lesions with a median size of 1.0 cm. Cancer
was present in 8 of 27 (30%) lesions. The large-
gauge vacuum-assisted motorized device rapidly
delivers multiple large samples after a single
probe insertion.

There is a crucial need for further refinement of
MR-compatible biopsy instrumentation. Current
systems require a "substitution" MR-compatible
needle or a plastic obturator to be inserted in lieu
of the trocar or biopsy device during imaging
because the susceptibility artifacts from the metal
trocar and the biopsy instrument are so large that
they unacceptably obscure and distort images of
the breast. Thus, although accuracy of sheath/
obturator placement can be confirmed by imaging, there is no guarantee that the biopsy device

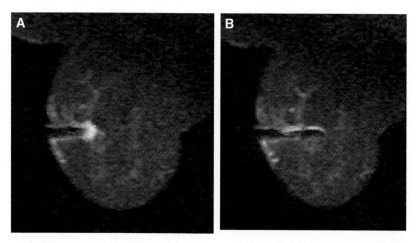

Fig. 5. Freehanded MR-guided large-gauge core needle biopsy. (*A*) Contrast-enhanced axial T1-weighted water-specific three-point Dixon fast-spin-echo image shows the tip of the 14-gauge titanium needle (Daum Medical USA, Chicago, Illinois) approaching a suspicious enhancing lesion lateral in the right breast. (*B*) After extending the inner trocar of the needle, the lesion is seen centered on the biopsy slot. This direct visualization of the biopsy instrument at the lesion provides critical imaging proof of accurate sampling.

position is identical, given the possibility of internal tissue motion as the large device is advanced through the sheath into the breast. In practice, this possible tissue motion caused by introduction of a biopsy device in breast tissue has limited the ability to sample small-sized (<1 cm) lesions. Ideally, breast biopsy apparatus should rapidly provide multiple large samples without needle artifacts obscuring the target and should provide vacuum to stabilize and draw in tissue and remove any hematoma. The lack of simple, satisfactory MR-guided core biopsy instruments has slowed widespread implementation of MR-guided large-gauge core needle biopsy. With surgical biopsy as the only alternative, wider use of diagnostic breast MR imaging, despite its great potential to improve breast cancer management, has been stifled for fear of finding lesions that cannot be worked up without surgery.

MR-guided tumor ablation

The introduction of screening mammography and the use of MR imaging of the breast have increased the detection rate of small-sized breast tumors [34]. As a consequence, there has been a major shift toward less invasive local treatment of breast cancer. Currently, the standard surgical treatment for T1 N0 M0 cancer is lumpectomy followed by radiation therapy [35]. The goal of breast-conservation surgery is complete removal of the malignant breast tumor and a surrounding

rim of normal breast tissue, with a secondary goal being improved cosmesis and reduced morbidity.

Technologic advances over the last decade have fueled interest in even less invasive local treatments for patients with limited-stage breast carcinoma. Several so-called "minimally invasive techniques" that allow percutaneous ablation of malignant breast tissue have been explored. Currently available techniques include radiofrequency ablation (RFA), cryoablation, laser irradiation, and focused ultrasound surgery. Different imaging modalities, including radiographic mammography, ultrasound, and MR imaging, can be used to guide the instruments, to monitor the therapeutic procedure, and for follow-up after treatment. The potential ability of MR imaging to reveal heating- or freezing-dependent signal changes combined with the high accuracy to reveal the three-dimensional extent of invasive tumors has spawned the nascent field of MR-guided minimal invasive therapy for treatment of breast cancer.

Radiofrequency ablation

RF energy heats tissue and causes in situ tumor cell destruction by thermal coagulation and protein denaturation. High-frequency (100–500 kHz) alternating current flows from the noninsulated electrode tip into the surrounding tissue. The electrical current causes ionic agitation, resulting in frictional heating of tissue surrounding the electrode [36,37]. Temperatures greater than

60°C produce coagulation necrosis. The shape of the ablated volume depends on the shape, size, and design of the RF electrode. There is a limit to the size of the thermal lesion that can be produced by using a single-needle electrode. Therefore, multiarray electrodes have been developed that, after they are fully deployed, give the device the shape of an umbrella and produce thermal lesions of 3 to 5 cm in diameter [38,39].

Although RFA is used in routine clinical practice to treat unresectable hepatic tumors, the experience of RFA in patients with breast carcinoma is limited. Furthermore, all previously reported studies assessing the feasibility of RFA of breast tumors used ultrasound to guide the instruments and monitor the RFA procedure; to date, there are no published studies on MR-guided RFA of breast lesions in patients. The first study on ultrasound-guided RFA treatment of breast tumors, reported by the authors' group in 1999, reported complete ablation in 4 of 5 patients [40]. Since then, several studies followed, all presenting promising results, with complete ablation rates varying from 86% to 100%. Izzo and colleagues [41] reported complete coagulation necrosis in 25 of 26 (96%) patients treated with RFA for small breast tumors. Another study by Singletary and colleagues [37] reported complete ablation in 86% of the patients treated with ultrasound-guided RFA because of small (T1) breast tumors. More recently, Burak and colleagues [42] reported on ultrasound-guided RFA of small breast tumors in 10 patients. In addition to ultrasound, they assessed the value of MR imaging performed in 9 patients before and after the ablation procedure for demonstration of ablation zone and for prediction of residual tumor after the RFA procedure. Postprocedural MR imaging detected no residual enhancement in 8 of 9 (86%) patients, which corresponded to the histologic findings. They concluded that ultrasound-guided RFA can be used to treat small breast tumors and that a postablation MR imaging scan appears to predict histologic findings. The most recent study on ultrasound-guided RFA was reported by Fornage and colleagues [43] who reported complete ablation of 20 of 21 (95%) lesions.

Despite these promising results, several concerns persist regarding the use of ultrasound for guiding and monitoring breast tumor RFA. One concern for ultrasound guidance of RFA is that it does not provide an accurate measurement of the tumor volume and may underestimate the true lesion size [36,44] compared with MR imaging or histopathology. Monitoring the progress of RFA is also difficult with ultrasound. The hyperechogenicity of the heated breast tissue and the ultrasonographic shadowing make it difficult to differentiate between necrotic ablated tissue and residual tumor. As a consequence, patient selection is critical to the success of the ablation procedure, with exclusion of patients suspected to have multifocal disease or tumors of uncertain size/shape. As the results of Burak and colleagues [42] showed, postprocedural MR imaging may be useful to assess when complete tumor ablation has been achieved by RFA therapy. Although there are still no published studies on "real time" MR-guided RFA of breast tumors, MR imaging is a logical choice for guiding probe placement because the procedure is similar to MR-guided needle placement for biopsy purposes (Fig. 6). A unique opportunity for MR imaging is the potential to directly image the electrical current paths in tissue [45] around the electrode. In theory, these paths could be used to predict the heat deposition anticipated from an RFA electrode, which is particularly critical for breast tissue because of the heterogeneous composition of the breast. Research is also underway into the use of MR imaging to monitor both temperatures achieved during RF ablation. Although MR imaging has been shown to depict temperature changes accurately using phase-difference images, additional refinements are necessary to enable accurate measurements in the presence of tissue motion, probe susceptibility artifacts, and in the heterogeneous mix of fat and water pixels. Lastly, postprocedure contrast-enhanced MR imaging yields more reliable information than ultrasound with respect to the size of the tumor necrosis. Recently, MR-compatible RFA probes have been developed for use within the magnet. Additional hardware modifications are necessary to prevent the RFA generator–produced RF noise from corrupting MR images.

Cryoablation

The cryoablation technique uses freezing to destroy tumor cells. Miniaturized argon-powered Joule-Thompson effect cryoprobes have been developed that rapidly reach tip temperatures approaching $-160°C$ (Endocare, Irvine, California; Galil Medical USA, Woburn, Massachusetts). After the probe is positioned under image guidance in the center of the tumor, expansion of high-pressure argon cools the probe tip and generates an iceball of frozen tissue surrounding the probe

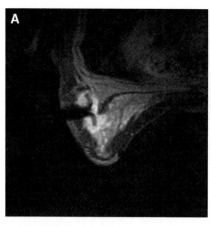
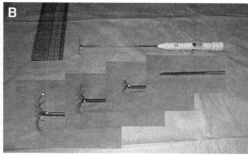

Fig. 6. MR-guided RFA. (*A*) Contrast-enhanced axial T1-weighted water-specific three-point Dixon gradient-echo image shows a deployed umbrella-shaped LeVeen needle electrode centrally in the mass. (*B*) The 15-gauge insulated multiple-needle electrode (LeVeen needle electrode, RadioTherapeutics Corp., Mountain View, California). Radially spaced stainless steel wires spread outward in an umbrella-shaped inverted arc with a tip-to-tip diameter of 2.5 cm.

tip [46]. The time required for each cycle depends on the probe's temperature and surface area, size of the iceball needed, and local tissue perfusion. Instant tumor necrosis is caused by protein denaturation; secondary cell death over the course of days is believed to be caused by ischemia because of disruption of microvasculature [46]. At least two freeze–thaw cycles are used to maximize the efficacy of the technique.

Stocks and colleagues [47] reported on a series of breast cancer patients treated with cryoablation followed by lumpectomy. These investigators showed promising results, with 90% of the breast tumors successfully ablated. More recently, Sabel and colleagues [48] reported the results of ultrasound-guided cryoablation of breast tumors in 27 patients. Cryoablation successfully destroyed 100% of the cancers <1.0 cm; however, for tumors >1.5 cm, cryoablation was not reliable. They concluded that cryoablation should be limited to patients with invasive ductal carcinoma <1.5 cm and with <25% ductal carcinoma in situ in core biopsy. Comparable results have been reported by Pfleiderer and colleagues [49] who reported on ultrasound-guided cryoablation in 16 breast cancer patients. Five tumors smaller than 16 mm did not show any remaining invasive cancer after treatment; however, in 11 patients with more extensive disease (ie, tumor diameter >23 mm or extensive ductal carcinoma in situ component), the cryoablation was incomplete. Recently, Kaufman and others [50,51] reported ultrasound-guided cryoablation to be a successful therapy for treatment of 63 benign breast lesions

(including 53 fibroadenomas). At 12 months' follow-up, these investigators found an overall tumor volume resorption of 88% and concluded that cryoablation was successful in treating core biopsy–proved benign breast lesions without any cosmetic deficit. Today, the Food and Drug Administration has approved the treatment of fibroadenomas with cryoablation without resection in a nonprotocol setting.

As with RFA, sonography has limitations for guiding and monitoring cryoablation in the breast. The marked impedance difference between frozen and nonfrozen tissue causes complete shadowing at the tissue–iceball interface. Only the most superficial boundary of the iceball can be accurately depicted. MR imaging is well suited as a guidance and monitoring modality for percutaneous cryosurgery. The cryosurgical iceball manifests as a signal void on most MR imaging sequences because of the marked reduction in free-water volume in the frozen tissue and because of T2* shortening in the frozen tissue. The iceball margins are clearly revealed in three dimensions without shadowing. MR imaging has recently been reported as a method for guiding cryosurgery in the breast [52].

Interstitial laser thermal therapy

Interstitial laser thermal therapy is a technique that uses laser light energy to heat and ablate tissue [53]. The laser light energy is delivered from the laser tip directly to the target by way of optical fibers inserted into the tissue. Of the several types of lasers that are commercially available, the most commonly used is the Nd-YAG laser (1064–1320 nm). The target tissue temperature is 80°C to 100°C, which is maintained for up to 15 to 20 minutes. Typically, an ablation zone in the form of a centric ring is produced, with one optic fiber producing burns of around 1.0 cm [54]. Thus, multiple fibers are used to cover one lesion. Macroscopically, the centric ablated zone consists of a central necrotic cavity surrounded by a ring of pale tissue, representing the "pseudoviability zone," and a peripheral hemorrhagic rim beyond which is representative of the limits of cancer destruction. The first study was reported by Mumtaz and colleagues [54] who treated 27 breast tumors with interstitial laser thermal therapy followed by surgical excision. They concluded that contrast-enhanced MR imaging is helpful in defining the extent of laser-induced necrosis and for residual tumor detection. Stereotactic-guided laser ablation of breast tumors has been reported in 36 patients by Dowlatshahi and colleagues [55]. They found complete ablation in 67% of the patients. More promising results were found by Bloom and colleagues [56], who reported complete ablation in all 40 patients with small localized (T1) breast cancer. These findings were supported by further research of Dowlatshahi and colleagues [57] who subsequently reported 93% to 100% successful ablation of small breast cancers in 54 patients. More recently, the same group reported a case report in which one patient was treated for breast cancer by interstitial laser thermal therapy and subsequently followed-up for 3 years with no signs of recurrence [58]. It can be concluded that small breast tumors can be completely ablated with negative tumor margins by interstitial laser thermal therapy.

Several imaging techniques (most commonly ultrasound) can be used for laser guidance; however, the potential advantages of using MR imaging guidance and monitoring are similar to the advantages of using MR imaging for RFA. Although the small size of the ablation zone from a single interstitial laser thermal therapy fiber is a limitation, the advantage of interstitial laser thermal therapy over RFA for MR-guided ablation is the complete lack of probe susceptibility artifacts and RF noise artifacts on MR images.

Focused ultrasound

Focused ultrasound therapy is a transcutaneous ablation method that is minimally invasive,

requiring only cutaneous anesthesia. The technique delivers high-power ultrasound energy (1–2 MHz) to the target point through the skin by using a large, focused transducer located in an external water bath that is in contact with the breast. At this target point, acoustic energy is converted into heat [59–61]. In general, a temperature elevation from 60°C to 90°C is produced during a 10- to 20-second sonication, resulting in protein denaturation, coagulation necrosis, and finally, irreversible cell damage of the target cells while sparing the surrounding tissue. Because only relatively small lesions (up to 7 mm^3) can be created, multiple lesions are overlapped to treat an entire tumor. Furthermore, although heating is rapid for each individual sonication, cooling is required between sonications, increasing the total procedure time sometimes up to 1 hour or more. MR imaging is the most suitable method to visualize the target lesion and to monitor the focused ultrasound procedure [62]. Several studies have examined the efficacy of MR-guided focused ultrasound for treatment of malignant invasive breast tumors and benign breast lesions such as fibroadenoma. The first study on MR-guided focused ultrasound for treatment of fibroadenomas was published by Hynynen and colleagues [62]. They treated 11 fibroadenomas in 9 patients under local anesthesia and reported that 8 of 11 (73%) lesions treated demonstrated complete or partial lack of contrast-material uptake on post-procedural T1-weighted images. The lack of effective treatment in three cases was most likely due to unanticipated patient movement during the ablation process that caused the overlapping ablation zones to no longer remain contiguous. No adverse side effects were reported. In the same year, the first case of successful MR-guided focused ultrasound ablation of invasive breast carcinoma was reported by Huber and colleagues [63]. More recently, Gianfelice and others [64–66] reported on MR-guided focused ultrasound treatment as an adjunct to chemotherapeutic regimen of tamoxifen in 24 female patients who were at increased risk for surgery or who had refused surgery. All patients had a follow-up of 6 months, and 19 of 24 (79%) patients had negative biopsy results after one or two treatment sessions. Only one minor complication, a second-degree skin burn, was reported. They concluded that MR-guided focused ultrasound is a promising method of focal tumor destruction. Wu and colleagues [67] reported focused ultrasound ablation in 23 breast cancer patients followed by modified radical mastectomy. In all cases, complete tumor necrosis was obtained, including a mean tumor margin of healthy tissue of 1.8 cm. More recently, Gianfelice and colleagues [66] reported the results of MR-guided focused ultrasound in 12 breast cancer patients before surgery. In 9 of the 12 patients treated with the latest available focused ultrasound system, a mean of 88.3% of cancer tissue was found to be necrotized. Residual tumor was predominantly identified at the periphery of the tumor mass. A major potential advantage of focused ultrasound therapy is that the shape of the ablation can be tailored to the shape of the lesion. Unlike RFA, cryosurgery, and interstitial laser thermal therapy, the ablation apparatus does not dictate the shape of the ablation zone, which is potentially very important for breast cancer ablation because breast tumors are often irregularly shaped.

Summary

Techniques and instrumentation are now widely available that enable interventional MR-guided preoperative needle localization and lesion marking. Minimally invasive MR-guided core biopsy techniques have been demonstrated but remain limited for small lesions and will be facilitated by the development of biopsy instruments that can be directly visualized using MR imaging.

MR-guided tumor ablation is beginning to be evaluated in a few centers. It holds promise as new treatment modality in the continuing trend toward greater breast conservation in the local therapy of breast cancer. Further studies are needed to document the ability of MR-guided ablation to control the margins of a tumor as effectively as surgery. Patients with an extensive in situ intraductal component may pose a significant hurdle because the extent of ductal carcinoma in situ may be underestimated on breast MR images. Ultimately, the success of MR-guided thermal ablation depends on the ability of MR imaging to map the extent of heating during the procedure so that the procedure can be performed to achieve complete control of the tumor margins. It is unfortunate that the conventional method for MR thermometry—the proton resonance frequency shift method—does not work in fat or in voxels with a mix of fat and glandular tissue and, hence, has limited applicability in the breast. Other methods, including measurement of T1 and T2, are being investigated as alternatives.

Acknowledgments

The authors thank Elizabeth Morris, MD, for providing figures on the grid localizing system.

References

[1] Bluemke DA, Gatsonis CA, Chen MH, et al. Magnetic resonance imaging of the breast prior to biopsy. JAMA 2004;292:2735–42.

[2] Berg WA, Gutierrez L, NessAiver MS, et al. Diagnostic accuracy of mammography, clinical examination, US, and MR imaging in preoperative assessment of breast cancer. Radiology 2004;233: 830–49.

[3] Harms SE, Flamig DP, Hesley KL, et al. MR imaging of the breast with rotating delivery of excitation off resonance: clinical experience with pathologic correlation. Radiology 1993;187:493–501.

[4] Daniel BL, Yen YF, Glover GH, et al. Breast disease: dynamic spiral MR imaging. Radiology 1998; 209:499–509.

[5] Hulka CA, Smith BL, Sgroi DC, et al. Benign and malignant breast lesions: differentiation with echo-planar MR imaging. Radiology 1995;197:33–8.

[6] Nunes LW, Schnall MD, Siegelman ES, et al. Diagnostic performance characteristics of architectural features revealed by high spatial-resolution MR imaging of the breast. AJR Am J Roentgenol 1997; 169:409–15.

[7] Knopp MV, Weiss E, Sinn HP, et al. Pathophysiologic basis of contrast enhancement in breast tumors. J Magn Reson Imaging 1999;10:260–6.

[8] Ikeda DM, Hylton NM, Kinkel K, et al. Development, standardization, and testing of a lexicon for reporting contrast-enhanced breast magnetic resonance imaging studies. J Magn Reson Imaging 2001;13:889–95.

[9] Liberman L, Morris EA, Dershaw DD, et al. MR imaging of the ipsilateral breast in women with percutaneously proven breast cancer. AJR Am J Roentgenol 2003;180:901–10.

[10] Fischer U, Kopka L, Grabbe E. Breast carcinoma: effect of preoperative contrast-enhanced MR imaging on the therapeutic approach. Radiology 1999; 213:881–8.

[11] Brekelmans KM, Brekelmans CT, Boetes C, et al. Efficacy of MRI and mammography for breast-cancer screening in women with a familial or genetic predisposition. N Engl J Med 2004;351:427–37.

[12] Orel SG, Schnall MD, Newman RW, et al. MR imaging-guided localization and biopsy of breast lesions: initial experience. Radiology 1994;193: 97–102.

[13] Daniel BL, Birdwell RL, Ikeda DM, et al. Breast lesion localization: a freehand, interactive MR imaging-guided technique. Radiology 1998;207: 455–63.

[14] Heywang-Köbrunner SH. Contrast-enhanced MRI of the breast. 1st edition. Basel (Switzerland): Karger; 1990.

[15] Heywang-Köbrunner SH, Heinig A, Schaumloffel U, et al. MR-guided percutaneous excisional and incisional biopsy of breast lesions. Eur Radiol 1999; 9:1656–65.

[16] Smith LF, Henry-Tillman R, Mancino AT, et al. Magnetic resonance imaging-guided core needle biopsy and needle localized excision of occult breast lesions. Am J Surg 2001;182:414–8.

[17] Morris EA, Liberman L, Dershaw, et al. Pre-operative MR imaging-guided needle localization of breast lesions. AJR Am J Roentgenol 2002;178: 1211–20.

[18] Heywang-Köbrunner SH, Huynh A, Vieweg P, et al. Prototype breast coil for MR-guided needle localization. J Comput Assist Tomogr 1994;18:876–81.

[19] Kuhl C, Elevelt A, Leutner C, et al. Interventional breast MR imaging: clinical use of a stereotactic localization and biopsy device. Radiology 1997;204: 667–75.

[20] Jackman RJ, Marzoni FA. Needle-localized breast biopsy: why do we fail? Radiology 1997;204:677–84.

[21] Kuhl CK, Leutner C, Mielcarek P, et al. Breast compression interferes with lesion enhancement in contrast-enhanced breast MR imaging. Radiology 1997;205P:538.

[22] Butts K, Pauly JM, Daniel BL, et al. Management of biopsy needle artifacts: techniques for RF-refocused MRI. J Magn Reson Imaging 1999;9:586–95.

[23] Daniel BL, Butts K, Glover GH, et al. Breast cancer: gadolinium-enhanced MR imaging with a 0.5-T open imager and three-point Dixon technique. Radiology 1998;207:183–90.

[24] Wald DS, Weinreb JC, Newstead G, et al. MR-guided fine needle aspiration of breast lesions: initial experience. J Comput Assist Tomogr 1996;20:1–8.

[25] deSouza NM, Kormos DW, Krausz T, et al. MR-guided biopsy of the breast after lumpectomy and radiation therapy using two methods of immobilization in the lateral decubitus position. J Magn Reson Imaging 1995;5:525–8.

[26] Doler W, Fischer U, Metzger I, et al. Stereotaxic add-on device for MR-guided biopsy of breast lesions. Radiology 1996;200:863–4.

[27] Nath ME, Robinson TM, Tobon H, et al. Automated large-core needle biopsy of surgically removed breast lesions: comparison of samples obtained with 14-, 16-, and 18-gauge needles. Radiology 1995;197: 739–42.

[28] Bedrosian I, Schlencker J, Spitz FR, et al. Magnetic resonance imaging-guided biopsy of mammographically and clinically occult breast lesions. Ann Surg Oncol 2002;9:457–61.

[29] Brenner RJ, Shellock FG, Rothman BJ, et al. Technical note: magnetic resonance imaging-guided pre-operative breast localization using "freehand technique." Br J Radiol 1995;68:1095–8.

[30] Daniel BL, Birdwell RL, Butts K, et al. Freehand iMRI-guided large-gauge core-needle biopsy: a new minimally invasive technique for diagnosis of enhancing breast lesions. J Magn Reson Imaging 2001;13:896–902.

[31] Liberman L, Morris EA, Dershaw DD, et al. Fast MRI-guided vacuum-assisted breast biopsy: initial experience. AJR Am J Roentgenol 2003;181: 1283–93.

[32] Viehweg P, Heinig A, Amaya B, et al. MR-guided interventional breast procedures considering vacuum biopsy in particular. Eur J Radiol 2002;42: 32–9.

[33] Perlet C, Heinig A, Prat X, et al. Multicenter study for the evaluation of a dedicated biopsy device for MR-guided vacuum biopsy of the breast. Eur Radiol 2002;12:1463–70.

[34] Liberman L, Morris EA, Lee MJ, et al. Breast lesions detected on MR imaging: features and positive predictive value. AJR Am J Roentgenol 2002; 179:171–8.

[35] Dowlatshahi K, Francescatti D, Bloom KJ, et al. Image guided surgery of small breast cancers. Am J Surg 2001;182:419–25.

[36] Singletary SE. Feasibility of radiofrequency ablation for primary breast cancer. Breast Cancer 2003;10: 4–9.

[37] Singletary SE, Fornage BD, Sneige N, et al. Radiofrequency ablation of early-stage invasive breast tumors: an overview. Cancer J 2002;8:177–80.

[38] Elliot R, Rice PB, Suits JA, et al. Radiofrequency ablation of a stereotactically localized non-palpable breast carcinoma. Am Surg 2002;68:1–5.

[39] Hayashi AH, Silver SF, van der Westerhuizen NG, et al. Treatment of invasive breast carcinoma with ultrasound-guided radiofrequency ablation. Am J Surg 2003;18:429–35.

[40] Jeffrey SS, Birdwell RL, Ikeda DM, et al. Radiofrequency ablation of breast cancer: first report of an emerging technology. Arch Surg 1999;134: 1064–8.

[41] Izzo F, Thomas R, Delrio P, et al. Radiofrequency ablation in patients with primary breast carcinoma: a pilot study of 26 patients. Cancer 2001;92: 2036–44.

[42] Burak WE, Agnese DM, Povoski SP, et al. Radiofrequency ablation of invasive breast carcinoma followed by delayed surgical excision. Cancer 2003; 98:1369–76.

[43] Fornage BD, Sneige N, Ross MI, et al. Small (<2 cm) breast cancer treated with US-guided radiofrequency ablation: feasibility study. Radiology 2004;231:215–24.

[44] Bohm T, Hilger I, Muller W, et al. Saline-enhanced radiofrequency ablation of breast tissue: an in vitro feasibility study. Invest Radiol 2000;35:149–57.

[45] Scott GC, Joy ML, Armstrong RL, et al. Rotating frame RF current density imaging. Magn Reson Med 1995;33(3):355–69.

[46] Edwards MJ, Broadwater R, Tafra L, et al. Progressive adoption of cryoablative therapy for breast fibroadenoma in community practice. Am J Surg 2004;188:221–4.

[47] Stocks LH, Chang HR, Kaufman CS, et al. Pilot study of minimally invasive ultrasound-guided cryoablation in breast cancer. Am Soc Breast Surg 2002.

[48] Sabel MS, Kaufman CS, Whitworth P, et al. Cryoablation of early-stage breast cancer: work-in-progress report of a multi-institutional trial. Ann Surg Oncol 2004;11:542–9.

[49] Pfleiderer SO, Freesmeyer MG, Marx C, et al. Cryotherapy of breast cancer under ultrasound guidance: initial results and limitations. Eur Radiol 2002;12:3009–14.

[50] Kaufman CS, Bachman B, Littrup PJ, et al. Office based ultrasound-guided cryoablation of breast fibroadenomas. Am J Surg 2002;184:394–400.

[51] Kaufman CS, Bachman B, Littrup PJ, et al. Cryoablation treatment of benign breast lesions with 12-month follow-up. Am J Surg 2004;188:340–8.

[52] Morin J, Traore A, Dionne G, et al. Magnetic resonance-guided percutaneous cryosurgery of breast carcinoma: technique and early clinical results. Can J Surg 2004;47(5):347–51.

[53] Harms S, Mumtaz H, Hyslop B, et al. RODEO MRI guided laser ablation of breast cancer. Soc Photo-Opt Instrum Eng Proc 1999;3590:484–9.

[54] Mumtaz H, Hall-Craggs MA, Wotherspoon A, et al. Laser therapy for breast cancer: MR imaging and histopathologic correlation. Radiology 1996;200:651–8.

[55] Dowlatshahi K, Fan M, Gould VE, et al. Stereotactically guided laser therapy of occult breast tumors, work in progress. Arch Surg 2000;135:1345–52.

[56] Bloom KJ, Dowlat K, Assad L. Pathologic changes after interstitial laser therapy of infiltrating breast carcinoma. Am J Surg 2001;182:384–8.

[57] Dowlatshahi K, Francescatti D, Bloom KJ. Laser therapy for small breast cancers. Am J Surg 2002;184:359–63.

[58] Dowlatshahi K, Dieschbourg JJ, Bloom KJ. Laser therapy of breast cancer with 3-year follow-up. Breast J 2004;10:240–3.

[59] Gianfelice DC, Mallouche H, Lepanto L, et al. MR-guided focused ultrasound ablation of primary breast neoplasms: works in progress. Radiology 1999;213P:106.

[60] Wu F, Chen WZ, Bai J, et al. Pathological changes in human malignant carcinoma treated with high-intensity focused ultrasound. Ultrasound Med Biol 2001;27:1099–106.

[61] Bohris C, Jenne JW, Rastert R, et al. MR monitoring of focused ultrasound surgery in a breast tissue model in vivo. J Magn Reson Imaging 2001;19:167–75.

[62] Hynynen K, Pomeroy O, Smith DN, et al. MR imaging-guided focused ultrasound surgery of fibroadenomas in the breast: a feasibility study. Radiology 2001;219:176–85.

[63] Huber PE, Jenne JW, Rastert R, et al. A new noninvasive approach in breast cancer therapy using magnetic resonance imaging-guided focused ultrasound surgery. Cancer Res 2001;61:8441–7.

[64] Gianfelice D, Khiat A, Boulanger Y, et al. Feasibility of magnetic resonance imaging-guided focused ultrasound surgery as an adjunct to tamoxifen therapy in high-risk surgical patients with breast carcinoma. J Vasc Interv Radiol 2003;14:1275–82.

[65] Gianfelice D, Khiat A, Amara M, et al. MR imaging-guided focused ultrasound surgery of breast cancer: correlation of dynamic contrast-enhanced MRI with histopathologic findings. Breast Cancer Res Treat 2003;82:93–101.

[66] Gianfelice D, Khiat A, Amara M, et al. MR imaging-guided focused US ablation of breast cancer: histopathologic assessment of effectiveness: initial experience. Radiology 2003;227:849–55.

[67] Wu F, Wang ZB, Cao YD, et al. A randomised clinical trial of high-intensity focused ultrasound ablation for the treatment of patients with localised breast cancer. Br J Cancer 2003;89:2227–33.

**ELSEVIER
SAUNDERS**

Magn Reson Imaging Clin N Am
13 (2005) 519–532

**MAGNETIC
RESONANCE
IMAGING CLINICS
of North America**

Musculoskeletal Interventional MR Imaging

Roberto Blanco Sequeiros, MD, PhD[a,b], John A. Carrino, MD, MPH[b,*]

[a]Department of Radiology, Oulu University Hospital, 90029, P.O. Box 50, Oulu, Finland
[b]Department of Radiology, Brigham and Women's Hospital, Harvard Medical School, ASB-1, LI, Room 003A,
75 Francis Street, Boston, MA 02115, USA

MR imaging is often the imaging modality of choice to investigate neoplastic, infectious, or degenerative processes of the musculoskeletal system. The reasons for this are numerous, including the capability to depict lesions exquisitely before they are detectable by most other modalities. This is of particular importance when medullary bone marrow lesions are considered [1,2]. Furthermore, MR imaging enables lesion detection before the development of irreversible damage to the structural coherence and support capability of the affected bone. This presents tremendous opportunities in the management of osseous musculoskeletal neoplasms and other disorders. Therefore, MR imaging can direct treatments not available by other modalities. MR imaging features not only superior tissue contrast but multiplanar primary imaging section orientation, lack of beam hardening artifacts, and absence of ionizing radiation [3–6] as opposed to fluoroscopy and CT. These characteristics make MR imaging particularly useful as a guidance modality in the musculoskeletal system. MR imaging guidance thus offers a less invasive and easier alternative to open surgical procedures but can also be used in conjunction with surgical techniques. The development of MR imaging technology, including the introduction of open-configuration scanners and dedicated interventional scanners and the adoption of high-field magnets for interventional applications (using an in/out CT scanner type paradigm), broadens the scope of MR-guided procedures that can be performed. New scanners providing relatively rapid imaging capabilities by means of hardware, software, and pulse sequence improvements enable real-time or near–real-time procedural guidance [3–7]. In principle, there are three broad interventional MR imaging categories of applications: biopsy, percutaneous minimally invasive therapy, and intraoperative use. All these can be applied to musculoskeletal procedures. As musculoskeletal interventional MR imaging applications have emerged, there are a multitude of factors to be assessed when performing these procedures. This article reviews the requisites and key applications of musculoskeletal interventional MR imaging.

Procedural components

As with any interventional procedure, the general rules of procedural agenda apply with musculoskeletal procedures. Contraindications to MR-guided biopsy are similar to those of other modalities in terms of patient factors, with some additional considerations attributable to the magnetic environment. The traditional contraindications include the classic "do not touch" lesions of benign origin, patients with bleeding diathesis, infection (unless the biopsy is to rule out infection), and site inaccessibility. Contraindications associated with MR imaging include cardiac pacemakers, large metallic foreign bodies, and noncompatible surgical clips at critical locations (eg, orbit, spinal cord). The unique element in interventional MR imaging is that a single imaging modality, MR imaging, can be used all the way through this agenda. When performing

---

* Corresponding author.

E-mail address: jcarrino@partners.org
(J.A. Carrino).

1064-9689/05/$ - see front matter © 2005 Elsevier Inc. All rights reserved.
doi:10.1016/j.mric.2005.04.010

interventions, MR imaging can be used to plan, guide, monitor, and control the procedure.

Setting up a musculoskeletal interventional MR imaging procedure

Planning

The assessment of the data on the procedural target should be thorough, because this dictates the approach, the route, and the action to be taken. The significance of preprocedural imaging data cannot be overemphasized. The most recent data should be readily available, including preprocedural MR imaging scans. This information should be gathered before the procedure to minimize procedural time, because the patient setup from a procedural perspective can be quite different than that required for diagnostic imaging. The diagnostic data assessment and procedural approach are truly two different entities, and, in this respect, interventional MR imaging is quite comparable to surgery.

To ensure safety during a possibly lengthy procedure, great effort should be aimed at patient positioning. The access route should be determined before the procedure, and patient positioning should be done accordingly. Padding and support should be used to maximize patient comfort and to prevent adverse events from extending or pressing the nerve structures on the extremities or other exposed areas. Draping of the patient and scanner should be thorough, because this gives the operator freedom of movement and enables focusing on the procedure instead of maintaining sterility. Patient monitoring should be arranged as determined by the procedural requirements. Because the procedure takes place in a magnetic environment, all instrumentation and devices used inside the field fringe should be safe or compatible with MR imaging.

Typically, "wrap around" type body coils or proximity surface coils are used for musculoskeletal interventions. The coils should be draped in such a fashion that no risk of possibly oozing body fluids entering the coil structures remains, because this provides a risk of coil malfunction and electrical shock. Coil preference depends on procedural requirements. If a superficial lesion is targeted, the surface coil obviously provides the best signal-to-noise ratio, and thus the best images. If an overall view of the area is to be appreciated and a deeper structure is to be targeted, however, a body coil might be advantageous depending on the field strength. When using low-field scanners, the use of a good surface coil

may overcome some of the inherent low signal attributable to the low-field strength. In general, with musculoskeletal procedures, a surface coil should be used. The surface coil should be positioned as close to the target area center as possible to maximize signal. Further interventional coil development and refinement are needed to address the wide range of musculoskeletal lesion locations and procedures. A crucial requirement for interventional coils is to provide a cut-out region for device placement or surgical incision.

Guiding

A suitable skin entry point and trajectory can be determined in a variety of fashions. Three main guidance methods exist for interventional MR imaging: externally referenced, self-referenced, and MR imaging tracking. Externally referenced (frameless stereotaxy) methods include optical guidance and radiofrequency guidance but are prone to distortion errors. With frameless stereotaxy, the image sections typically can be prescribed according to the data on instrument's location and direction provided by the system (Fig. 1). In one method, images can be generated centered on the position of the instrument tip in the conventional axial-coronal-sagittal planes. In another method, a tool can be used, such as an ultrasound (US) transducer, and images can be generated along the axis in any orthogonal plane about the optically tracked tool. One-step localization and targeting using image guidance are the essential features of frameless stereotaxy. The near–real-time imaging during needle advancement offers an opportunity for trajectory correction and depth measurement. Sophisticated tracking software providing real-time scanner guidance according to the instrument position enables easy determination of puncture site and puncture control during the whole procedure. This type of software is usually a scanner manufacturer–installed option for interventional use. Self-referenced methods include using anatomic landmarks and fiducial markers and tend to minimize but not to eliminate distortion errors. Fiducial markers or a grid can be attached to the skin over the region of interest, and subsequent localizer imaging determines the entry point. A marker (liquid- or fat-containing capsule) or grid (TargoGrid; MRI Devices, Daum, Wisconsin) can be used for this purpose. Because the MR imaging environment is safe and nonionizing, the operator can hold an instrument to the point of interest and thus provide the localization. For palpable lesions

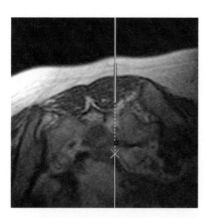

Fig. 1. Externally referenced guidance method of localization. Frameless stereotaxy using optical triangulation localizes the biopsy needle holder, which can be used for interactive image plane acquisition. Axial T2-weighted, three-dimensional, completed balanced steady-state image (repetition time = 8.4 milliseconds, echo time = 4.2 milliseconds, flip angle of 45°) of the pelvis illustrates tracking software–generated virtual graphic overlay over the needle, providing real-time guidance for access to the S1 foramen. The needle icon (*solid blue line*) is superimposed on the image during the intervention and indicates the current location of the needle (*thicker solid blue line, red outline* denotes introduction into the patient), whereas the continued trajectory of the needle is displayed as the yellow line (*dotted line, in-plane; solid line, out of plane*). For a needle completely within the section plane, the yellow line would be completely dashed and flashing. The distal continued trajectory is displayed as the thinner yellow line. The needle exits the image plane at X. The red dot represents an operator-defined target end point.

or lesions near identifiable surface anatomy, an elegant yet simple method is to scan with the operator's finger pointing to the presumed puncture site and to use this as a reference (Fig. 2). MR imaging tracking uses the MR imaging hardware for guidance and is considered to be "distortion-free." This is more commonly used for intravascular catheter applications. It is customary to obtain at least two views of the target area (three planes are often acquired) to identify the target and surrounding anatomic structures before the insertion of the instrument. With MR imaging, this corresponds to imaging in two different planes.

Percutaneous bone access

Currently, there is a paucity of MR imaging–compatible bone needle products. As musculoskeletal applications expand, however, it is anticipated

that more options will become available. We have used trephine sets (Fig. 3A) of 3- and 6-mm inner diameter (MRI Devices). The advantage of this biopsy set is that it is autoclavable and thus can be used several times (up to approximately 10 times). This set is completely compatible with MR imaging and can be used with an accessory piezoelectrically driven drill to enhance penetration of sclerotic lesions (see Fig. 3B). There is also an accessory spiral drill that further enhances the penetration capability of the device.

Monitoring and controlling

Imaging protocols and artifact considerations

Interventional MR imaging sequences can differ substantially from routine MR imaging sequences. The divergent goals are to keep imaging time at a minimum while trying to maximize resolution (contrast, spatial, or temporal). The sequences are typically structured with short repetition time (TR) gradient echo (GE) images. GE images provide good visualization of the instruments from susceptibility artifact, but the signal voids can be large. Typically, lower flip angles, associated with less T1 weighting and a shorter TR, diminish the contrast resolution. T1-weighted fast spin echo (FSE) sequences provide good anatomic conspicuity but poorer visualization of instruments, which can be almost invisible when T2-weighted FSE is used. True fast imaging with steady-state precession (FISP) type sequences are a good compromise because they combine reasonable anatomic resolution and instrument conspicuity with good speed.

Currently, for most pulse sequence types, the imaging speed of near–real-time image updates can be achieved but at a cost of lower spatial resolution. It is more practical to use a longer imaging time to achieve good image resolution and facilitate better control. Contrast resolution can be further augmented with breath-hold or induced apnea during imaging, because this diminishes the artifact caused by breathing motion. This technique is especially applicable for the spine. When performing procedures in the thoracic region, respiratory movement may hinder the image quality in low-field MR imaging scanners, thus generating the need for apnea periods during imaging. In these circumstances, general anesthesia is a viable choice. In the future, parallel imaging may aid in satisfying the requirement for faster imaging. This entails the development of open-structure coils for interventional purposes as

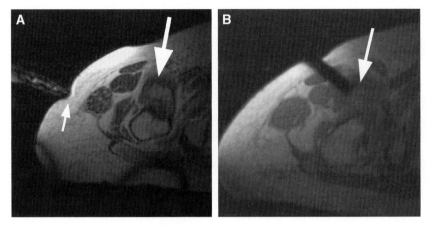

Fig. 2. Self-referenced guidance method of localization. (*A*) Axial T2-weighted, three-dimensional, completed balanced steady-state image (repetition time [TR] = 8.4 milliseconds, [TE] echo time = 4.2 milliseconds, flip angle of 45°) just below the hip joint shows an intermediately bright-signal lesion emanating from the femur with extraosseous extension anterior to the lesser trochanter (*large arrow*). Self-referenced techniques are defined by placing MR imaging visible markers close to a target. In this case, the lesion is being localized by the operator's finger (*small arrow*); user exposure is not an issue in the MR imaging environment. The trajectory is calculated from the position of the target relative to the marker (fingertip location). (*B*) Axial T1-weighted gradient echo imaging (TR = 130 milliseconds, TE = 11 milliseconds, flip angle of 90°) shows a biopsy needle with the tip at the lesion margin (*arrow*). Percutaneous core needle biopsy yielded the diagnosis of lymphoma.

well as software and user interface development to control continuous imaging.

Pulse sequence development for rapid imaging is an active area of development for interventional MR imaging. Interventional MR imaging poses some of the greatest demands on the temporal and spatial resolution of imaging technology because of a combination of factors: the changing orientation of the imaging plane; surgical and therapeutic events occurring within the field of view (FOV); physiologic motion near and within the FOV; intensity changes in the FOV attributable to the introduction of contrast agents, deposition of heat, or other therapy effects; and the need for three-dimensional (3D) volume information to apply, monitor, and control therapies safely and effectively. MR-guided interventions require imaging methods that prescribe, acquire, reconstruct, and display a series of images dynamically. Dynamic imaging differs from standard MR imaging in that continually updating or reacquiring image data forms a large number of images successively and rapidly.

There are special technical considerations when imaging procedural activity with interventional MR imaging. Because of the nature of MR imaging, we are not able to see the instrument used directly; what is visualized is the artifact caused by magnetic susceptibility, the disturbance

to the image acquisition. In general, the signal void artifact is larger than the actual size of the instrument. It must be noted that the artifact is not necessarily symmetric with respect to the instrument. The instrument can also lie in the center of the artifact, near either side, or somewhere in between. Usually, it is possible by windowing and/or leveling the image to infer the exact position of the instrument. Windowing must be such that the gray scale variation within the artifact is seen.

When performing an MR-guided biopsy, it must be recognized that the size of the needle artifact used for needle locale information in MR imaging is dependent on several factors [8], which should be familiar to the operator. The size of the susceptibility artifact is mostly dependent on the strength of the main magnetic field (B_0), instrument position with respect to the main field, instrument material, imaging sequence, and frequency- or phase-encoding direction (Fig. 4). One should understand these factors and their role in successfully performing MR-guided procedures near critical structures, such as neurovascular bundles. In general, the stronger B_0 is, the larger is the artifact caused by the instrument. The more perpendicular the instrument is with respect to the B_0, the more pronounced is the artifact from the instrument. The instrument material is one of

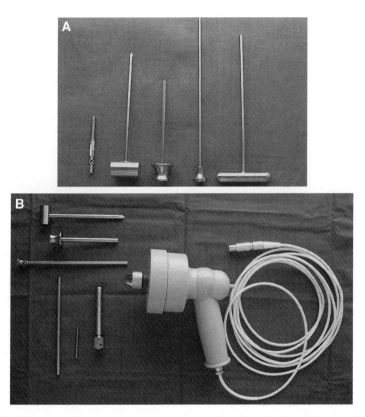

Fig. 3. Musculoskeletal biopsy needles and bone access equipment. Photographs show (*A*) a bone biopsy set with 6 mm of inner diameter (MRI Devices, Daum, Wisconsin) used for cortical penetration and sample procurement and (*B*) a piezoelectrically driven drill with a trephine attached (MRI Devices) that can be used for penetration through normal intact cortex in the diaphysis. (Courtesy of Intermagnetics Companies, Orlando, Florida; with permission.)

the most important factors affecting the size of the artifact; the more ferromagnetic the instrument is, the larger is the susceptibility artifact. Typically, when using a GE sequence, the artifact is larger than that seen with an FSE sequence because of the multiple refocusing pulses that characterize FSE and are absent with GE. The frequency- or phase-encoding direction affects the directional features of instrument artifact. Depending on the stage of the procedure, it may be advantageous to select a frequency- or phase-encoding direction that turns the artifact away from the target area and instrument path. The needle thickness also affects artifact size; the removal of a mandrel (eg, stylet, obturator) diminishes the artifact size in MR imaging.

When operating on the extremities, pelvis, and lumbar spine, the musculoskeletal structures mostly remain stationary. A strap or tape is useful for distal extremity work so that the patient does not need to focus effort on remaining still.

When operating on the upper spinal segments, however, especially at the thoracic level, the image quality may be hindered on low-field magnets because of respiratory and cardiac motion. This can be controlled to some extent by changing the phase-encoding direction to align with the patient's head-to-feet axis. Alignment with the head-to-feet axis is also beneficial in avoiding possible artifacts caused by cerebrospinal fluid flow.

Musculoskeletal MR-guided procedures

Interventional procedures in the musculoskeletal region are, in effect, minimally invasive procedures of a surgical nature. These procedures have been performed under several radiologic imaging modalities, with MR imaging being the most recent addition to the armamentarium. The information available on procedural strategies and indications for musculoskeletal MR-guided interventions is limited but growing. We discuss

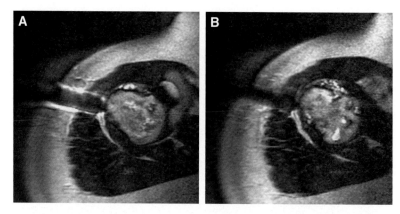

Fig. 4. Effect of frequency-encoding direction on bone need artifact in a proximal humerus biopsy with a 4-mm bone needle (MRI Devices, Daum, Wisconsin). Axial T2-weighted images (repetition time = 2000 milliseconds, echo time = 108 milliseconds, echo train length = 12) show that with a frequency-encoding direction relatively perpendicular to the long axis of the needle (*A*), the susceptibility artifact makes the needle appear wider (note susceptibility artifact at margins) than with a frequency-encoding direction relatively parallel to the needle (*B*). Biopsy of this heterogeneous lesion yielded the diagnosis of fibrous dysplasia.

biopsies, aspirations, spinal injections, and some future trends, including tumor ablation.

MR-guided musculoskeletal biopsy

Correct assessment of lesions that could be infectious, malignant, or benign in origin is essential for the selection of effective treatment in musculoskeletal diseases. Although surgical biopsy is often considered the method of choice to obtain a diagnosis in bone lesions, a substantial proportion of biopsy samples obtained at surgical biopsies may be unsatisfactorily diagnosed [9]. The percutaneous biopsy technique reduces the cost of the procedure, the anesthetic requirements, and the risk of complications compared with the surgical biopsy technique [10]. Percutaneous biopsy is performed by inserting a trephine needle through the skin to the desired location under imaging guidance. Forwarding the trephine drill to the lesion through the working tube collects the sample. The drill is then removed, and a cylindrical biopsy sample is collected. Almost any location in the human body can be reached with percutaneous biopsy techniques.

MR imaging is considered to be the superior modality for detecting musculoskeletal neoplasms and for defining the anatomic properties within bone and soft tissue. Assessment of diagnosis in bone and especially soft tissue neoplasms is particularly challenging because of the variable spectra of imaging findings and overlap between benignancy and malignancy. Biopsy is often the procedure of choice to obtain definitive information on the nature of a neoplastic or tumor type lesion investigated before the institution of specific therapy.

Indications for MR-guided musculoskeletal biopsy

Bone or musculoskeletal biopsy is used to characterize a suspicious lesion, such as a primary malignancy, metastatic deposit, or infectious process. Cross-sectional imaging modalities, such as CT and MR imaging, can be more time-consuming but provide better contrast resolution and visualization of the bone and soft tissue lesion than fluoroscopy [11]. A percutaneous approach using x-ray fluoroscopy or CT guidance is feasible, with a reported success rate of 87% to 100% [12–15]. The complication rate is low, with no significant incidents reported [14–16]. US provides a good means to assess musculoskeletal pathologic findings, but its role in detecting cortical bone–encapsulated or deeply situated pathologic findings is limited.

MR imaging has several features that favor its use as a guidance method. Because of its good sensitivity, MR imaging is able to detect lesions not seen at all in other modalities. In particular, edematous lesions often seen only by MR imaging as a signal increase of bone marrow in heavily fluid-sensitive sequences can be reliably visualized and readily biopsied [2,17,18]. MR imaging also provides superior tissue contrast, often without the need for contrast medium for osseous lesions.

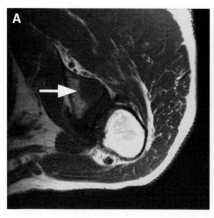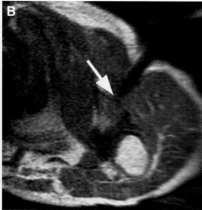

Fig. 5. Bone biopsy in a 61-year-old man with a history of lung cancer and a solitary positron emission tomography-positive bone focus. The patient is in the prone position. (*A*) Axial T1-weighted conventional spin echo image (repetition time [TR] = 500 milliseconds, echo time [TE] = 10 milliseconds) through the shoulder girdle shows a low-signal lesion in the scapula in a subarticular location relative to the glenohumeral joint (*arrow*). (*B*) Axial T1-weighted fast spin echo (FSE) image (TR = 300 milliseconds, TE = 8 milliseconds, echo train length = 2) image shows a biopsy needle placed from a posterior approach through the infraspinatus muscle approximating the lesion (*arrow*). Biopsy of this lesion yielded metastatic small cell carcinoma.

Another target for MR-guided biopsies is the patient with a recurrent musculoskeletal neoplasm, particularly soft tissue sarcomas. These tumors are typically visualized morphologically only in follow-up MR imaging scans. Without MR imaging guidance, the localization for biopsy would be difficult or potentially inaccurate, making interpretation of a negative pathologic sample problematic. Contrast enhancement can be used to characterize a soft tissue lesion and to target the most viable part of it.

There are several nonrandomized retrospective case series that have established the feasibility and safety of MR-guided musculoskeletal biopsies and show a diagnostic yield similar to other modalities. The technique is effective when established interventional MR imaging programs exist and is sufficiently applicable for use in clinical practice. In our practice, MR-guided musculoskeletal biopsy is used for specific instances and problematic lesions. The categories of usefulness that we consider are for [19] lesions not visible by other modalities (Fig. 5), a postoperative collection or lesion adjacent to hardware (particularly if concerned about sarcoma recurrence), targeting a specific portion of a lesion (eg, based on signal intensity or contrast enhancement characteristics), and in pregnant patients desiring to minimize ionizing radiation exposure. In our view, MR-guided biopsy, when available, is a viable option for performing musculoskeletal biopsies on soft

tissue elements (Fig. 6) and synovial-based lesions (Fig. 7).

General considerations

It is important to recognize that the rules generally concerning all diagnostic procedures performed under imaging guidance also apply when performing MR-guided procedures. It is advisable to obtain preoperative MR imaging scans of the region of interest before the planned procedure, because the event of planning the procedure may require a certain effort and time as well as the services of an orthopedic oncologic surgical consultant to determine an approved route. The patient preparation must be done accordingly so as to minimize complication risks. Biopsy procedures can usually be performed under local anesthesia and intravenous conscious sedation (IVCS). Musculoskeletal biopsy may also be performed with regional, monitored, or general anesthesia, however, depending on the clinical situation.

MR-guided bone biopsy: procedural aspects

The lesion should be identified reliably before initiation of the procedure. This can usually be achieved with the fast GE–based sequences used in MR imaging interventions, such as true FISP [20]. The time frame to achieve acceptable image

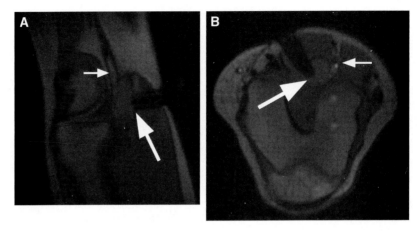

Fig. 6. Soft tissue biopsy in a 26-year-old woman with a history of posterior knee ache and fullness presenting with a popliteal fossa mass. Sagittal oblique (*A*) and axial (*B*) gradient echo MR imaging scans (repetition time = 20 milliseconds, echo time = 9.8 milliseconds, flip angle of 90°) of the knee show an intermediate-signal soft tissue lesion in the popliteal fossa with a biopsy needle within the lesion (*large arrows*). Real-time imaging facilitates needle placement while avoiding critical structures, such as the main neurovascular bundle (*small arrows*). Biopsy of this lesion yielded the diagnosis of solitary fibrous tumor (a benign lesion).

quality for interventional use ranges between near real-time and 40 seconds, depending on scanner field strength, software, and sequence construction. Contrast enhancement can help in identification of the viable part of the lesion [21]. As mentioned previously, the biopsy route should be planned ahead based on previous diagnostic studies. In our practice, the lesions that are principally chosen for MR-guided biopsy are selected because they are only or best visualized by MR imaging. MR imaging also enables a trajectory that avoids critical anatomic structures during biopsy. The patient should be positioned in such a way so as to enable the easiest, safest, or best surgical access route. The advantage of open-configuration scanners is that the patient does not need to be moved with a couch or gantry during the procedure.

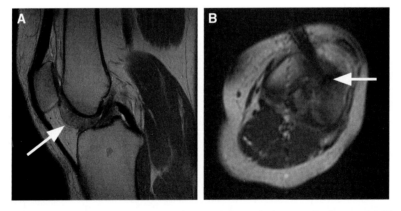

Fig. 7. Intra-articular biopsy in a 41-year-old woman with patellofemoral symptoms for 3 years. (*A*) Diagnostic sagittal T2-weighted fast spin echo (FSE) image (repetition time [TR] = 3000 milliseconds, echo time [TE] = 108 milliseconds, echo train length [ETL] = 8) revealed an intermediate-signal synovial proliferative process with some low-signal foci extending predominantly into the infrapatellar fat pad region (*arrow*) and patellofemoral articulation. Real-time MR imaging guidance facilitated an inferior-to-superior subpatellar approach via the anterior knee. (*B*) Axial T2-weighted FSE image (TR = 2000 milliseconds, TE = 80 milliseconds, ETL = 12) shows a biopsy needle tip in the lesion (*arrow*). Biopsy of this lesion yielded the diagnosis of pigmented villonodular synovitis.

A trephine is most commonly used when performing bone biopsies. The mechanical properties of the MR imaging–compatible biopsy sets are different from those of the regular ones used for CT, US, or fluoroscopy. The metal alloy is dominantly titanium based; this makes the instrument durable, and it is also softer and lacks the hardness of steel. It is often the case that more than one drill or set is needed to collect one sample. Targets containing hard cortical type bone structures may especially pose a problem because of high frictional stress to the instrument. Instruments may also snap (break) because of friction stress. If a high-pitched creaking frictional sound is heard while revolving the drill manually, the drill should be replaced immediately. In addition, bending in the instrument is sometimes observed, and the instrument may need to be replaced. Instrument bending must be taken into account, because the correct position should be unambiguously ascertained. In practice, this means confirmatory images where the needle artifact or injected contrast agent is clearly visible. If necessary, instrument bending is more easily identified by thicker sections. When using rigid instrumentation (4- and 6-mm trephine sets), bending is usually not a problem unless the bone is especially sclerotic or when attempting access through normal diaphyseal cortex in a long bone, such as the humerus or femur.

Underneath the hard cortical bone, intramedullary lesions are sometimes predominantly of soft tissue structure, and as in soft tissue lesions, it may be difficult to obtain a biopsy with a trephine. A true-cut or aspiration type biopsy needle can thus be used. There are several manufacturers that provide MR imaging–compatible true-cut and aspiration needles (eg, E-Z-EM, Cook Medical, MRI Devices, Somatex). Cytologic sampling can also be useful, yielding a faster diagnosis for certain lesions, such as metastatic neoplasm, because there is no need for decalcification as with bone samples [12,16].

MR-guided spinal injections

Low-back disorders are prevalent in all societies. Minimally invasive procedures are an emerging option to relieve pain and to minimize the risk of disability. Spine injections, such as selective nerve blocks, are minimally invasive procedures that have been used to diagnose a variety of causes of back pain and sciatica and to treat radicular pain.

Indications for MR-guided selective nerve blocks

Selective nerve blocks and epidural injections are used to control radicular and low-back pain. Increasingly, they are used as a nonsurgical option for treatment of disk degeneration and herniation. Selective nerve injections are used to confirm the segmental nerve level origin of symptoms when other diagnostic means fail to provide a definitive answer or as presurgical confirmation. The evaluation of the effectiveness of epidural injections and selective nerve blocks in treating radicular pain is beyond the scope of this article, but these procedures have variable efficacy, in part, related to the symptomatology (axial versus radicular) and patient selection. Nevertheless, it can be stated that contained disk herniation–generated radicular pain responds reasonably well to spine injection treatments [22–24]. Nerve blocks also have value in predicting the success of surgery [25]. Patients referred for spinal injections have varying manifestations of clinical and imaging findings, including patients with equivocal or minimal imaging findings, patients with disk herniation declining surgical treatment, patients with good results from a previous nerve block, patients with multiple-level symptoms, and postsurgical patients with recurrent or persistent symptoms.

There are few if any absolute contraindications, but the following should be considered as relative contraindications: uncontrollable bleeding diathesis, systemic or local infection at the puncture site, allergy to a corticosteroid or local anesthetic, and pregnancy. When using MR imaging, there is no risk of ionizing radiation; thus, the procedure is safe to perform after the first trimester of pregnancy if essential. Risks and complications include cerebrospinal fluid leak, nerve laceration, infection, bleeding, adverse medication effects, pneumothorax at thoracic-level blocks, and vascular events at the cervical level.

MR imaging guidance provides an excellent roadmap of vertebral column pathologic anatomy and affects the performance of MR-guided nerve blocks. Superb visualization of nerve root structures can be obtained. Obscure anatomy caused by degeneration or pathologic change is readily identified, and procedures are planned accordingly [22,26]. In the lumbosacral area, the symptomatic ventral root of the nerve can be assessed with ease. With fluoroscopy, the sacral foramen is sometimes difficult to access; MR imaging overcomes this problem. As a single modality, MR imaging facilitates the diagnosis and treatment of radicular pain caused by degenerative disease.

MR-guided selective nerve blocks: procedural aspects

Because a nerve root block is a minimally invasive procedure with little associated risk, neither admission nor sedation is usually needed. Patients should be positioned to achieve easy entry into the nerve root, which typically entails a prone or semioblique prone position. The prone position is suitable for open-bore scanners. If a clamshell or C-arm type scanner is used, it may be advisable to position the patient in a semioblique prone position (affected side up) so as to improve access by the operator. Periradicular nerve infiltration is particularly suited for MR-guided interventions, because the root sheath forms a structure easily detectable in MR imaging scans and saline can be used as a contrast agent [26].

Sterile conditions should be secured, and a surface coil should be used. Needle insertion can be achieved in the same manner as in bone biopsies. Needles that are used for spinal injections need to be thin to minimize patient discomfort and the potential for neurologic injury. Typically, 20- to 25-gauge needles are used. Because the needles are thin, they inevitably bend, and it is beneficial to use multiple planes to localize the needle tip reliably during the procedure; thicker sections can also be used. Manufacturers that provide biopsy instruments also have a wide variety of needles appropriate for MR-guided nerve root blocks.

Before inserting the needle, local anesthesia (1% lidocaine) should be administered. When inserting the needle, soft tissue anatomic landmarks can be readily and directly visualized with diminished importance of osseous structures, which are vital in fluoroscopy. With MR imaging, the segmental exiting spinal nerve itself can be targeted. A slightly oblique approach is usually most beneficial. The needle should be placed adjacent to the nerve root (Fig. 8A). At this point, the patient may also report paresthesias that are similar in distribution but not necessarily in character as the index symptomatology. It is important to stop advancing the needle and to perform a control scan. The needle position at the nerve root sheath can be controlled most

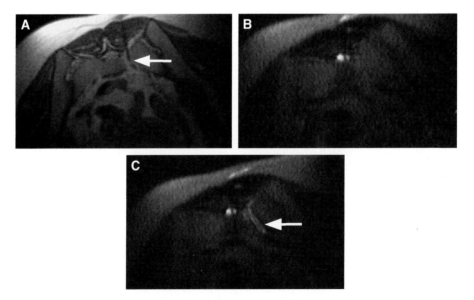

Fig. 8. Nerve block spine injection in a 28-year-old man with an L5–S1 disk extrusion causing S1 nerve compression and radicular pain. (*A*) Axial three-dimensional completed balanced steady-state sequence (repetition time [TR] = 8.4 milliseconds, echo time [TE] = 4.2 milliseconds, flip angle of 45°) shows a 21-gauge needle positioned adjacent to the S1 exiting segmental nerve (*arrow*). Single-shot fast spin echo images (TR = 9000 milliseconds, TE = 274 millliseconds) images taken from the corresponding level without saline (*B*) and with saline injected (*C*) show the needle tip adjacent to the exiting nerve and subsequent periradicular deposition of fluid confirming the location (*arrow*).

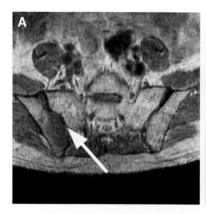 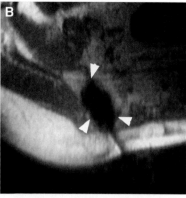

Fig. 9. Cryotherapy tumor ablation in a 47-year-old man with a history of colon cancer and unilateral right-sided low-back pain referable to the sacroiliac joint region. (*A*) Axial T1-weighted spin echo image (repetition time [TR] = 500 milliseconds, echo time [TE] = 8 milliseconds) shows an intermediate-signal lesion in the posterior ilium extending to the sacroiliac joint (*arrow*), reflecting a metastatic deposit. (*B*) Axial T1-weighted fast spin echo image gradient (TR = 300 milliseconds, TE = 10 milliseconds, echo train length = 2) through the pelvis with patient in the prone position (image inverted) shows the susceptibility artifact of a needle placed from a posterior approach into the right ilium. Routine sequences are suitable to demonstrate an elliptic signal void representing the cryolesion (also referred to as the "ice ball") covering the entire region of the metastatic deposit (*arrowheads*).

practically with MR imaging. For this purpose, a heavily T2-weighted sequence with a long echo time (TE) is needed (eg, single-shot fast spin echo [SSFSE], five slices, 7 mm × 7 mm, TR = 9000 milliseconds, TE = 274 milliseconds, 380 × 380 FOV, 256 × 256 matrix). When anatomic imaging data suggest that the final point of needle position is achieved, a quick half-Fourier SSFSE sequence is applied (see Fig. 8B). After this, the needle mandrel is removed and saline (up to 2 mL) is injected through the needle. The SSFSE sequence is then repeated, and the saline should be visualized in a periradicular space distribution (see Fig. 8C). If saline is not visualized, the needle tip may be located in a vessel. In this case, gentle aspiration should be performed; if blood emerges, the needle should be repositioned slightly. Arterial structures are identifiable during the initial approach, however, and can be avoided easily. When the needle position is secured with a positive saline control, the therapeutic agent can be distributed. Typically, a mixture of a corticosteroid and lidocaine is used.

Other-guided therapeutic and diagnostic injections

The musculoskeletal system also includes other pain sources that can be diagnosed and treated under MR imaging guidance. Ligamentous and small joint structure pathologic findings are often identified as the cause of pain. Depending on the condition, these can be assessed and treated with MR-guided injections or penetrative procedures [7]. Benign and malignant conditions can be targeted. Benign lesions include developmental, infectious, degenerative, and posttraumatic lesions. As a guidance modality, MR imaging often stands above the traditional modalities, because these lesions are commonly more conspicuous with MR imaging. Typically, cysts or cyst-like structures are good targets because of the sensitivity of MR imaging to detect fluid. Cysts can be situated in practically any musculoskeletal location. These typically occur in relation or proximity to joint structures because they often form as extensions of joint cavity recesses. Infectious cysts can be targeted and drained for treatment and culture. Depending on the cause and volume of the cyst, whether synovial or of other origin, corticosteroids are the most commonly used drugs to treat noninfectious conditions. The overall procedural pattern in interventional MR imaging follows that of a periradicular injection. If the cyst is associated with bone, the removal procedure with trephination is more akin to a bone biopsy.

Simple bone cysts are currently being treated with percutaneous techniques under CT and fluoroscopy [27]. A typical technique includes introducing two needles into the cyst, after which lavage is performed. This treatment can be amplified with percutaneous curettage, alcohol

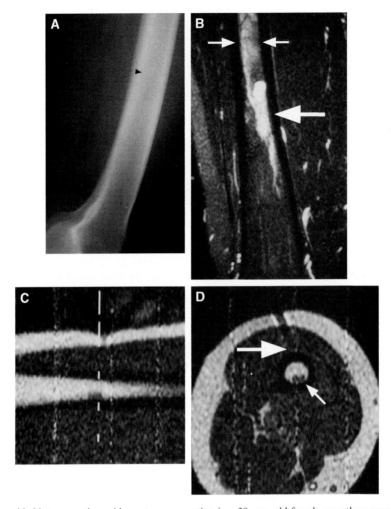

Fig. 10. Image-guided intraoperative guidance tumor resection in a 39-year-old female marathon runner with a history of breast cancer presenting with a solitary mid-diaphyseal femur lesion exhibiting positive bone scintigraphy but not visualized by radiography (region of the lesion shown by *arrowhead* in *A*) or CT imaging (not shown). The orthopedic oncologic surgeon requested image-guided assistance for localization and to minimize the risk of fracture by limiting the amount of bone resected in this weight-bearing location. (*B*) Preprocedural coronal short tau inversion recovery fast spin echo (FSE) image (repetition time [TR] = 3500 milliseconds, echo time [TE] = 30 milliseconds, inversion time = 110 milliseconds, echo train length [ETL] = 6) shows a high-signal intensity endosteal lesion (*large arrow*) with adjacent marrow edema-like signal (*small arrows*). (*C*) Sagittal T1-weighted FSE image (TR = 300 milliseconds, TE = 10 milliseconds, ETL = 2) shows the needle icon passing through the lesion (*dashed line*) from the opposite cortical margin. (*D*) Axial T1-weighted FSE image (TR = 300 milliseconds, TE = 10 milliseconds, ETL = 2) shows localization needle placement (*large arrow*) with the lesion present along the opposite endosteal surface (*small arrow*). This allowed the surgeon to use a small drill hole rather than a larger 1-cm corticotomy if this had been done as a non–image-guided procedure. Presagittal (*E*) and postsagittal (*F*) T1-weighted spin echo images (TR = 500 milliseconds, TE = 8 milliseconds) show the limited extent of resection with maximal preservation of the cortex. Biopsy of this lesion yielded the diagnosis of enchondroma.

ablation, or introduction of corticosteroids into the cyst cavity. Furthermore, bone augmentation material can be added to the cyst to retain structural coherence. This material can be autologous bone, demineralized bone matrix, hydroxyapatite or bone cement, or polymethyl methacrylate (PMMA). This type of more complex procedure is well suited for MR imaging guidance if MR imaging–compatible instruments are available for therapy.

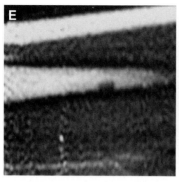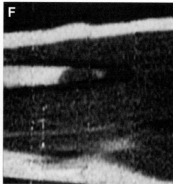

Fig. 10 (*continued*)

One of the most recent MR-guided applications to control the source of pain in the spine is to use thermal methods to ablate nerve structures and benign lesions. These methods can potentially be performed by MR imaging with superb control because MR imaging provides a platform to measure temperature (MR thermometry) quantitatively. Treatment of degenerative facet pain, osteoid osteoma, and vertebral disk disease is possible by these thermoablative methods, which include laser, cryotherapy, and radiofrequency ablation [28,29].

Percutaneous techniques can also be used to approach malignant lesions of bone. This aims not only to diagnose but to apply therapy to achieve palliation and debulking of the tumor mass [30,31]. Common metastases affecting bone tissue include those arising from prostate and breast carcinoma. Because MR imaging is sensitive in detecting these tumors, it is conceivable that MR imaging guidance could play a major role in the focal ablative treatment of bone involvement from these entities. In cryotherapy, the "ice ball" lesion created by the probe is seen as a signal void; in effect, the margins define the tumor "kill zone" (Fig. 9). Therefore, the treatment can be monitored by routine spin echo, FSE, or GE sequences. Control is achieved by placing numerous probes and by creating lesions of various sizes (a process the authors refer to as "ice sculpting").

Intraoperative musculoskeletal interventional MR imaging

As opposed to MR-guided neurosurgery, MR-guided musculoskeletal surgery is in its infancy, but there are several potential indications that could be applied as cutting-edge techniques should MR imaging guidance be used. The foremost application would be tumor and reparative pediatric musculoskeletal surgery, where MR imaging can provide the operator with unsurpassed insight to the target area (Fig. 10). Developmental bone disorders, whether posttraumatic or congenital, are a potential target. MR imaging can detect the newly formed cortical bridging when an unwanted union has occurred and potentially guide the surgeon to correct the condition without difficulty or ionizing radiation to the patient and operator.

Summary

MR imaging guidance has great potential to direct the management of diagnostic and therapeutic procedures performed in the musculoskeletal region. To take full advantage of this excellent diagnostic tool, radiologists should also embrace the minimally invasive techniques available for MR imaging. This can be achieved by cooperation with clinical colleagues, multidisciplinary integration, and the development of efficient techniques for MR-guided procedures. By combining the excellent ability to recognize pathologic findings and the feasibility of performing interventional procedures, MR imaging is emerging as a powerful tool in diagnosing and treating musculoskeletal neoplasms and in performing minimally invasive procedures, such as spine injections.

References

[1] Ghanem N, Altehoefer C, Hogerle S, et al. Comparative diagnostic value and therapeutic relevance of magnetic resonance imaging and bone marrow scintigraphy in patients with metastatic solid tumors of the axial skeleton. Eur J Radiol 2002;43(3):256–61.

[2] Hoane BR, Shields AF, Porter BA, et al. Detection of lymphomatous bone marrow involvement with magnetic resonance imaging. Blood 1991;78(3): 728–38.

[3] Silverman SG, Collick BD, Figueira MR, et al. Interactive MR-guided biopsy in an open-configuration MR imaging system. Radiology 1995;197(1): 175–81.

[4] Lewin JS, Petersilge CA, Hatem SF, et al. Interactive MR imaging-guided biopsy and aspiration with a modified clinical C-arm system. AJR Am J Roentgenol 1998;170(6):1593–601.

[5] Lewin JS, Duerk JL, Jain VR, et al. Needle localization in MR-guided biopsy and aspiration: effects of field strength, sequence design, and magnetic field orientation. AJR Am J Roentgenol 1996;166(6): 1337–45.

[6] Ojala R, Sequeiros RB, Klemola R, et al. MR-guided bone biopsy: preliminary report of a new guiding method. J Magn Reson Imaging 2002;15(1): 82–86.

[7] Genant JW, Vandevenne JE, Bergman AG, et al. Interventional musculoskeletal procedures performed by using MR imaging guidance with a vertically open MR unit: assessment of techniques and applicability. Radiology 2002;223(1):127–36.

[8] Butts K, Pauly JM, Daniel BL, et al. Management of biopsy needle artifacts: techniques for RF-refocused MRI. J Magn Reson Imaging 1999;9(4):586–95.

[9] Mankin HJ, Lange TA, Spanier SS. The hazards of biopsy in patients with malignant primary bone and soft-tissue tumors. J Bone Joint Surg Am 1982;64(8): 1121–7.

[10] Fraser-Hill MA, Renfrew DL, Hilsenrath PE. Percutaneous needle biopsy of musculoskeletal lesions. 2. Cost-effectiveness. AJR Am J Roentgenol 1992; 158(4):813–8.

[11] Neuerburg J, Adam G, Bucker A, et al. A new MR-(and CT-) compatible bone biopsy system: first clinical results. Rofo Fortschr Geb Rontgenstr Neuen Bildgeb Verfahr 1998;169(5):515–20 [in German].

[12] Tikkakoski T, Lahde S, Puranen J, et al. Combined CT-guided biopsy and cytology in diagnosis of bony lesions. Acta Radiol 1992;33(3):225–9.

[13] Settle WJ, Ebraheim NA, Coombs R, et al. CT-guided biopsy of metastatic sacral tumors. Orthopedics 1990;13(7):753–8.

[14] Leffler SG, Chew FS. CT-guided percutaneous biopsy of sclerotic bone lesions: diagnostic yield and accuracy. AJR Am J Roentgenol 1999;172(5): 1389–92.

[15] Jelinek JS, Kransdorf MJ, Gray R, et al. Percutaneous transpedicular biopsy of vertebral body lesions. Spine 1996;21(17):2035–40.

[16] Blanco Sequeiros R, Klemola R, Ojala R, et al. MRI-guided trephine biopsy and fine-needle aspiration in the diagnosis of bone lesions in low-field (0.23 T) MRI system using optical instrument tracking. Eur Radiol 2002;12(4):830–5.

[17] Adam G, Bucker A, Nolte-Ernsting C, et al. Interventional MR imaging: percutaneous abdominal and skeletal biopsies and drainages of the abdomen. Eur Radiol 1999;9(8):1471–8.

[18] Kaplan GR, Saifuddin A, Pringle JA, et al. Langerhans' cell histiocytosis of the spine: use of MRI in guiding biopsy. Skeletal Radiol 1998;27(12):673–6.

[19] Khurana B, Carrino JA, Winalski CS, et al. MR-guided musculoskeletal interventions: a valuable tool in certain contexts. Presented at the International Society for Magnetic Resonance in Medicine 10th Scientific Meeting and Exhibition. Honolulu (HI), May 20–24, 2002.

[20] Duerk JL, Lewin JS, Wendt M, et al. Remember true FISP? A high SNR, near 1-second imaging method for T2-like contrast in interventional MRI at .2 T. J Magn Reson Imaging 1998;8(1):203–8.

[21] Parkkola RK, Mattila KT, Heikkila JT, et al. Dynamic contrast-enhanced MR imaging and MR-guided bone biopsy on a 0.23 T open imager. Skeletal Radiol 2001;30(11):620–4.

[22] Sequeiros RB, Ojala RO, Klemola R, et al. MRI-guided periradicular nerve root infiltration therapy in low-field (0.23-T) MRI system using optical instrument tracking. Eur Radiol 2002;12(6):1331–7.

[23] Weiner BK, Fraser RD. Foraminal injection for lateral lumbar disc herniation. J Bone Joint Surg Br 1997;79(5):804–7.

[24] Karppinen J, Malmivaara A, Kurunlahti M, et al. Periradicular infiltration for sciatica: a randomized controlled trial. Spine 2001;26(9):1059–67.

[25] Riew KD, Yin Y, Gilula L, et al. The effect of nerve-root injections on the need for operative treatment of lumbar radicular pain. A prospective, randomized, controlled, double-blind study. Bone Joint Surg Am 2000;82-A(11):1589–93.

[26] Ojala R, Vahala E, Karppinen J, et al. Nerve root infiltration of the first sacral root with MRI guidance. J Magn Reson Imaging 2000;12(4):556–61.

[27] Dormans JP, Dormans NJ. Use of percutaneous intramedullary decompression and medical-grade calcium sulfate pellets for treatment of unicameral bone cysts of the calcaneus in children. Orthopedics 2004;27(1 Suppl):S137–9.

[28] Sequeiros RB, Hyvonen P, Sequeiros AB, et al. MR imaging-guided laser ablation of osteoid osteomas with use of optical instrument guidance at 0.23 T. Eur Radiol 2003;13(10):2309–14.

[29] Skjeldal S, Lilleas F, Folleras G, et al. Real time MRI-guided excision and cryo-treatment of osteoid osteoma in os ischii–a case report. Acta Orthop Scand 2000;71(6):637–8.

[30] Aschoff AJ, Merkle EM, Emancipator SN, et al. Femur: MR imaging-guided radio-frequency ablation in a porcine model-feasibility study. Radiology 2002;225(2):471–8.

[31] Posteraro AF, Dupuy DE, Mayo-Smith WW. Radiofrequency ablation of bony metastatic disease. Clin Radiol 2004;59(9):803–11.

ELSEVIER
SAUNDERS

Magn Reson Imaging Clin N Am
13 (2005) 533–543

MAGNETIC
RESONANCE
IMAGING CLINICS
of North America

Intraoperative MR Imaging

Walter A. Hall, MD[a,*], Charles L. Truwit, MD[b]

[a]University of Minnesota School of Medicine, MMC #96,
420 Delaware Street SE, Minneapolis, MN 55455, USA
[b]University of Minnesota School of Medicine, MMC #292,
420 Delaware Street SE, Minneapolis, MN 55455, USA

MR imaging has been used extensively for the evaluation of neurosurgical patients for more that 20 years. Over this same period, frame-based stereotaxy has been replaced by the use of frameless neuronavigational systems, with a few minor exceptions such as for the placement of deep brain stimulators (DBS) for movement disorders. With the rapid evolution of technologic advances in neurosurgery, it is no surprise that the use of MR imaging to guide the performance of safe and effective surgical procedures is at the forefront of development. The performance of intraoperative MR imaging has the distinct advantage over frameless neuronavigational systems in that it allows the surgeon to make adjustments dynamically for brain shift, which can occur after the cranium is opened and cerebrospinal fluid is drained.

As the field of intraoperative MR imaging has progressed, it has become uncertain what magnetic field strength magnet is most appropriate for neurosurgery. The first operational intraoperative MR system used a 0.5-T double-coil design (Signa SP, General Electric Medical Systems, Milwaukee, Wisconsin) whereby the surgeon performs the procedure between the coils, and imaging can be performed in a continuous fashion (Fig. 1). Magnet designs for image-guided surgery have varied from 0.12-T to 3-T in strength, with the image quality and advanced functionality depending on the field strength. Many of the imaging techniques that are routinely used during diagnostic MR imaging such as MR angiography, MR

venography, diffusion-weighted imaging, MR spectroscopy (MRS), and brain activation studies known as functional MR imaging are only available using magnets of 1.5-T or higher field strength. The ability to obtain this information expeditiously at the time of the planned procedure allows the neurosurgeon to make pre- and intraoperative decisions that enhance the safety of the surgery and assure that the surgery is accomplished successfully. Although few 1.5-T or higher intraoperative MR imaging systems are operational, it is clear that sites using this technology are attempting to take full advantage of the information available to safely and effectively perform neurosurgery. This article highlights the current capabilities of intraoperative MR-guided surgery for a variety of neurosurgical procedures and traces the evolution of the field to its present level of technical sophistication.

Intraoperative MR imaging systems

Image quality in intraoperative MR imaging is directly related to the strength of the magnetic field of the system and the stability of the static and gradient magnetic fields. The optimal features for an intraoperative MR imaging system are in direct conflict with the requirements for high image quality. High-resolution imaging is best achieved using a "closed" MR imaging system, whereas the ideal configuration for an intraoperative MR imaging system allows maximal access to the patient. Although most intraoperative MR imaging systems incorporate lower field strength (<1.5-T) magnets, high-field (1.5-T) intraoperative systems are now becoming increasingly

* Corresponding author.
E-mail address: hallx003@umn.edu (W.A. Hall).

1064-9689/05/$ - see front matter © 2005 Elsevier Inc. All rights reserved.
doi:10.1016/j.mric.2005.04.001

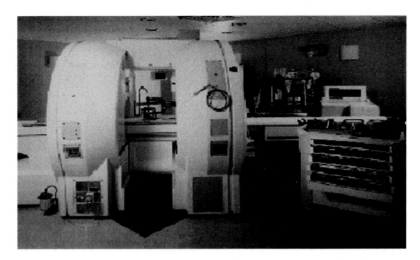

Fig. 1. The 0.5-T double-coil design intraoperative MR system whereby the surgeon performs surgery between the coils and imaging can be performed continuously. (Courtesy of General Electric Medical Systems, Milwaukee, Wisconsin; with permission.)

popular because of their advanced functional imaging capabilities.

A low field strength (0.12-T) intraoperative MR imaging system (Odin Polestar, Odin Medical Technologies, Yokne'am, Israel) allows for partial imaging of the head during surgery, with the entire procedure being performed within the magnetic field using standard surgical instrumentation (Fig. 2).

Low-field intraoperative MR imaging systems use magnets whose strength is less than 0.5 T. These systems have a biplanar or vertical gap design (Fonar Corporation, Melville, New York; Hitachi Medical Corporation, Twinsburg, Ohio) that has

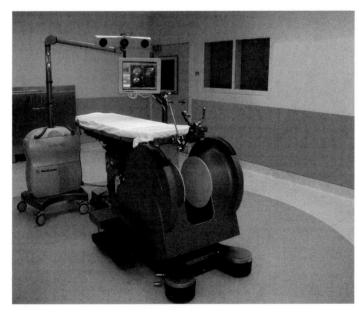

Fig. 2. A 0.12-T intraoperative MR imaging system allows for neurosurgery to be performed entirely within the magnetic field using standard surgical instrumentation. (Courtesy of Odin Medical Technologies, Yokne'am, Israel; with permission.)

been used for diagnostic and intraoperative MR imaging. The patient is placed between two flat magnetic poles, 25 to 40 cm in diameter, that allow for access from the side. A modification of the biplanar design is the C-arm design (Siemens Medical Solutions, Erlangen, Germany; Marconi Medical, Highland Heights, Ohio) whereby a single column on one side supports the upper magnetic pole and allows for 240° of side access that enables biopsies of the neck and high cervical spine lesions. The limited space of 40 cm between the biplanar magnetic pole and the operating table limits the utility of this intraoperative MR system for patients of all sizes. Some low-field systems are located adjacent to an operating room where the surgery is performed, and the patient is shuttled to and from the magnet. Although seemingly more open, the head is generally at least as far from the surgeon in these systems as in high-field, closed bore systems. Other low-field systems such as the Odin Polestar allow for maximal patient access; however, even in this system there are limitations due to the inter-magnet distance, thus limiting patient positioning and girth. The principal advantage of the lower magnetic field strength relates to the less strict requirements for MR-compatible surgical instru-mentation. In addition, in these systems, unlike the GE Signa system, the surgeon is not required to stand in the gap between the magnets. All low-field systems are constrained by signal-to-noise ratios and thus afford reduced temporal resolution and reduced spatial resolution per unit time compared with higher field intraoperative MR systems. Clin-ically, these limitations mandate increased imaging time to achieve image quality that is sufficient for accurate surgical decision making [1].

The 0.5-T "double-donut" design intraoper-ative MR imaging system introduced in 1994 is the prototypic midfield strength system. This imaging system design removed the central por-tion of a standard cylindric magnet and was the first system developed specifically for interven-tional use. The magnetic field generated by this magnet configuration is inhomogeneous and 30 cm in diameter [1]. The inhomogeneous magnetic field results because the magnetic field generated by each superconducting magnet is considerably greater than the 0.5-T field strength that is present at isocenter. This magnet configuration allows for vertical and lateral access to the imaging isocenter, and the individual supercon-ducting magnets are separated by a 56-cm gap in which the surgeon stands during procedures. This gap between the magnets creates the need

for special gradient radiofrequency coils that limit the field of view and reduce the gradient strength. The lowered isocenter field strength results in longer imaging times, less signal-to-noise ratio, decreased spatial resolution, and limited physiologic and functional imaging capa-bilities [2]. The advantage afforded by improved patient access in this imaging system is over-shadowed by the sacrifice that is made in the image quality at the imaging isocenter. Because all surgery is performed within the magnetic field, the system requires all nonferromagnetic instrumentation.

High-field intraoperative MR systems have the advantage over low- and midfield systems of having full diverse functional capabilities such as MR angiography, MR venography, diffusion-weighted imaging, MRS, MR thermometry, fat suppression, and brain activation and perfusion studies [3]. Initially, a principal disadvantage of midfield and high-field intraoperative MR imag-ing systems was the inability to use conventional surgical instrumentation near the magnet. As a result, most surgical procedures using a high-field intraoperative MR system have been performed outside the 5-G line; to obtain intraoperative scans in these systems, the patient needed to be transported into the magnet for scanning or the magnet needed to be transported to the patient. With the authors' initial interventional MR unit (ACS-NT, Philips Medical Systems, Best, The Netherlands), the patient was placed on an angiography table that could swivel and dock with the MR-imaging gantry that permitted rapid transit into and out of the scanner. Patient access in this short-bore magnet was enhanced with 100-cm diameter flared openings. For cranioto-mies, the surgery was performed outside the 5-G line because there was no need for frequent imaging; however, brain biopsies were performed entirely within the magnet because of the need for rapid, repetitive imaging as the biopsy needle was passed through the brain to the target. Using a similar approach to patient access, several other sites (University of Erlangen, Erlangen, Germany and University of California Los Angeles, Los Angeles, California) have installed systems where-by a rotating operating surgical table was adapted to a 1.5-T Magnetom Sonata Maestro Class scanner (Siemens Medical Solutions) that allows the table to be turned into the axis of the scanner [4]. Recently, the authors updated their scanner (Intera I/T, Philips Medical Systems), and using this new intraoperative MR system, they

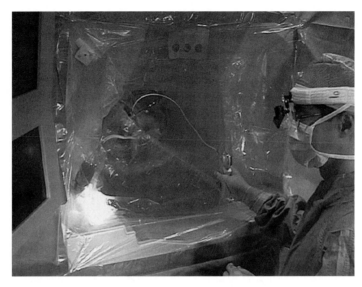

Fig. 3. A 1.5-T high field intraoperative MR system whereby craniotomies can be performed entirely within the magnetic field due to the availability of MR imaging–compatible instrumentation and monitoring equipment. (Courtesy of Philips Medical Systems, Best, The Netherlands; with permission.)

have performed craniotomies entirely within the magnetic field due to the availability of all MR-compatible instrumentation and monitoring equipment (Fig. 3).

In contrast to the authors' intraoperative MR imaging system whereby the operating table is mobile, an alternative high-field system design uses a mobile, 92-cm bore diameter, 1.5-T magnet (Magnex Scientific, Abingdon, Oxon, United Kingdom) that moves on a ceiling-mounted track to the stationery operating table. Disadvantages of this system are the need to reposition local radio-frequency shielding during imaging to maintain a high signal-to-noise ratio and the need to remove all instrumentation that is not MR-compatible from the operative field at the time of scanning. The initial implementation of this design did not permit any access to the patient during imaging so that minimally invasive procedures under MR imaging guidance were not possible. A more recent implementation of this system has adopted the approach of surgical access to the patient's head from the now-open back end of the scanner, thus enabling minimally invasive, MR-guided intra-operative neurosurgical procedures.

Finally, at the authors' new, second site (Hennepin County Medical Center, Minneapolis, Minnesota), an intraoperative MR-capable, 3-T MR scanner (Intera, Philips Medical Systems) has been established, whereby minimally invasive and open craniotomy procedures are performed solely at the rear of the scanner. Although this limits patient positioning to some degree, the rapid acquisition of high-field images offers significant improvement in patient flow and throughput, particularly with respect to surgical draping. This advance has been made possible by the much wider availability of MR-compatible instruments and equipment.

Brain shift

Neuronavigational systems lack spatial accuracy because of the brain deformation known as brain shift that occurs during neurosurgery after the skull is opened. No neuronavigational device, whether it is guided by mechanical arms, ultrasound, electromagnetism, or optical probes, has the ability to compensate for intraoperative brain shift. Intraoperative imaging is the only technique currently available that can detect the deformation of the brain surface and displacement of deeper intracranial structures. Brain shift has been evaluated in an intraoperative MR system, and the only structures found to have shifted during surgery were those located directly over or within a 1-cm radius of the lesion being resected [1]. The average degree of surface displacement has been found to be 1 cm, with gravity acting as the main shifting force. This degree of brain shift can result in incomplete tumor resection and possible encroachment on normal brain parenchyma. When using neuronavigation intraoperatively to guide brain tumor surgery, it has been reported that intraoperative reregistration on MR imaging data is necessary because of the extent of the brain shift in 11% of resections [5].

Brain biopsy

Early MR-guided brain biopsies were performed in a freehand manner in much the same way that the early CT-guided brain biopsies were accomplished. Initially, there was no ability to direct the brain biopsy needle toward the target or to stabilize the needle after the tissue of interest had been accessed. Within a short interval, the need for needle stabilization devices (MRI Devices Corp., Waukesha, Wisconsin; Snapper-Stereo-Guide, MagneticVision, Zurich, Switzerland) became apparent, and they were rapidly designed and developed simultaneously. The authors' site developed a disposable trajectory guide (Navigus, Image-Guided Neurologics, Melbourne, Florida) that the authors have combined with a unique targeting technique known as prospective stereotaxy to perform brain biopsy in near real time using a 1.5-T high-field intraoperative MR imaging system. To this day, the authors still perform all of their brain biopsies under general anesthesia to prevent the inadvertent displacement of the needle after it has reached the target tissue and for patient comfort when the procedure lasts longer than anticipated [1].

Prospective stereotaxy represents a novel way to determine the pathway for the brain biopsy needle. It uses a trajectory guide that starts at the target and then moves away from the target toward the distal end of an alignment stem, which functions in some ways like a joystick [6]. After the neurosurgeon has chosen the location for the biopsy (target point), two additional points are necessary to establish an appropriate trajectory that will enable the brain biopsy to be performed safely and successfully. The second point is at the tip of the alignment stem and represents the pivot point. The third point is at a location in space that represents where the alignment stem should be to establish the exact trajectory necessary to reach the target. The alignment stem can be pivoted around the pivot point until all three points are collinear, which will ensure that when the biopsy needle is passed through the trajectory guide, the target will be encountered.

Depending on the imaging characteristics of the target tissue, the alignment stem is filled with saline or a saline/contrast mixture so that it can be visualized during prospective stereotaxy. After the alignment stem is inserted into the guide tube, it is pivoted freely in space until all three points are aligned; generally, this requires a total of 2 to 5 minutes using near real time MR imaging updates. Imaging along the entire length of the alignment stem in two different orientations, depending on the location of the target, visually verifies that the trajectory for brain biopsy is accurate and safe. After the proper alignment has been established, the guide tube is locked in place and the biopsy needle is passed in a stepwise fashion through the brain to the target tissue. While the biopsy sample is being examined by the pathologist to confirm that diagnostic tissue is present, a series of three scans are performed (most commonly in the axial projection) to exclude the presence of intraoperative hemorrhage resulting from the biopsy. Because these scans are typically obtained before significant conversion of intracellular oxyhemoglobin to deoxyhemoglobin could occur, the authors' acquire and compare a combination of imaging sequences including half-Fourier acquisition single-shot turbo spin echo (HASTE), gradient echo T2*, and turbo fluid-attenuated inversion recovery (FLAIR).

To enhance their diagnostic yield for brain biopsy, the authors have combined their intraoperative MR-guided brain biopsies with MRS. The MRS techniques they have used are single-voxel spectroscopy (SVS) and turbo spectroscopic imaging (TSI). SVS (1.5 cm^3 × 1.5 cm^3 × 1.5 cm^3 voxel; 1-Hz spectral resolution; echo time/repetition time, 136 ms/2000 ms; 4.5-minute acquisition) was performed on the region of interest in the brain and compared with a contralateral control area [6]. TSI (32 mm × 32 mm grid of spectra in a single plane; 0.66 cm^3 × 0.66 cm^3 × 2.0 cm^3 spatial resolution; 4.4-Hz spectral resolution; echo time/repetition time, 272 ms/2000 ms, turbo factor, 3; 11-minute acquisition) was performed on a single axial brain slice to measure the brain metabolites phosphocholine, creatine, N-acetyl aspartate, and lactate/lipid [6]. The regions of elevated phosphocholine on SVS and TSI, believed to represent areas of increased cellular density due to rapid membrane turnover, should correspond to tumor tissue and are thus targeted for brain biopsy (Fig. 4). N-acetyl aspartate is

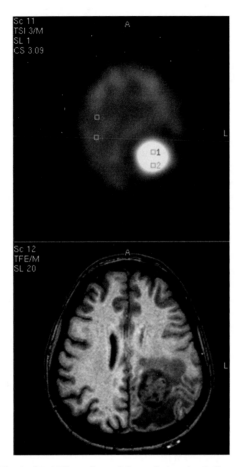

Fig. 4. (*Top*) The regions of elevated phosphocholine on TSI are believed to represent areas of increased cellular density due to rapid membrane turnover that should correspond to tumor tissue when targeted for brain biopsy. (*Bottom*) This patient was found to have a glioblastoma multiforme on pathologic examination.

a neuronal marker and is elevated in areas of normal brain tissue.

Brain biopsy results

Of the first 140 cases treated using the 0.5-T MR imaging system, 63 were brain biopsies. Biopsies of lesions were performed in all areas of the brain and only 1 patient sustained an intraoperative hemorrhage that was detected and emergently evacuated, leading the authors to conclude that the intraoperative MR imaging system allowed for rapid evaluation of the surgical site and the ability to intervene dynamically [6]. In a series of 27 patients, another group performed 10

brain biopsies using a 0.2-T MR imaging scanner and concluded that they could adjust for brain shift by obtaining updated imaging sets [6]. Using the same 0.2-T system to operate in the fringe fields, 16 brain biopsies were performed, with 15 yielding diagnostic tissue. A biopsy could not be performed safely in one patient with a brain stem tumor, and no hemorrhages were detected [6]. Over a 1-year period, 12 brain biopsies were performed in a 0.2-T vertical gap system. The authors of this study had several technical problems during surgery that included poor image quality in 5 patients, an inability to visualize at the probe in 3 cases, and instrumentation concerns in 2 cases. They found benefit in being able to visualize the biopsy needle in the region of interest and in the ability to exclude the presence of hemorrhage during the procedure [6].

In the authors' first 35 brain biopsies performed after January 1997 but before the development of the trajectory guide, all samples yielded diagnostic tissue, of which most was primary brain tumor tissue [6]. One patient with a brain stem tumor sustained a temporary hemiparesis that resolved with physical therapy. Another patient experienced a scalp cellulitis that was successfully treated with antibiotics. In this preliminary series of patients, SVS was performed in 6 patients and was believed to correlate well with the pathologic findings. The trajectory guide was used in 40 brain biopsies beginning in January 1999. All biopsies were diagnostic and there were no clinically or radiographically significant hemorrhages detected in any patient. Neurologic morbidity in the form of a hemiparesis was seen after biopsy of a lesion near the motor cortex. Another patient sustained a fatal cardiac event despite preoperative clearance. Over a concurrent 12-month period, MRS was coupled with the trajectory guide in 17 patients and it was believed that the MRS data enhanced the diagnostic yield of brain biopsy [6]. Using MRS in a group of 26 patients undergoing brain biopsy, it was believed that there was more spectral contamination with TSI than with SVS due to the low spatial resolution associated with the technique [6]. In a series of 140 brain biopsies in which the influence of the imaging on surgical decision making was analyzed, MRS guidance was used in 42 (30%) patients. Twenty-one (48%) patients had TSI alone, 13 (31%) had SVS alone, and 8 (19%) had TSI and SVS. There was excellent correlation between the phosphocholine levels seen in those patients who had SVS and TSI.

Craniotomy for tumor

Patients are induced with general anesthesia before being transported to the intraoperative MR imaging suite. All appropriate invasive monitoring lines are placed after intubation. A carbon fiber head holder is applied to secure the head in the operative position to facilitate repeat intraoperative imaging. MR imaging visible markers are placed around the operative field to localize the site for cranial opening before prepping and shaving the scalp. Preoperative imaging is obtained for intraoperative comparison after the tumor has been partially resected. The authors currently use HASTE (scan time, 14 seconds; 16 slices) or turbo FLAIR (scan time, 2 minutes, 6 seconds; 42 slices) imaging to visualize low-grade primary brain tumors that do not enhance after the administration of intravenous contrast [1]. In enhancing brain tumors, the administration of intravenous contrast is reserved until after the tumor has been resected to prevent the subsequent spread of contrast to the surrounding edematous brain parenchyma where the blood-brain barrier has been disrupted by the tumor. Even with repeat administration of contrast, it is difficult to interpret intraoperative images because of the continued diffusion of contrast throughout the brain. Another explanation for the continued diffusion of contrast around the tumor resection cavity is the direct surgical trauma that results from the use of electrocautery or ultrasonic aspiration, which can alter peritumoral vasculature [1].

After the baseline MR imaging scans are completed, the patient is transported to the surgical side of the intraoperative MR suite outside the magnetic field and the surgery commences. Most tumor resections require at least three imaging sets: one before the start of surgery, another to evaluate the extent of the tumor resection, and one final set after the craniotomy has been closed to exclude the presence of an intraoperative hematoma that resulted during closure. Imaging may be obtained at any time during the procedure, however, although there is a 5-minute delay to ensure the sterility of the surgical field and to remove any instruments that are not MR imaging–compatible before transport into and out of the scanner. MR images can be obtained in any projection to allow surgeons to visualize areas of the brain that may harbor residual tumor and may be obscured by the collapse or shift of the brain into the resection cavity that occurs during tumor resection.

On completion of the tumor resection, the three previously mentioned "hemorrhage" scans (HASTE, turbo FLAIR, and T2*) are obtained (Fig. 5). After more than 300 tumor resections, the authors have not yet detected a clinically or radiographically significant hematoma that has required reopening the craniotomy for evacuation. When there is a concern that an ischemic event or infarction has occurred during surgery, the authors perform diffusion-weighted MR imaging at the time of the hemorrhage scans. After the last set of scans is obtained, the patient is transported to the recovery room for extubation. Because each set of scans may extend surgery by 10 to 15 minutes, imaging updates are rarely performed within an hour of the previous acquisition. In the authors' first years, the average time for a craniotomy with resection of tumor was likely to be increased by one third or less [1].

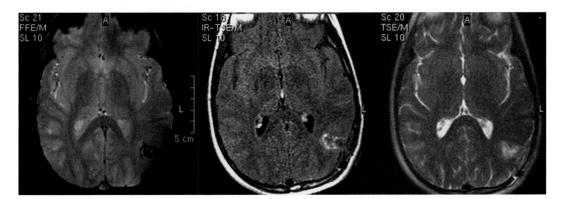

Fig. 5. The difficulty in detecting hyperacute blood (before the conversion of intracellular oxyhemoglobin to deoxyhemoglobin) on MR imaging necessitates the acquisition and comparison of this combination of image sequences. (*Left*) Gradient echo T2*. (*Middle*) Turbo FLAIR. (*Right*) HASTE.

Craniotomy for tumor results

Of the first 92 patients who underwent craniotomy at the authors' institution, 89 had brain tumor resections. There were no complications in those patients related to the instrumentation or monitoring equipment. A surgical resection was considered complete when the entire preoperative lesion was absent on subsequent intraoperative MR imaging. In the authors' initial review of the first 30 tumor resections performed using intraoperative MR imaging guidance, 24 (80%) were believed to be complete on review by the radiologist. Reasons for incomplete resection were the proximity of the lesion to eloquent cortex, extensive cerebral edema, and excessive intraoperative hemorrhage [2]. Using the mobile 1.5-T magnet for tumor resections, the operative management in 11 of 40 patients was changed, which resulted in smaller craniotomies and maximal tumor resection [7]. In the authors' first 200 patients who had surgery at high-field strength, there were 77 pituitary tumor resections and 100 craniotomies in which the surgical resection was extended in 39% [3]. There were no complications related to MR imaging, and 2% of patients developed wound infections. Similarly, the authors have had no complications related to MR imaging and experienced two infections in their first 319 procedures (0.6%) [1]. To the authors' knowledge, there have been no complications related to patient transport in high-field intraoperative MR-guided surgical systems when there is movement of the surgical field into and out of the scanner.

Functional MR-guided tumor resection

The authors have applied several of the high-field functional MR imaging capabilities to the planning of intraoperative MR-guided tumor resections. The acquisition and processing of brain activation studies adds approximately 15 minutes to the length of the surgical procedure. Brain activation imaging is performed immediately before the induction of general anesthesia in cases in which the tumor for resection is in close proximity to eloquent cortex. Eloquent cortex is defined as cortex that results in a neurologic deficit if it is inadvertently injured during the tumor resection. The areas of brain activation that the authors have been able to map safely and successfully are those for motor function, language, and working memory (Fig. 6). The

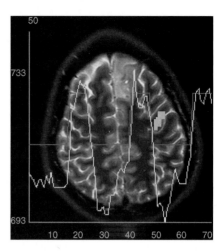

Fig. 6. This brain activation study shows that the motor cortex was activated with finger tapping.

motor cortex can be activated with finger, tongue, and toe tapping. The functional MR imaging protocol is a single-shot echo planar imaging scan (echo time/repetition time, 40 ms/3000 ms; field of view, 210 mm) with a 64 mm × 64 mm image matrix and 7-mm–thick slices with a 1-mm intersection gap that is repeated 72 times in a sequential fashion over an imaging interval of 4 minutes [8]. The accuracy of the test is measured by a waveform that is superimposed on a graph that indicates when the patient is performing the task. After acquisition, areas of blood oxygen level–dependent activation are immediately calculated on the scanner console and then demonstrated on high-quality anatomic images. These images are displayed on the liquid crystal display screens and reviewed by the neurosurgeon before beginning the procedure. By assessing short- and long-term recall using list retention, memory function can be localized in patients with medial temporal lobe lesions in the dominant hemisphere. Language mapping is performed by testing silent speech where patients think of the names of animals beginning with the first letter of the alphabet. In the authors' first 348 MR-guided surgical procedures, there were 103 tumor resections [8]. Functional MR imaging of eloquent cortex was necessary in 14 patients (14%). Speech function was localized in 3 cases, memory function in 3 cases, and motor function in 11 cases. In only 1 case in which the motor function of the tongue was intimately involved with a low-grade glioma was a surgical resection not attempted [8]. In all cases, data obtained by brain activation studies were accurate, and no patient sustained a neurologic deficit following tumor resection.

Diffusion tensor imaging–guided tumor resection

Diffusion tensor imaging uses the diffusion energy of water to map white matter tracts as they pass through the brain [9]. This technique was first used intraoperatively to map out the optic radiations in two pediatric patients with low-grade gliomas in order to avoid their inadvertent injury which would result in a visual field deficit. In both cases, the tumors were radiographically completely resected and no change in visual fields was sustained after surgery [9]. When preoperative and intraoperative white matter tractography was compared using diffusion tensor imaging in 37 patients having glioma resection, the maximum white matter shifting ranged from −8 to +15 mm (+2.7 ± 6.0 mm; mean ± SD) [10]. The shifting of the white matter tracts was inward in 30% of patients and outward in 62% [10].

Deep brain stimulator placement

The placement of DBS for movement disorders such as Parkinson's disease refractory to medications is an ideal application for intraoperative MR imaging guidance because of the ability to confirm that the electrodes are in the proper position before leaving the operating room. Because of the need for exquisite accuracy in placing the DBS in the subthalamic nuclei, trajectory selection and electrode passage was first performed using an MR imaging–compatible stereotactic head frame (Radionics, Burlington, Massachusetts). A unique imaging pulse sequence (three-dimensional stimulation) has been developed and implemented to reduce the metal artifact generated by the DBS lead [1].

Local anesthesia and mild sedation are used for DBS placement because of the necessity to perform microelectrode recording of hyperactivity in single cells during the operative procedure, which confirms accurate localization within the subthalamic nuclei. Thin-slice T1-weighted imaging is the most useful imaging sequence for planning target selection and electrode placement. The procedure is currently performed outside the 5-G line using standard surgical instrumentation. After both electrodes are placed in the subthalamic nuclei, the position is confirmed using multiplanar imaging using three-dimensional stimulation sequences. The patient returns to the operating room at some point in the future to have both leads attached to the subcutaneous pulse generators. Because placement of the DBS can result in clinical improvement known as impact effect, the pulse generators are usually

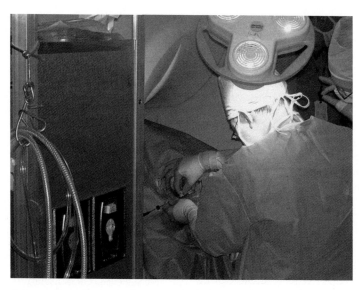

Fig. 7. Brain biopsy being performed using an intraoperative 3-T MR system. (Courtesy of Philips Medical Systems, Best, The Netherlands; with permission.)

activated and programmed 2 weeks after surgery [1]. Because of the cumbersome nature of the stereotactic head frame, the trajectory guide has been adapted for placement of DBS in the subthalamic nuclei, with successful clinical outcomes, although these results have not yet been published (Philip Starr, MD, personal communication, 2005).

Costs

There is very little information published on the costs and benefits of intraoperative MR-guided neurosurgery. Early analysis based on cost suggested that the technology was not ready for widespread installation [11]. At that time, it was believed that there would be much more substantial data available for analysis within 1 to 2 years [11]. The authors retrospectively compared the costs and benefits of brain tumor resection in the main operating room with the intraoperative MR suite [12]. In adult brain tumor resections, length of stay for MR-guided resection was 55% shorter for first-time resections and 31% shorter for repeat resections than length of stay for resections in the main operating room. Total hospital costs were 14% lower for first resections and 3% lower for repeat resections performed using MR imaging guidance compared with conventional resections [12]. In pediatric patients having brain tumor resections, the average length of stay using MR imaging guidance was 10 days shorter for first resections and 5 days shorter for repeat resections compared with conventional surgery. The costs for MR-guided surgery were 46% lower for first resections and 44% lower for repeat resections compared with those in the main operating room. No repeat resections were reported after first resections performed with MR-guidance compared with a 20% repeat resection rate in adults and 30% in children treated with conventional surgery. Intraoperative MR-guided surgery was believed to improve net health outcomes by reducing hospital length of stay, repeat resection rate, and hospital costs [12].

Future directions

Intraoperative MR-guided surgery at 1.5-T clearly offers advantages over surgery performed using lower field strength systems. Because of the enhanced functionality that is capable at 1.5-T, the question of whether surgery at even higher field strength would offer any potential clinical advantage has been proposed. To address the application of higher field strength MR-guided neurosurgery, the authors adapted a 3-T diagnostic MR scanner (Philips Medical Systems) for intraoperative neurosurgical use (Fig. 7). To date, they have performed three brain biopsies at 3-T, of which all yielded diagnostic tissue and none had untoward events related to the MR environment. Metallic artifact associated with the brain biopsy needle was more pronounced at the higher, 3-T field strength, which confounded the interpretation of the intraoperative imaging.

Intraoperative MR-guided neurosurgery has been performed for over 10 years. The safety and efficacy of operating in an MR environment is no longer a proof of concept and is generally accepted by those involved in the development of this surgical technique. Widespread dissemination of this technology has been limited by rising medical costs and the up-front expenditure that is necessary to establish an intraoperative MR surgical program. Most groups have concluded that 1.5-T MR-guided neurosurgery provides the optimal imaging strength for intraoperative scan interpretation and enhanced functionality. Investigation is underway to determine whether intraoperative MR imaging at a field strength higher than 1.5-T is clinically beneficial.

References

[1] Chu RM, Tummala RP, Hall WA. Intraoperative magnetic resonance imaging-guided neurosurgery. Neurosurg Q 2003;13:234–50.

[2] Martin AJ, Hall WA, Liu H, et al. Brain tumor resection: intraoperative monitoring with high-field strength MR imaging-initial results. Radiology 2000;215:221–8.

[3] Hall WA, Liu H, Martin AJ, et al. Safety, efficacy and functionality of high-field strength interventional MR imaging for neurosurgery. Neurosurgery 2000;46:632–41.

[4] Nimsky C, Ganslandt O, von Keller B, et al. Intraoperative high-field strength MR imaging: implementation and experience in 200 patients. Radiology 2004;233:67–78.

[5] Nimsky C, Ganslandt O, Hastreiter P, et al. Intraoperative compensation for brain shift. Surg Neurol 2001;56:357–65.

[6] Hall WA, Truwit CL. 1.5 T: spectroscopy-supported brain biopsy. Neurosurg Clin N Am 2005;16: 165–72.

[7] Sutherland GR, Kaibara T, Louw D, et al. A mobile high-field magnetic resonance system for neurosurgery. J Neurosurg 1999;91:804–13.

[8] Hall WA, Liu H, Maxwell RE, et al. Influence of 1.5-tesla intraoperative MR imaging on surgical decision making. Acta Neurochir Suppl 2003;85:29–37.

[9] Tummala RP, Chu RM, Liu H, et al. Application of diffusion tensor imaging to magnetic resonance-guided brain tumor resection. Pediatr Neurosurg 2003;39:39–43.

[10] Nimsky C, Ganslandt O, Hastreiter P, et al. Preoperative and intraoperative diffusion tensor imaging-based fiber tracking in glioma surgery. Neurosurgery 2005;56:130–8.

[11] Kucharczyk W, Bernstein M. Do the benefits of image guidance in neurosurgery justify the costs? From stereotaxy to intraoperative MR. AJNR Am J Neuroradiol 1997;18:1855–9.

[12] Hall WA, Kowalik K, Liu H, et al. Costs and benefits of intraoperative MR-guided brain tumor resection. Acta Neurochir Suppl 2003;85:137–42.

ELSEVIER
SAUNDERS

Magn Reson Imaging Clin N Am
13 (2005) 545–560

**MAGNETIC
RESONANCE
IMAGING CLINICS**
of North America

MR Imaging–Controlled Focused Ultrasound Ablation: A Noninvasive Image-Guided Surgery

Ferenc A. Jolesz, MD[a],*, Kullervo Hynynen, PhD[b],
Nathan McDannold, PhD[b], Clare Tempany, MD[a]

[a]Division of MRI and Image-Guided Therapy Program, Department of Radiology,
Brigham and Women's Hospital, Harvard Medical School, 75 Francis Street, Boston, MA 02115, USA
[b]Focused Ultrasound Laboratory, Department of Radiology, Brigham and Women's Hospital,
Harvard Medical School, 221 Longwood Avenue, LMRC, 5th Floor, Boston, MA 02115, USA

Acoustic energy has been used medically for a wide range of applications from imaging to therapy. The concept of using focused ultrasound waves to thermally coagulate tumors as a noninvasive alternative to surgery was first proposed in 1942 [1]. It was recognized that localized high temperatures (greater than 56°C) generated by the sonications could induce cell damage as a result of heat-induced protein denaturation and coagulation necrosis. Focused ultrasound is essentially a thermal ablative therapy that denatures the diseased tissue. If correctly targeted by imaging, it can be used for the treatment of deep-lying tumors that can be destroyed with "surgical precision" without damaging the surrounding normal tissue.

Ideally, to accomplish this type of noninvasive surgery, the targeted tissue and the heat induced by the focused ultrasound beam should be accurately localized. The development of ultrasound-induced tissue coagulation as a noninvasive soft tissue ablation method has been delayed due to the lack of an imaging method that can correctly define tumor margins and a temperature-sensitive

imaging technique that can identify focal temperature elevation. Recent advances in MR imaging technology have provided noninvasive imaging for guiding focused ultrasound treatment. MR imaging has good anatomic resolution, has high sensitivity for tumor definition, and most important, can be used for real-time monitoring of tissue temperature elevation and for the detection of the subsequent process of thermal coagulation. Specifically, MR imaging has the ability to display "maps" of temperature with a few degrees of sensitivity. The integration of MR imaging and focused ultrasound surgery (FUS) has resulted in real-time, image-controlled, noninvasive thermal ablation systems [2–4]. The major advantage of MR imaging guidance over other imaging modalities is its ability to achieve accurate targeting of tumors while avoiding thermal injury of normal tissues. MR imaging also offers the unique potential for closed-loop feedback control of tissue heating and for direct measurement of the deposited thermal dose, which significantly enhances the safety and efficacy of FUS in the treatment of tumors.

The goal of this article is to provide an overview of the principles of MR-guided and MR imaging–controlled FUS. To this end, the authors (1) provide a comprehensive introduction to a novel "disruptive" technology that will arguably revolutionize the current practice of surgery, interventional radiology, and radiation therapy; (2) present a retrospective review of the technology and the

This work was sponsored by National Institutes of Health grants P01CA067165, R25CA089017, R01EB003268, and R33EB000705, and by InSightec, Ltd.

* Corresponding author.

E-mail address: jolesz@bwh.harvard.edu
(F.A. Jolesz).

literature that supports it; (3) compare MR-guided FUS with other ablation methods; (4) describe the current treatment paradigm; and (5) discuss existing and future clinical applications.

History of focused ultrasound surgery

In the 1930s, ultrasound was first proposed for use in cancer treatments. The intensity and the exposure time were used as the measures of the ultrasound exposure, the hypothesis being that the propagating wave had preferential lethal effects on cancer cells. The ability to focus ultrasound energy through soft tissues so that focal tissue volumes could be noninvasively destroyed was discovered and first proposed by Lynn and colleagues [1]. This technique was later modified and used in the destruction of small tissue volumes in the central nervous system in animals and in humans [5–7]. Burov [8] used high-intensity pulsed ultrasound and produced resorption of rabbit carcinomas and human malignant melanomas [9,10]. This high-intensity approach was subsequently tested in the treatment of human breast and brain tumors [11].

Despite promising results from these studies, high-intensity ultrasound therapy has not been widely used. A possible reason for this is that the size of the destroyed tissue volume depends on the applied power, the duration of the sonication, and the tissue type [12]. Thus, extensive experimental studies have been necessary to determine the correct power settings required for ablation in different clinical settings. Moreover, in the early studies, it was difficult to accurately aim the beam and to evaluate the response to the treatment.

During the 1990s, several commercial companies began to develop clinical FUS devices that are currently being used in clinical trials or in early stages of clinical practice. These prototypes use single-focus transducers that are mechanically moved to aim the beam. The targeting is based on ultrasound images [13–16]. The same principle was also applied for prostate tumor treatments with intracavitary applicators consisting of a mechanically targeted, single-element transducer and an ultrasound imaging transducer that were inserted into the rectum [17,18]. Both of these approaches have been extensively tested in clinical trials and are currently commercially available outside of the United States.

The major breakthrough in the field has been the introduction of MR imaging guidance and MR imaging–based temperature control [2–4]. For MR-guided FUS, a mechanically targeted, single-element, focused ultrasound device was first developed and tested clinically for breast tumor treatments [4,19–21].

Driven by a need to electronically steer the focus, to have control over the focal spot size and shape, and to compensate for beam distortions induced by overlaying tissues, phased-array applicators have been developed for ultrasound surgery [22–26]. These applicators have many small ultrasound sources, each driven by a separate and individually controllable radiofrequency (RF) driver that effectively allows the phase and amplitude of the ultrasound wave of each element to be individually controlled. Thus, the ultrasound field is also controlled electronically. Limited phased-array applicators (with approximately 200 array elements) are currently used in a commercially available MR-guided ultrasound surgery system (ExAblate 2000, InSightec, Haifa, Israel) that controls the focal spot depth and the size of the focus. A larger, 500-element phased-array system has also been constructed for transcranial brain surgery and allows for corrections of skull-induced distortions of the ultrasound field [27]. This device, ready for the first clinical tests, uses acoustic modeling of the ultrasound field and information from the skull bone obtained from CT scans for correction of these distortions [27,28].

Comparison with other thermal ablations

Thermal ablations use localized high temperature to heat beyond 57°C to 60°C—the threshold for protein denaturation sufficient to produce coagulation necrosis. Thermal ablative treatment, unlike hyperthermia, is not selective, and normal and neoplastic tissues sustain irreversible cellular damage when the tissue is heated above this critical level. As opposed to heat-induced damage, freezing may not result in definitive cell death unless freezing cycles are repeated at a relatively low temperature. Depositing heat or transferring cold usually involves the invasive insertion of various types of heat-conducting probes into the targeted tissue with relatively minor injury. The thermal convection or diffusion that distributes the heat from the probes, however, largely depends on the physical and physiologic properties of the tissue and is further influenced by vascularity and tissue perfusion. As a consequence, the size and shape of the treatment volume may not accurately correspond to the three-dimensional extent of the tumor. This disparity may result in overtreatment (damage of normal tissue beyond the tumor margin) or undertreatment (tissue remains untreated within the tumor margin). In the case of larger tumors, most of the probe-delivered thermal ablation requires the use of multiple probes, which increases the invasiveness of the treatment.

To optimize the treatment and to limit the coagulation to the targeted tumor, imaging is necessary. The primary role of imaging is to correctly localize the target volume, which can be accomplished by using various diagnostic imaging methods that can define (within their limit of spatial and contrast resolution) the full three-dimensional extent of the tumor. The secondary role of imaging is to monitor the heating of the tissue using temperature-sensitive imaging. If this monitoring has the appropriate spatial, temporal, and temperature resolution, then temperature-sensitive imaging can also be used to control the procedure. To achieve complete coverage of the tumor without complications, an image-based control system for thermal ablative therapies must be used. Probe-delivered thermal ablation methods such as interstitial laser therapy, RF heating, and cryoablation have only limited ability to deposit a uniform energy dose within the entire volume of the tumor. There is an unavoidable thermal gradient extending from the probe to the periphery of the treatment zone. Depending on the size and position (and in the case of multiple probes, the number and location of the probes), the size and the shape of the treatment volume vary. Treatment volume is also influenced by tissue properties, vascularization, and the temporal sequence of the energy delivery. Preoperative three-dimensional treatment planning may help in optimizing energy delivery [29]; however, it does not eliminate the need for intraprocedural monitoring of heat deposition.

Studies suggest that the best solution to optimizing the match between the targeted tumor volume and the heat treatment zone is to use temperature-sensitive MR imaging [30–32]. By showing more or less accurate (within few degrees of Celsius) temperature values, thermal imaging can demonstrate the thermal gradient around the probe and thus help define the demarcation zone within which irreversible tissue death occurs and outside of which tissue damage is reversible. The reversible thermal tissue damage is consistent with

cell survival and postoperative tumor recurrence. Real-time MR imaging monitoring is also valuable in depicting inhomogeneous tissue treatment (cold spots in heat treatments and hot spots in cryoablation). These inhomogeneities are due to the variability of microvasculature and the presence of larger blood vessels. Without imaging, these anomalies cannot be found. Monitoring can also provide input for potential closed-loop feedback control methods that can optimize energy deliveries [33]. Since 1988, when the advantages of MR imaging monitoring and control of laser–tissue interactions were fist described [30], MR-guided RF, microwave, and cryoablation methods have been accepted and minimally invasive treatment options have been established [34–37].

The most attractive thermal ablation method with the greatest clinical potential is FUS [38,39]. Using this noninvasive method, most of the limitations of probe-delivered thermal ablations are eliminated. FUS is a nonincisional method that requires no probe insertion. After appropriate image-guided targeting (achieved by locating spots with subthreshold thermal doses), the focused acoustic energy beam is applied but causes no tissue damage beyond the target volume. Within the treatment zone, the results are more homogenous and the effects of tumor vascularity and tissue heterogeneity are minimal. The ablation is controlled, precise, predictable, reproducible, and repeatable (unlike radiosurgery). The coagulated lesions develop instantaneously and are sharply demarcated and distinct.

MR imaging–based temperature imaging

Most of the parameters measured in an MR image (eg, T1 and T2 relaxivity, the diffusion coefficient, the equilibrium magnetization, and the water proton resonant frequency [PRF]) are sensitive to temperature changes. This characteristic makes MR imaging an attractive modality for monitoring focused ultrasound or other heating methods for thermal therapy. Indeed, this trait was realized quickly, and in the early days of MR imaging, numerous studies were performed that tested the temperature sensitivity of MR imaging sequences [40–43].

Most attention has been focused on the use of T1 relaxivity and the PRF shift for temperature monitoring. Due to its relative insensitivity to motion and ability to acquire T1-weighted images with standard sequences but without postprocessing,

T1-weighted imaging has been used clinically in hundreds of patients for visualizing heating progression during interstitial ablative therapies in liver with laser [44]. The main weaknesses of this method are twofold: (1) the temperature sensitivity is dependent on tissue type and (2) the temperature sensitivity changes as tissue is heated and coagulated [30]. It is unfortunate that these restrictions severely limit the usefulness of the method.

In contrast, the water PRF shift does not have these problems [45–48]. In addition, it has been found to be the most sensitive MR imaging–based thermometry method [45] and images can be acquired rapidly with standard pulse sequences [46]. With these special features, it can be used over the large range of temperatures encountered during FUS, from visualizing the subthreshold exposures needed to localize the focal spot before ablation occurs [47] to quantifying temperature changes above the coagulation threshold. This capacity allows for accurate on-line prediction of regions that have achieved a sufficient thermal exposure [48] and for fully automated closed-loop feedback control [49,50]. A growing number of studies are experimentally demonstrating that MR imaging–based thermometry can accurately predict (on average) the threshold for thermal damage [51–54] and the spatial extent of the ablated

area during focused ultrasound thermal ablation or other thermal ablation therapies [55,56]. Fig. 1 shows an example of such agreement after focused ultrasound treatment of a VX2 tumor implanted in rabbit thigh muscle [57].

The two major weaknesses of the PRF shift thermometry method are its motion sensitivity and its lack of temperature sensitivity in fat. The motion sensitivity stems from the need for image subtractions to create the temperature maps. Several strategies have been proposed that would allow for temperature monitoring in moving organs, such as using navigator echoes; acquiring multiple baseline images over various points in the breathing cycle [58]; referencing the water PRF shift to a temperature-insensitive PRF such as lipid [59,60] (instead of just a baseline [preheated] image); or using unheated areas surrounding the heated zone instead of baseline subtractions [61]. A suitable method should be available soon to allow for water PRF shift–based thermometry in moving organs. The lack of temperature sensitivity in lipid arises from its lack of hydrogen bonds (such bonds are responsible for the temperature dependence of the water PRF temperature sensitivity). The inability to monitor temperature in fat limits the usefulness of the method in breast [19–21] and makes it difficult to detect the low-level heating that can occur in the subcutaneous

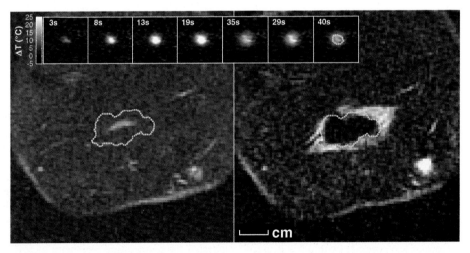

Fig. 1. Contrast enhanced T1-weighted images of an implanted VX2 tumor in rabbit thigh muscle acquired before (*left*) and after (*right*) focused ultrasound thermal ablation. The image on the right shows thermal dose contours superimposed, which agree superbly with the nonperfused area induced by the ablation—typically what has been found in animal studies. The inset shows a time series of temperature images of the focal heating during a 20-second sonication (imaging performed perpendicular to the direction of the ultrasound beam direction). This treatment was performed with an MR-guided focused ultrasound system that uses a phased-array transducer. (Details of this study are described in reference [57].)

fat over the course of multiple, overlapping sonications during focused ultrasound ablation in abdominal organs, which may be an issue in future focused ultrasound treatments.

Closed-loop feedback control in a clinical focused ultrasound system

Much of the research that has been performed over the last decade in MR imaging–based thermometry control of focused ultrasound thermal ablation and ultrasound phased-array technology has been implemented using a clinical focused ultrasound device, the ExAblate 2000. This device consists of a phased-array transducer, mechanical positioning device, and an RF amplifier that is incorporated into a standard 1.5-T General Electric MR imaging patient table, along with a control unit and operator PC. This system is fully integrated with the MR unit. It prescribes and triggers the temperature-sensitive sequences, reconstructs them, and calculates the accumulated isoeffective thermal dose [62] to estimate (on-line) the ablated volume.

At the outset of the MR-guided FUS procedure with this device, the radiologist prescribes the treatment volume using treatment planning images that are obtained in multiple orientations. The skin is also outlined. The treatment consists of multiple sonications that are delivered sequentially (with a cooling period in between) to treat a prescribed volume. For benign tumors such as uterine fibroids, these sonications do not need to overlap. A preliminary grid of sonication targets is displayed on the treatment plan and the ultrasound beam path is displayed for each target. When the beam path for any individual target passes through any critical structure or when the target itself is too close to a critical structure, it can be moved or the transducer can be angled so that the target and the beam path are safe.

After the treatment plan is determined, the coordinates of the ultrasound device and the MR imaging system are aligned. This procedure is performed first by roughly indicating the location of the transducer on the images. Next, sonications are delivered that are below the threshold for tissue damage. During the sonication, a time series of MR imaging–based temperature images are acquired and displayed for the user. If the location of the heating does not overlap with the target location, then the user clicks on the true location of the heating, and the system updates the

alignment. This procedure is first performed with imaging in a plane perpendicular to the ultrasound beam direction and then repeated with imaging parallel to the direction because the beam direction is longer along its direction of propagation.

After the system coordinates are aligned with the MR imaging coordinates, the treatment begins. Typically, the power is increased stepwise to the treatment level to verify that the patient is not experiencing discomfort. The treatment power level and other acoustic parameters are initially determined by the system based on acoustic simulations to which the treatment depth is inputted (treatment depth was determined when the user drew the outline of the skin). During treatment, the parameters are continuously modified as needed based on the feedback obtained by the temperature mapping. After each sonication, the system calculates the accumulated isoeffective thermal dose for that sonication, which is displayed on top of the imaging for the user to inspect. This dose is added to the dose that has accumulated for the whole treatment. If the peak temperature or the size of the thermal dose region that is achieved is unacceptable, then the user can adjust the sonication parameters and repeat the sonication as necessary until the result is as desired. If the accumulated dose does not cover a sufficient volume after multiple sonications, then more targets can be added. Fig. 2 shows the treatment progression during a typical uterine fibroid progression with the ExAblate 2000 system, illustrating this closed-loop feedback control based on the MR imaging–based thermal dosimetry.

In the authors' experience, substantial variations occur in the measured temperature rise from patient to patient and even from location to location with a single treatment, so this closed-loop control is essential for control of focused ultrasound thermal ablation. Even when the same acoustic parameters are used, the authors have observed temperature variations from patient to patient and within individual patients that have a magnitude as high as a factor of two. From the authors' perspective, verbal feedback from patients during treatments has perhaps been as important as the thermometry feedback. During treatment, the patients are awake and under conscious sedation, and they can tell the user whether they are experiencing any discomfort due to the sonications. They can also halt the sonication if necessary. This additional feedback is

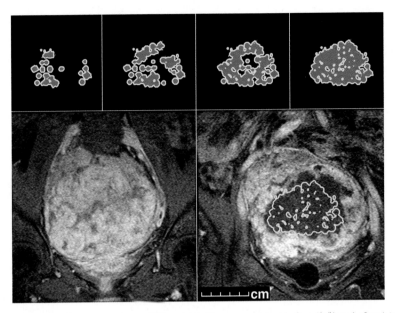

Fig. 2. Thermal dosimetry and contrast enhanced T1-weighted images acquired before (*left*) and after (*right*) MR-guided focused ultrasound thermal ablation of a uterine fibroid treatment with the Exablate 2000 system. The four maps on the top show the accumulated thermal dose at four points during the treatment. After each sonication, these maps are updated, allowing the user to gauge the progress of the treatment. The user has complete freedom to choose the order of the sonication targets; in this case, they were delivered in a somewhat random pattern so that heat would not accumulate in overlying tissues. As the treatment progressed, the volume was filled in. Because this tumor was benign, it was not necessary to completely fill in the target volume; the goal was to treat as much volume as possible within the time limits allowed by the study guidelines. Note that the nonperfused volume was somewhat larger than the accumulated thermal dose volume, perhaps due to vascular occlusion within the fibroid volume.

critical to avoiding any adverse side effects to the treatments.

Clinical applications

Breast

The first clinical application of MR-guided FUS was performed in the breast, a location where the access is simple and no bony or air-containing structure is present. There is a need to develop a minimally invasive or noninvasive breast-saving solution for tumor removal. Open surgery of breast lesions can result in complications including anesthesia-related complications, hemorrhage, infection, scarring, and disfigurement. These complications have motivated the introduction of minimally invasive percutaneous or ablative procedures that offer an alternative for tumor control. Laser, RF, and cryosurgery have been tested as alternatives to lumpectomy [37]. Hirose and colleagues [63] reported on MR-guided lumpectomy for patients with an invasive

breast cancer diagnosed by core needle biopsy and demonstrated that MR imaging can define tumor margins intraoperatively better than the surgeon. These preliminary results have motivated the testing of MR-guided FUS for treating breast fibroadenomas and breast cancers.

The feasibility of guiding FUS treatments with MR imaging has thus far been shown with biopsy-proven fibroadenoma [19] and breast cancer [20,21]. Hynynen and colleagues [19] reported on nine women with 11 lesions (mean volume 1.9 cm^3) who underwent partial ablation of their lesions. Partial or total success was reported in 73% of treatments. Problems included motion, under-treatment due to conservatively low power settings in early cases, beam reflection due to cavitation, or injection of local anesthetic. Additional challenges include difficulty in monitoring temperature and dose in perilesional fat using phase-difference techniques [63]; thus, tumor margin treatment cannot be verified intraprocedurally. Treatment was assessed with contrast-enhanced long-term follow-up images. Surrounding edema was visible up to 2 days following therapy. After 3 years, the lesion was visible as only a small hypointense area of reduced signal intensity on nonenhanced T1-weighted images.

Huber and colleagues [64] reported on FUS treatments in a core biopsy–proven patient who had invasive breast cancer. Immunohistochemistry of the resected specimen demonstrated that FUS homogeneously induced lethal and sublethal tumor damage with consecutive upregulation of p53 and loss of proliferative activity.

Gianfelice and colleagues [20] reported on 12 patients with invasive breast carcinomas who underwent FUS. Correlation between histopathologic analysis of resected tumor sections and MR imaging revealed that 95.6% of the tumor was within the targeted zone; a mean of 88.3% of the cancer tissue was necrosed in their later series. Residual tumor was identified predominantly at the periphery of the tumor mass. The group concluded treatment area should be increased. In more recent work, Gianfelice and colleagues [21] assessed the value of dynamic, contrast-enhanced MR imaging to monitor residual tumor. They treated 17 patients with small breast tumors (diameter <3.5 cm). The lesions were surgically resected and the presence of residual tumor was determined by histopathology. There was good correlation between residual tumor and dynamic, contrast-enhanced MR imaging, suggesting that MR-guided FUS could provide a reliable non-invasive method for the treatment of breast tumors. With the exception of minor skin burns, no complications occurred in these studies. Currently, there has been improvement of the breast treatment system, including cooling of the skin and a phased-array system. These improvements have resulted in almost complete ablation within the MR imaging–defined margins and in decreased incidence of minor skin burns.

MR-guided focused ultrasound surgery for treatment of uterine leiomyomas

The most successful clinical application of MR-guided FUS to date is the treatment of women who have symptomatic uterine leiomyomas. In the following sections, the authors describe the procedure, including the methods used and the study design of the phase I/II and phase II trials that led to Food and Drug Administration (FDA) approval of the ExAblate 2000 system in October 2004.

Clinical features of leiomyomas

Uterine leiomyomas are extremely common and occur in up to 25% of women. When they are symptomatic, they can cause symptoms due to bulk/pressure, bleeding, or disruption of fertility. Pathologically, they are neoplasms of the myometrium, composed of whorled arrangements of smooth muscle in the uterus. They can exist in many different forms (classic, hypercellular, hypervascular, and degenerative), with cystic necrosis or red/hemorrhagic degeneration. MR imaging can identify most of these different forms. They can be located in several sites (ie, in the uterus intramurally [submucosal or subserosal], outside the uterus in the broad ligament or adnexa, or arising from other organs with smooth muscle capsules).

MR imaging of leiomyomas

MR imaging has been used for many years to diagnose, classify, and characterize leiomyomas. It is clearly the best imaging modality for (1) establishing the full definition of the burden of disease, (2) determining the volume of every leiomyoma in the uterus, and (3) following patients on medical therapy. More recently, it is being used with greater frequency in treatment planning and monitoring, especially since the introduction and widespread adaptation of uterine artery embolization as a minimally invasive treatment option for women with symptomatic leiomyomas. The value of MR imaging in such planning is to define the volume, location, and perfusion status of the leiomyomas. The typical imaging protocol would consist of multiplanar T2-weighted images (Fig. 3) and T1-weighted images before and after the injection of gadolinium contrast (Fig. 4). The latter is essential in defining perfusion status and particularly essential in detecting areas of necrosis. Using magnetic resonance angiography techniques, it is also possible to define the uterine and ovarian arteries and determine whether there are collateral channels and branches of the uterine arteries perfusing the ovaries. In such situations, uterine artery embolization may cause embolization of the ovary and should be avoided. Direct application of the MR-guided FUS technique for leiomyomas is described by Tempany and colleagues [65]. MR-guided focused ultrasound in the context of leiomyomas is clearly an excellent illustration of the power of imaging in delineating a target and directly monitoring the treatment delivery and its effect. The T2-weighted images of the leiomyoma show its location, the relationship of all adjacent structures,

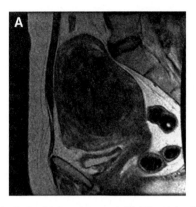
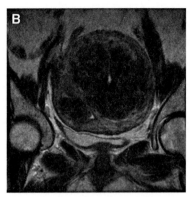

Fig. 3. Sagittal (*A*) and coronal (*B*) T2-weighted images show a large left intramural leiomyoma.

the beam path as it passes through the tissues, and the distal beam path after it has passed through the focal point. The pretreatment imaging assists in selecting the optimal leiomyoma for treatment

Patient selection for MR-guided focused ultrasound treatment

In the phase I/II and phase III clinical trials performed to date, which took place before FDA approval of the ExAblate 2000 device, the authors used the following enrollment criteria: (1) women who had symptomatic leiomyomas (as defined by the so-called "UF-QOL" [uterine fibroid quality of life] questionnaire developed by Spies and colleagues [66]); (2) women who had completed their families; and (3) women who had a uterine size less than that of a 20-week gestation. All patients had pelvic MR imaging examinations, as described previously, with intravenous contrast. MR imaging had to demonstrate at least one leiomyoma over 5 cm; further, the leiomyoma had

to be solid (ie, enhanced with gadolinium). It also had to be in a safe and accessible location for FUS, which meant that the leiomyoma meeting the selection criteria had to be anterior in the pelvis, with no intervening bowel loops between them and the anterior abdominal wall. The patient's clinical history and images were then reviewed and the target leiomyoma or leiomyomas were identified for treatment.

The procedure, patient preparation, and postprocedure follow-up

The patient prepares for the procedure by fasting the night before and by shaving the skin of the lower abdomen to allow safe passage of the ultrasound beam. Any scars are identified on the skin. The procedure is performed with intravenous conscious sedation (typically this means intravenous fentanyl and midazolam), and a Foley catheter is placed to prevent distention of the

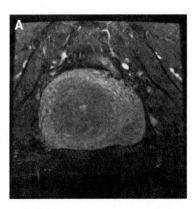
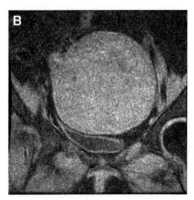

Fig. 4. Coronal precontrast (*A*) and axial postcontrast (*B*) images show homogeneous enhancement of the leiomyoma before MR-guided FUS treatment.

urinary bladder and consequent uterine motion during the procedure.

The treatments were performed using the ExAblate 2000 system, which consists of a phased-array transducer (~200 elements; frequency: 0.96–1.14 MHz); a computer-controlled positioning system; a multichannel RF amplifier system; and a user interface—all integrated with a standard 1.5-T clinical MR imaging unit (General Electric Medical Systems, Milwaukee, Wisconsin). The xy (lateral) position and angle of the transducer were mechanically controlled and the focusing depth and size of the focal zone were controlled by the phased array by way of beam steering. Imaging was performed with a custom pelvic coil (USA Instruments, Aurora, Ohio). The system controlled the MR imaging scanner, automatically prescribing and starting the temperature-sensitive imaging sequence.

The patient is positioned prone over the transducer, which is in water bath and has a gel pad placed anteriorly. Skin coupling is achieved with the pad and the addition of degassed water around it. The patient is also connected to the EKG and blood pressure monitors that are required to follow her vital signs during the administration of the intravenous conscious sedation. The treating radiologist remains outside the room while a nurse performs the monitoring inside; both are present for the entire procedure. The nurse also assists in all communications between the patient and the treating physician.

Initial images are obtained in three dimensions with T2-weighted pulse sequences. These images are then used to redefine the target leiomyoma and define the subvolume for treatment. Under current FDA guidelines, (1) the volume for a single treatment must be no more than 100 mL per leiomyoma or 150 mL total, (2) the border of the treatment volume must be within 15 mm of the outer serosal surface of the uterus, and (3) the total treatment time must not exceed 3 hours. With these factors in mind, the volume is defined and the treatment begins.

Treatment. Initially a low-power sonication (30–50 W) is delivered into the center of the target and simultaneous phase imaging is performed. The resultant images must show the focal spot and its location must be correct before moving up to higher therapeutic power sonications (90–100 W). After each sonication is delivered, the patient is questioned about any sensations she may have felt. It is critical that the patient provide accurate

and prompt feedback. The patient may feel heat, warmth, or even burning pain in her skin, uterus, or back. The treatment parameters are all adjusted to ensure these are avoided as much as possible. Prolonged and repeated pain or burning can lead to serious adverse events such as skin damage or nerve injury. It is normal for the patient to "feel" the sonication in the uterus; the feeling is often described as a mild cramp or localized warmth.

As the sonications are delivered, temperature imaging provides immediate and direct feedback on the temperature change at the focal point. The goal is to achieve temperatures above 55°C and ideally between 70°C to 80°C. This range ensures thermal coagulation and necrosis of the tissue.

After all planned sonications are delivered, the treatment concludes with postintravenous contrast imaging of the treatment volume. The nonenhancing tissue volume can then be immediately delineated (Fig. 5) and followed along with the patient's symptomatic response over the following months and years. The patient is taken from the room, recovers for a brief period of time (usually 1–2 hours), and then goes home with an escort or family member. The patient is usually well enough to return to normal activities later that day or the next day.

Postprocedure complications

Over 600 women have been treated worldwide with this device and there have been no treatment-related deaths, life-threatening events, unintended second procedures, separate interventional treatments, or patients discharged with a urinary

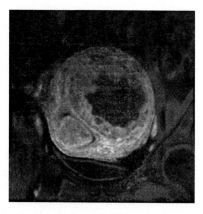

Fig. 5. Coronal postcontrast image shows focal nonenhancement in the center of the leiomyoma in the area of MR-guided FUS, which represents the thermally ablated tissue.

catheter. The most serious complication following MR-guided FUS to date was the development of sciatic nerve palsy in one woman due to absorption of energy by bone in the far field of the sonication. The results of electromyography and MR-neurography were negative. The subject's weakness and numbness clinically resolved by her 12-month follow-up visit. Review of all treatment images suggest that the nerve itself was not directly sonicated, but that heat transfer from the sacrum likely led to indirect injury of the nerve. Subsequently, the assessment of energy parameters beyond the focus and particularly near the bony pelvis has been incorporated into all protocols, and a safety margin of 4 cm from the sacrum has been mandated.

Treatment outcomes

The ability of MR imaging to document the immediate post-treatment results is the first step in assessing the treatment effect. By using the rapid, dynamic intravenous contrast enhancement with gadolinium, the physician can immediately measure the size and volume of the necrotic lesion. The gadolinium is administered in the standard clinical fashion through an intravenous line using a rapid manual or pump administration; the typical dose is 20 mL. Thus, by comparing the images acquired before treatment with those immediately after, the change is clearly evident. Not only can the treatment volume be evaluated but also any nontargeted necrosis or damage can be seen.

The effect of MR-guided FUS on uterine leiomyomas has been evaluated in the following ways:

1. Post-treatment nonenhancing tissue volume. This measurement is the volume of nonenhancing tissue (as defined after the injection of intravenous gadolinium) compared with a precontrast, pretreatment set of images.
2. Pathologic findings. These findings were evaluated in the phase I/II trials after the hysterectomy.
3. Patient symptom response as measured on the UF-QOL. The UF-QOL allows assessment of all fibroid symptoms and calculates a symptom severity score for the patients. The symptom severity score assesses menorrhagia and bulk-related symptoms on a single 100-point scale, whereby higher scores indicate greater symptom severity.

The UF-QOL is currently the only validated instrument for assessing uterine fibroid symptoms and their impact on health-related quality of life. It was evaluated in an ethnically diverse population and has demonstrated reliability and validity [66].

4. Volume changes in the overall uterus and in the individually treated leiomyoma. These changes are currently being evaluated at 6, 12, 24, and 36 months after treatment.

The authors used the UF-QOL in the trials performed to assess the safety and efficacy of MR-guided FUS. In the early phase I/II trial, Tempany and colleagues [65] reported on the early safety and feasibility, where all patients had hysterectomy after MR-guided FUS, the size and volume of the area of necrosis, and cellular changes. Stewart [67] reported the results of the larger group in the phase I/II trials, showing safety and a high level of acceptance among patients and doctors. Subsequently, in the phase III trial, the response in symptom severity scores was reported by Hindley and colleagues [68]. When these data were presented to the FDA in 2004, of the 109 subjects undergoing MR-guided FUS, 77 (70.6%) achieved at least a 10-point reduction in their symptom severity score at 6 months following treatment ($P < .0001$). The mean decrease in score was 23.8 points, almost threefold greater than was postulated (symptom severity score change score from 61.7 ± 16.3 at baseline to 37.3 ± 21.0 at follow-up, $P < .0001$). As a result of these data and all data collected over the trials, in October 2004, the FDA approved MR-guided FUS for the treatment of symptomatic leiomyomas.

Brain

Although the original vision of FUS primarily involved applications for brain tumor treatment [5–7], the lack of accurate targeting and control of energy deposition prevented its clinical use in the central nervous system. Applying FUS in the brain has also been hampered by the presence of the bony skull, which distorts the ultrasound beam and may cause excessive heating due to its high absorption. The authors recently developed a technique that uses large ultrasound phased-array and CT-derived skull thickness information to correct for the wave propagation and to allow for transcranial focusing without overheating the skull [27,28]. Based on this array technology, InSightec developed a complete system designed for clinical FUS (Fig. 6). Although this technique has been tested in primates to establish the clinical feasibility of the approach, due to the small size of the primate head, these experiments can only establish the maximum intensity levels that could be delivered through the living skull bone.

These and other results [54,69] continue to support that ultrasound-induced, completely non-invasive thermal ablation of brain lesions may be feasible. By cooling the coupling water, the outer skull surface temperatures can be kept acceptably low, and the brain surface temperatures become the limiting factor. When the results are scaled to human size, it appears focal coagulation is possible without damaging the brain surface, bone, or skin. Using a phased array of ultrasound transducers, it is now possible to precisely target and thermocoagulate brain tumors through the intact skull under MR imaging guidance. Recent studies conducted by the authors' group have also demonstrated that focused ultrasound, administered in doses lower than those necessary to coagulate tissue, produces a localized and transient opening of the blood-brain barrier [70–73].

This approach could prove to be an even more significant clinical application than tumor ablation because it theoretically should enable the delivery of macromolecules such as antibodies, chemotherapeutic agents, and neuroprotective substances through the blood-brain barrier to the site of treatment. For example, neurotoxin-attached antibodies that can recognize tumor cells may be delivered through the blood-brain barrier, where they will proceed to home and destroy the tumor cells in a cell-specific manner. Indeed, the localized, "immunotargeting" of the brain may bring a completely new treatment concept to a wide range of central nervous system diseases including malignant brain tumors, epilepsy, Parkinson's disease, and other maladies that may be amenable to management with selective, anatomically targeted large molecules.

Targeted drug and gene delivery

The ability (under MR imaging guidance) to concentrate acoustic energy into a targeted anatomic or functional location deep in the body can be used for other interventions beyond thermal coagulation. A mild temperature elevation (a few degrees Celsius below the tissue coagulation threshold) induced by ultrasound can be used to activate genes for gene therapy [73]. Similarly, such exposures could be used to increase the circulation and the leakage of blood vessels, thereby increasing the uptake of targeted agents in blood stream. This mild temperature elevation could also be used to release drugs from temperature-sensitive liposomes circulating in the bloodstream [74,75]. With the ability of MR imaging to accurately quantify the temperature rise, such low-level exposures can be precisely controlled; it may also be possible to monitor the released drug concentration [76]. Furthermore, the same

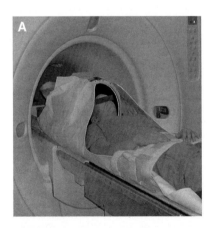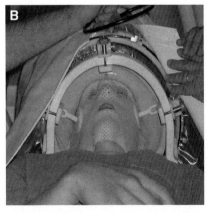

Fig. 6. Photographs of a volunteer in a clinical prototype MR-guided FUS designed for transcranial exposures. (*A*) Volunteer lying in the device, which consists of a 30-cm diameter hemispherical phased-array transducer with 500 elements. The large size of the transducer allows it to distribute the energy over as much surface of the head as possible to avoid overheating the skull. (*B*) After a flexible membrane is attached around the volunteer's forehead and to the transducer, the resulting enclosed space around the head is filled with degassed water. A thermoplastic mask is used to fix the head in place.

devices developed for thermal ablation can be used for this purpose.

By using short bursts at high-pressure amplitudes, thermal effects can be minimized or eliminated and the nonthermal effects of cavitation can be used. Various mechanical effects have been observed with such exposures. Histologic studies have shown that cavitation can disrupt the blood-brain barrier [77,78], cause selective vascular damage, generate tissue necrosis, and produce complete tissue disintegration [77]. In addition, animal tumor studies have shown that focused ultrasound–induced cavitation can activate certain chemicals [79]. The disruption of arteriosclerotic plaques and thrombi are also thought to be cavitation-mediated events [80,81]. Finally, high-amplitude focused ultrasound beams can also be distorted to create shock waves at the focus, which in turn might influence cell membrane permeability [82]. An increase in blood vessel permeability has been demonstrated in muscle tissue in vivo after ultrasound exposures [89] and may be useful for gene therapy [83–88]. Cavitation effects can be amplified further by injecting preformed microbubbles into the vasculature. Although these bubbles have been developed for imaging, they have also been shown to reduce the power required for inducing tissue effects by at least two orders of magnitude [89]. It may also be possible to include therapeutic agents in the shell of the microbubbles so that they break and release their contents in the target location when exposed to ultrasound [90].

The use of these microbubbles may be especially useful in the brain, where the delivery of therapeutic agents by way of the blood supply is often impossible to achieve because the blood-brain barrier prevents many large molecules from penetrating into the brain tissue through the endothelium layer of brain capillaries. The normal blood-brain barrier limits the passage of ionized water-soluble compounds to those with a molecular weight smaller than 180 d. Most currently available, effective chemotherapeutic agents, however, have a molecular weight between 200 d and 1200 d and cannot reach the tumor cells in areas of the brain where the blood-brain barrier is intact. The impenetrability of the blood-brain barrier is often identified as a major factor in the relative inefficiency of chemotherapy in treating central nervous system metastases of systemic cancers, even in cases in which complete remission of these tumors occurs in locations outside of the central nervous system.

The authors have shown that when preformed microbubbles are first injected into the blood stream, low-power ultrasound bursts can be used to open the blood-brain barrier without damaging the surrounding neurons [70–72]. These bubbles expand and contract in the acoustic field inside of the capillaries, effectively making the blood-brain barrier permeable to large-molecular MR imaging contrast agents. This defect heals itself in approximately 6 hours. The blood-brain barrier opening is induced only at the focal spot of the ultrasound field. The authors demonstrated that when MR imaging guidance is used to target specific brain locations, the opening of the blood-brain barrier can be achieved with minimal damage to surrounding tissues.

Summary

The history of MR-guided FUS demonstrates the need for merging advanced therapy technology with advanced imaging. Without the ability of MR imaging to localize the tumor margins and without the temperature-sensitive imaging that provides the closed-loop control of energy deposition, this method is inadequate for most clinical applications. Given these limitations, high-intensity focused ultrasound initially appeared to have a narrow application area and was not able to compete with other surgical or ablation methods. Today, MR imaging–guided FUS has become a safe and effective means of performing probe-delivered thermal ablations and minimally invasive surgery. Moreover, it has the potential to replace treatments that use ionizing radiation such as radiosurgery and brachytherapy. Although the cost of integrating "big ticket" MR imaging systems with complex and expensive phased arrays is high, this expenditure will largely be offset by eliminating hospitalization and anesthesia and by reducing complications. In effect, an investment in this emerging technology will ultimately redound to the benefit of the health care delivery system and, most important, to the patient.

The FUS system provides a safe, repeatable treatment approach for benign tumors (eg, uterine fibroid and breast fibroadenoma) that do not require an aggressive approach. MR-guided FUS can also be used for debulking cancerous tissue. It has already been tested as a breast cancer treatment; its application for other malignancies in the brain, liver, and prostate is under development [91–93]. MR-guided FUS offers an attractive alternative to conventional surgery because it incorporates intraoperative MR imaging, which provides far more precise target definition than is possible with the surgeon's direct visualization of the lesion.

MR-guided FUS is undeniably the most promising interventional MR imaging method in the field of image-guided therapy today. It is applicable not only in the thermal coagulative treatment of tumors but also in several other medical situations for which invasive surgery or radiation may not be treatment options. The use of FUS for treating vascular malformation [94] or functional disorders of the brain is also exciting. It is uniquely applicable for image-guided therapy using targeted drug delivery methods and gene therapy. Further advances in this technology will no doubt improve energy deposition and reduce treatment times. In the near future, FUS will offer a viable alternative to conventional surgery and radiation therapy; in the longer-term, it may also enable a host of targeted treatment methods aimed at eradicating or arresting heretofore intractable diseases such as certain brain malignancies and forms of epilepsy.

References

[1] Lynn JG, Zwemer RL, Chick AJ, et al. A new method for the generation and use of focused ultrasound in experimental biology. J Gen Physiol 1942; 26:179–93.

[2] Cline HE, Schenck JF, Hynynen K, et al. MR-guided focused ultrasound surgery. J Comput Assist Tomogr 1992;16(6):956–65.

[3] Cline HE, Hynynen K, Watkins RD, et al. Focused US system for MR imaging-guided tumor ablation. Radiology 1995;194(3):731–7.

[4] Hynynen K, Freund WR, Cline HE, et al. A clinical, noninvasive, MR imaging-monitored ultrasound surgery method. Radiographics 1996;16(1):185–95.

[5] Fry WJ, Barnard JW, Fry FJ, et al. Ultrasonic lesions in the mammalian central nervous system. Science 1955;122:517–8.

[6] Fry WJ, Fry FJ. Fundamental neurological research and human neurosurgery using intense ultrasound. IRE Trans Med Electron 1960;7:166–81.

[7] Lele PP. A simple method for production of trackless focal lesions with focused ultrasound: physical factors. J Physiol 1962;160:494–512.

[8] Burov AK. High intensity ultrasonic oscillations for the treatment of malignant tumors in animal and man. Dokl Akad Nauk SSSR 1956;106:239–41.

[9] Burov AK, Adreevskaya G. The effect of ultra-acoustic oscillation of high intensity on malignant tumors in animals and man. Dokl Akad Nauk SSSR 1956;106:445–8.

[10] Oka M. Surgical application of high-intensity focused ultrasound. Clin All Round (Jpn) 1960;13:1514.

[11] Heimburger RF. Ultrasound augmentation of central nervous system tumor therapy. Indiana Med 1985;78:469–76.

[12] Frizzell LA, Linke CA, Carstensen EL, et al. Thresholds for focal ultrasonic lesions in rabbit kidney, liver and testicle. IEEE Trans Biomed Eng 1977; 24:393–6.

[13] Vallancien G, Harouni M, Veillon B, et al. Focused extracorporeal pyrotherapy: feasibility study in man. J Endourol 1992;6:173–80.

[14] Visioli AG, Rivens IH, ter Haar GR, et al. Preliminary results of a phase I dose escalation clinical trial using focused ultrasound in the treatment of localised tumours. Eur J Ultrasound 1999;9(1):11–8.

[15] Wu F, Chen WZ, Bai J, et al. Pathological changes in human malignant carcinoma treated with high-intensity focused ultrasound. Ultrasound Med Biol 2001;27(8):1099–106.

[16] Kohrmann KU, Michel MS, Gaa J, et al. High intensity focused ultrasound as noninvasive therapy for multilocal renal cell carcinoma: case study and review of the literature. J Urol 2002;167(6):2397–403.

[17] Chapelon JY, Ribault M, Vernier F, et al. Treatment of localized prostate cancer with transrectal high intensity focused ultrasound. Eur J Ultrasound 1999; 9(1):31–8.

[18] Sanghvi NT, Hawes RH. High-intensity focused ultrasound. Gastrointest Endosc Clin N Am 1994; 4(2):383–95.

[19] Hynynen K, Pomeroy O, Smith DN, et al. MR imaging-guided focused ultrasound surgery of fibroadenomas in the breast: a feasibility study. Radiology 2001;219(1):176–85.

[20] Gianfelice D, Khiat A, Amara M, et al. MR imaging-guided focused US ablation of breast cancer: histopathologic assessment of effectiveness—initial experience. Radiology 2003;227(3):849–55.

[21] Gianfelice DC, Mallouche H, Lepanto L, et al. MR-guided focused ultrasound ablation of primary breast neoplasms: works in progress. Radiology 1999;213(P):106–7.

[22] Cain CA, Umemura SA. Concentric-ring and sector vortex phased array applicators for ultrasound hyperthermia therapy. IEEE Trans Microw Theory Tech 1986;34:542–51.

[23] Ebbini ES, Cain CA. A spherical-section ultrasound phased array applicator for deep localized hyperthermia. IEEE Trans Biomed Eng 1991;38:634–43.

[24] Fan X, Hynynen K. A study of various parameters of spherically curved phased arrays for noninvasive ultrasound surgery. Phys Med Biol 1996;41:591–608.

[25] Hong W, VanBaren P, Ebbini ES, et al. Ultrasound surgery: comparison of strategies using phased array

systems. IEEE Trans Ultrason Ferroelectr Freq Contr 1996;43(6):1085.

[26] Fjield T, Hynynen K. The combined concentric-ring and sector-vortex phased array for MRI guided ultrasound surgery. IEEE Trans Ultrason Ferroelectr Freq Contr 1997;44(5):1157–67.

[27] Hynynen K, Clement GT, McDannold N, et al. 500-element ultrasound phased array system for noninvasive focal surgery of the brain: a preliminary rabbit study with ex vivo human skulls. Magn Reson Med 2004;52(1):100–7.

[28] Clement GT, Hynynen K. A non-invasive method for focusing ultrasound through the human skull. Phys Med Biol 2002;47(8):1219–36.

[29] Silverman SG, Sun MR, Tuncali K, et al. Three-dimensional assessment of MRI-guided percutaneous cryotherapy of liver metastases. Am J Roentgenol 2004;183(3):707–12.

[30] Jolesz FA, Bleier AR, Jakab P, et al. MR imaging of laser-tissue interactions. Radiology 1988;168: 249–53.

[31] Bleier AR, Jolesz FA, Cohen MS, et al. Real time magnetic resonance imaging of laser heat deposition in tissue. Magn Res Med 1991;21:132–7.

[32] Matsumoto R, Mulkern RV, Hushek SG, et al. Tissue temperature monitoring for thermal interventional therapy: comparison of TI-weighted MR sequences. J Mag Res Imaging 1994;4:65–70.

[33] McDannold NJ, King RL, Jolesz FA, et al. Usefulness of MR imaging-derived thermometry and dosimetry in determining the threshold for tissue damage induced by thermal surgery in rabbits. Radiology 2000;216(2):517–23.

[34] Lewin JS, Connell CF, Duerk JL, et al. Interactive MRI-guided radiofrequency interstitial thermal ablation of abdominal tumors: clinical trial for evaluation of safety and feasibility. J Mag Res Imaging 1998;8:40–5.

[35] Silverman SG, Tuncali K, Adams DF, et al. MR imaging-guided percutaneous cryotherapy of liver tumors: initial experience. Radiology 2000;217: 657–64.

[36] Morikawa S, Inubushi T, Kurumi Y, et al. Feasibility of respiratory triggering for MR-guided microwave ablation of liver tumors under general anesthesia. Cardiovasc Intervent Radiol 2004;27(4):370–3.

[37] Harms SE. MR-guided minimally invasive procedures. Magn Reson Imaging Clin N Am 2001;9: 381–92.

[38] Jolesz FA, Hynynen K. Magnetic resonance image-guided focused ultrasound surgery. Cancer J 2002; 8(Suppl 1):S100–12.

[39] Jolesz F, Hynynen K. Focused ultrasound. In: DeVite VT, Hellman S, Rosenberg SA, editors. Cancer, principles and practice of oncology. 7th edition. Philadelphia: Lipincott Williams and Wilkins; 2005. p. 2883–91.

[40] Parker DL. Applications of NMR imaging in hyperthermia: an evaluation of the potential for localized tissue heating and noninvasive temperature monitoring. IEEE Trans Biomed Eng 1984;31(1):161–7.

[41] Le Bihan D, Delannoy J, Levin RL. Temperature mapping with MR imaging of molecular diffusion: application to hyperthermia. Radiology 1989;171(3): 853–7.

[42] Bleier AR, Jolesz FA, Cohen MS, et al. Real-time magnetic resonance imaging of laser heat deposition in tissue. Magn Reson Med 1991;21(1):132–7.

[43] Kuroda K, Miki Y, Nakagawa N, et al. Noninvasive temperature measurement by means of NMR parameters—use of proton chemical shift with spectral estimation technique. Med Biol Eng Comput 1991;29:902.

[44] Vogl TJ, Straub R, Eichler K, et al. Malignant liver tumors treated with MR imaging-guided laser-induced thermotherapy: experience with complications in 899 patients (2,520 lesions). Radiology 2002;225(2):367–77.

[45] Kuroda K, Chung AH, Hynynen K, et al. Calibration of water proton chemical shift with temperature for noninvasive temperature imaging during focused ultrasound surgery. J Magn Reson Imaging 1998; 8(1):175–81.

[46] Ishihara Y, Calderon A, Watanabe H, et al. A precise and fast temperature mapping using water proton chemical shift. Magn Reson Med 1995;34(6): 814–23.

[47] Hynynen K, Vykhodtseva NI, Chung AH, et al. Thermal effects of focused ultrasound on the brain: determination with MR imaging. Radiology 1997; 204(1):247–53.

[48] Chung AH, Jolesz FA, Hynynen K. Thermal dosimetry of a focused ultrasound beam in vivo by magnetic resonance imaging. Med Phys 1999;26(9): 2017–26.

[49] Vimeux FC, de Zwart JA, Palussiere J, et al. Real-time control of focused ultrasound heating based on rapid MR thermometry. Invest Radiol 1999; 34(3):190–3.

[50] Smith NB, Merilees NK, Hynynen K, et al. Control system for an MRI compatible intracavitary ultrasound array for thermal treatment of prostate disease. Int J Hyperthermia 2001;17(3):271–82.

[51] Graham SJ, Chen L, Leitch M, et al. Quantifying tissue damage due to focused ultrasound heating observed by MRI. Magn Reson Med 1999;41(2):321–8.

[52] McDannold NJ, King RL, Jolesz FA, et al. Usefulness of MR imaging-derived thermometry and dosimetry in determining the threshold for tissue damage induced by thermal surgery in rabbits. Radiology 2000;216(2):517–23.

[53] Chen L, Wansapura JP, Heit G, et al. Study of laser ablation in the in vivo rabbit brain with MR thermometry. J Magn Reson Imaging 2002;16(2): 147–52.

[54] McDannold N, Vykhodtseva N, Jolesz FA, et al. MRI investigation of the threshold for thermally induced blood-brain barrier disruption and brain

tissue damage in the rabbit brain. Magn Reson Med 2004;51(5):913–23.

[55] Hazle JD, Stafford RJ, Price RE. Magnetic resonance imaging-guided focused ultrasound thermal therapy in experimental animal models: correlation of ablation volumes with pathology in rabbit muscle and VX2 tumors. J Magn Reson Imaging 2002; 15(2):185–94.

[56] Stafford RJ, Price RE, Diederich CJ, et al. Interleaved echo-planar imaging for fast multiplanar magnetic resonance temperature imaging of ultrasound thermal ablation therapy. J Magn Reson Imaging 2004;20(4):706–14.

[57] McDannold N, Martin H, Jolesz FA, et al. Long-term survival after focused ultrasound surgery in tumors guided by MRI: preliminary results. Presented at the 10th Scientific Meeting and Exhibition of the International Society for Magnetic Resonance in Medicine. Honolulu (HI), 2002.

[58] Vigen KK, Daniel BL, Pauly JM, et al. Triggered, navigated, multi-baseline method for proton resonance frequency temperature mapping with respiratory motion. Magn Reson Med 2003;50(5): 1003–10.

[59] Kuroda K, Oshio K, Chung AH, et al. Temperature mapping using the water proton chemical shift: a chemical shift selective phase mapping method. Magn Reson Med 1997;38(5):845–51.

[60] Kuroda K, Mulkern RV, Oshio K, et al. Temperature mapping using the water proton chemical shift: self-referenced method with echo-planar spectroscopic imaging. Magn Reson Med 2000;43(2):220–5.

[61] Rieke V, Vigen KK, Sommer G. Referenceless PRF shift thermometry. Magn Reson Med 2004;51(6): 1223–31.

[62] Sapareto SA, Dewey WC. Thermal dose determination in cancer therapy. Int J Radiat Oncol Biol Phys 1984;10(6):787–800.

[63] Hirose M, Kacher DF, Smith DN, et al. Feasibility of MR imaging-guided breast lumpectomy for malignant tumors in a 0.5-T open-configuration MR imaging system. Acad Radiol 2002;9(8):933–41.

[64] Huber PE, Jenne JW, Rastert R, et al. A new noninvasive approach in breast cancer therapy using magnetic resonance imaging-guided focused ultrasound surgery. Cancer Res 2001;61(23):8441–7.

[65] Tempany CM, Stewart EA, McDannold N, et al. MR imaging-guided focused ultrasound surgery of uterine leiomyomas: a feasibility study. Radiology 2003;226(3):897–905.

[66] Spies JB, Coyne K, Guaou N, et al. The UFS-QOL, a new disease-specific symptom and health-related quality of life questionnaire for leiomyomata. Obstet Gynecol 2002;99(2):290–300.

[67] Stewart EA, Gedroyc WM, Tempany CM, et al. Focused ultrasound treatment of uterine fibroid tumors: safety and feasibility of a noninvasive thermoablative technique. Am J Obstet Gynecol 2003; 189(1):48–54.

[68] Hindley J, Gedroyc WM, Regan L, et al. MRI guidance of focused ultrasound therapy of uterine fibroids: early results. AJR Am J Roentgenol 2004; 183(6):1713–9.

[69] McDannold N, King RL, Hynynen K. MRI monitoring of heating produced by ultrasound absorption in the skull: in vivo study in pigs. Magn Reson Med 2004;51(5):1061–5.

[70] Hynynen K, McDannold N, Vykhodtseva N, et al. Non-invasive opening of BBB by focused ultrasound. Acta Neurochir Suppl 2003;86:555–8.

[71] Sheikov N, McDannold N, Vykhodtseva N, et al. Cellular mechanisms of the blood-brain barrier opening induced by ultrasound in presence of microbubbles. Ultrasound Med Biol 2004;30: 979–89.

[72] Hynynen K, McDannold N, Sheikov N, et al. Local and reversible blood-brain barrier disruption by noninvasive focused ultrasound at frequencies suitable for trans-skull sonications. Neuroimage 2005; 24(1):12–20.

[73] Rome C, Couillaud F, Moonen CT. Spatial and temporal control of expression of therapeutic genes using heat shock protein promoters. Methods 2005;35(2):188–98.

[74] Magin RL, Niesman MR. Temperature-dependent drug release from large unilamellar liposomes. Cancer Drug Deliv 1984;1(2):109–17.

[75] Needham D, Dewhirst MW. The development and testing of a new temperature-sensitive drug delivery system for the treatment of solid tumors. Adv Drug Deliv Rev 2001;53(3):285–305.

[76] Viglianti BL, Abraham SA, Michelich CR, et al. In vivo monitoring of tissue pharmacokinetics of liposome/drug using MRI: illustration of targeted delivery. Magn Reson Med 2004;51(6):1153–62.

[77] Vykhodtseva NI, Hynynen K, Damianou C. Histologic effects of high intensity pulsed ultrasound exposure with subharmonic emission in rabbit brain in vivo. Ultrasound Med Biol 1995;21(7): 969–79.

[78] Mesiwala AH, Farrell L, Wenzel HJ, et al. High-intensity focused ultrasound selectively disrupts the blood-brain barrier in vivo. Ultrasound Med Biol 2002;28(3):389–400.

[79] Umemura S, Yumita N, Nishigaki R, et al. Sonochemical activation of hematoporphyrin: a potential modality for cancer treatment. Presented at the 1989 IEEE Ultrasonics Symposium. Montreal (Canada), October 3–6, 1989.

[80] Siegel RJ, Cumberland DC, Myler RK, et al. Percutaneous ultrasonic angioplasty: initial clinical experience. Lancet 1989;2(8666):772–4.

[81] Rosenschein U, Bernstein JJ, DiSegni E, et al. Experimental ultrasonic angioplasty: disruption of atherosclerotic plaques and thrombi in vitro and arterial recanalization in vivo. IEEE Trans Ultrason Ferroelectr Freq Contr 1990;43(6): 1043–105.

[82] Kim HJ, Greenleaf JF, Kinnick RR, et al. Ultra-sound-mediated transfection of mammalian cells. Hum Gene Ther 1996;7:1339–46.

[83] Bednarski MD, Lee JW, Yuh EL, et al. In vivo target-specific delivery of genetic materials with MR-guided focused ultrasound. Ultrasonics 1998; 30(5):325–30.

[84] Amabile PG, Waugh JM, Lewis TN, et al. High-efficiency endovascular gene delivery via therapeutic ultrasound. J Am Coll Cardiol 2001;37(7):1975–80.

[85] Huber PE, Pfisterer P. In vitro and in vivo transfection of plasmid DNA in the Dunning prostate tumor R3327–AT1 is enhanced by focused ultrasound. Gene Ther 2000;7(17):1516–25.

[86] Unger EC, Hersh E, Vannan M, et al. Gene delivery using ultrasound contrast agents. Echocardiography 2001;18(4):355–61.

[87] Kondo I, Ohmori K, Oshita A, et al. Treatment of acute myocardial infarction by hepatocyte growth factor gene transfer: the first demonstration of myocardial transfer of a "functional" gene using ultrasonic microbubble destruction. J Am Coll Cardiol 2004;44(3):644–53.

[88] Huber PE, Mann MJ, Melo LG, et al. Focused ultrasound (HIFU) induces localized enhancement of

reporter gene expression in rabbit carotid artery. Gene Ther 2003;10(18):1600–7.

[89] Miller DL, Quddus J. Diagnostic ultrasound activation of contrast agent gas bodies induces capillary rupture in mice. Proc Natl Acad Sci U S A 2000; 97(18):10179–84.

[90] Unger EC, Hersh E, Vannan M, et al. Local drug and gene delivery through microbubbles. Prog Cardiovasc Dis 2001;44(1):45–54.

[91] Jolesz FA, Hynynen K, McDannold N, et al. Noninvasive thermal ablation of hepatocellular carcinoma by using magnetic resonance imaging-guided focused ultrasound. Gastroenterology 2004;127(5 Suppl 1):S242–7.

[92] Smith NB, Merrilees NK, Dahleh M, et al. Control system for an MRI compatible intracavitary ultrasound array for thermal treatment of prostate disease. Int J Hyperthermia 2001;17(3):271–82.

[93] McDannold N, Moss M, Killiany R, et al. MRI-guided focused ultrasound surgery in the brain: tests in a primate model. Magn Reson Med 2003;49(6). 1188–91.

[94] Hynynen K, Colucci V, Chung A, et al. Noninvasive arterial occlusion using MRI-guided focused ultrasound. Ultrasound Med Biol 1996;22(8):1071–7.

ELSEVIER
SAUNDERS

Magn Reson Imaging Clin N Am
13 (2005) 561–581

**MAGNETIC
RESONANCE
IMAGING CLINICS**
of North America

Radiofrequency Thermal Ablation: The Role of MR Imaging in Guiding and Monitoring Tumor Therapy

Sherif Gamal Nour, MD[a,b,c],*, Jonathan S. Lewin, MD[d,e]

[a]Department of Radiology, University Hospitals of Cleveland, 11100 Euclid Avenue, Cleveland, OH 44106, USA
[b]Departments of Radiology and Biomedical Engineering, Case Western Reserve University School of Medicine,
319 Wickenden Building, Cleveland, OH 44106, USA
[c]Department of Diagnostic Radiology, Cairo University Hospitals, Cairo, Egypt
[d]Department of Radiology, The Johns Hopkins Hospital, 600 North Wolfe Street,
Baltimore, MD 21287, USA
[e]The Russell H. Morgan Department of Radiology and Radiological Science,
The Johns Hopkins University School of Medicine, 720 Rutland Avenue, Baltimore, MD 21205, USA

Advances in tumor therapy continue to explore numerous exciting fields, including gene therapy [1–3]; targeted drug delivery monitoring [4,5]; control of angiogenesis [6]; and the delivery of various forms of thermal energy, such as radiofrequency (RF) [7,8], laser [9], focused ultrasound [10], microwave [11], and cryotherapy [12] for tumor ablation. Innovations in medical imaging, particularly in MR imaging and its subset of interventional applications, represent an integral part of this continued progress of oncologic therapy beyond the traditional treatment options. Although the ability to image vital processes at the cellular and molecular levels is promisingly progressing in the development phase, detection of the instant tissue changes associated with thermal damage is a reality that constitutes the basis for using MR imaging to monitor thermal ablation procedures.

This article briefly describes the principle of radiofrequency ablation (RFA), discuss the rationale and technical aspects of performing ablation procedures under MR imaging, introduces the setup and equipment used for MR-guided RFA, explains the tissue basis of imaging thermally induced necrosis, and illustrates the scope of the current applications and future directions in the field of MR-guided thermal ablation.

Radiofrequency thermal ablation: the principle

The idea of using direct heat to eradicate tumors dates back to the early Egyptian and Greek medical scriptures in which superficial tumors were subjected to cautery [13]. RFA entails the deployment of RF current into the target tissue through an electrode connected to an RF generator. As the current flows from the source to the return (grounding pad) electrode placed on the patient's skin, the ions in the tissues surrounding the monopolar source electrode begin to agitate, resulting in frictional (resistive) heating with consequent formation of a zone of coagulation necrosis surrounding the RF electrode tip (Figs. 1 and 2). Reproducible tissue destruction has been observed in a variety of tissues. In contrast to cryoablation, where malignant cells are more resistant to lethal damage from freezing compared with normal cells, cancer cells demonstrate increased sensitivity to hyperthermic damage over that of normal tissues [14,15]. Furthermore, studies in human subjects and animal models have shown that thermal ablation zone shape and size can be controlled through the electrode design as well as the duration and magnitude of the energy delivered [16–20]. Energy deposition is easy to control with RFA and allows gradual tissue heating [16]. The presence of

* Corresponding author. Department of Radiology, University Hospitals of Cleveland, 11100 Euclid Avenue, Cleveland, OH 44106.
E-mail address: nour@uhrad.com (S.G. Nour).

1064-9689/05/$ - see front matter © 2005 Elsevier Inc. All rights reserved.
doi:10.1016/j.mric.2005.04.007

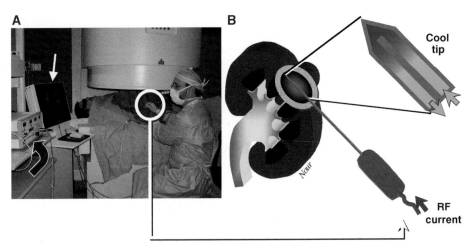

Fig. 1. Illustration of the typical paradigm used for MR-guided and monitored RF-tumor ablation. (*A*) The interventional MR imaging suite setup during thermal ablation procedures. The open MR imaging system configuration facilitates proper access to the patient during the procedure. The in-room RF-shielded liquid crystal display monitor (*straight arrow*) equipped with a computer mouse and foot pedal (not shown), along with the ability to control fast gradient echo sequences from the scanner side, facilitates interactive near–real-time navigation of the RF electrode into the targeted tumor in a safe and time-efficient manner. The RF generator (*curved arrow*) is also operated at the scanner side. (*B*) Once the electrode is positioned within the targeted renal tumor, the RF generator is switched on to start the ablation procedure while pumping iced water through special channels within the RF electrode shaft to prevent charring at the electrode-tumor interface that would stop further RF deposition and interfere with adequate tumor destruction. The development of the ablation zone is monitored through intermittent MR imaging (fast spin echo [FSE] T2-weighted and/or FSE short tau inversion recovery) during the ablation session. (*From* Lewin JS, Nour SG, Connell CF, et al. Phase II clinical trial of interactive MR-guided interstitial radiofrequency thermal ablation of primary kidney tumors: initial experience. Radiology 2004;232(3):837; with permission.)

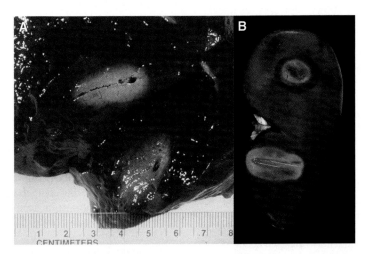

Fig. 2. Gross pathologic specimens demonstrate bisected zones of coagulation necrosis after RFA within rabbit's liver (*A*) and porcine kidney (*B*). The pale coagulated tissues are surrounded by darker rims of reactive tissue response consisting of hyperemia, hemorrhage, and edema. RF electrode tracts are visible in the centers of the ablated zones and usually demonstrate some hemorrhage and edema as well. (*A, Modified from* Boaz TL, Lewin JS, Chung YC, et al. MR monitoring of MR-guided radiofrequency thermal ablation of normal liver in an animal model. J Magn Reson Imaging 1998;8(1):65; with permission. *B, Modified from* Merkle EM, Shonk JR, Duerk JL, et al. MR-guided RF thermal ablation of the kidney in a porcine model. AJR Am J Roentgenol 1999;173(3):649; with permission.)

a thermistor in the electrode tip gives continuous temperature feedback, and impedance measurements provide another parameter related to tissue changes at the ablation site. These features are of particular importance when destroying tumors adjacent to neurovascular structures. Unlike radiation therapy but like other thermal ablative therapies, interstitial RFA can be repeated multiple times without concern for the cumulative dose.

Rationale for image guidance

Although RFA of localized malignancies has been practiced under direct surgical [21,22] and laparoscopic [23] visualization, much of the excitement over expanding the therapeutic uses of RF energy beyond the neurosurgical and cardiac fields has been provoked by the advancements in imaging technology. The ability to perform thermal treatment of cancer percutaneously under image guidance has changed RFA from an adjuvant surgical technique to a minimally invasive alternative to surgery that is more suited to the large sector of poor surgical candidates. The primary contribution of image guidance to needle-based thermal treatment is securing safe and precise electrode delivery into the targeted pathologic finding. Not surprisingly, the ideal electrode trajectory during actual procedure execution is sometimes significantly different from that suggested on the preprocedural imaging data because of the frequent shift of anatomic structures when using modified patient positions during treatment. In addition, the guided approach provides updated information regarding the development of new pathologic conditions that may alter treatment decision making, such as the appearance of new tumor foci or the accumulation of ascites. Once the RF electrode is successfully delivered into the targeted tumor, image guidance adds to the efficacy of the procedure by optimizing the electrode position within the pathologic tissue and by showing the thickness of intact tissue between the targeted tumor and adjacent vital structures, such as the gallbladder, bowel loops, or renal pelvis, thereby enabling confident inclusion of an adequate "safety margin" to the ablated volume.

Role of MR imaging

RFA procedures can be performed under ultrasound (US), CT, or MR imaging guidance, all of which usually allow the accurate placement of the RF electrode into the targeted tumor. The major contribution of MR imaging to interstitial RF thermotherapy, however, is its outstanding ability to monitor the zone of thermal tissue destruction during the procedure, and thus to provide real-time guidance for deposition of the RF energy. Through MR imaging monitoring, thermal ablation zone size and configuration can be directly controlled by the operator and adjusted during the procedure to compensate for deviations from the preoperative predictions and to define the treatment end point without moving the patient from the interventional suite (Fig. 3). This is an attribute of MR imaging that cannot be reliably duplicated by any other currently used imaging modality. MR imaging is exceptionally well suited for this purpose because of the absence of ionizing radiation, excellent soft tissue discrimination, spatial resolution, multiplanar capabilities, and its sensitivity to temperature and blood flow [24–26]. This not only permits accurate tumor destruction, including the margins, but extends the application of RFA to the safe destruction of tumor within the visceral organs and adjacent to vital neurovascular structures. Furthermore, MR imaging is not hampered by the difficulties caused by changes in tissue imaging characteristics brought about by RFA, as has been described by some authors using US guidance [27]. During RFA, gas microbubbles begin to accumulate in the tissues, thus creating progressively increasing echogenic areas that cast posterior acoustic shadowing, which masks the exact margins of the tumor being ablated under US guidance (Fig. 4). When monitored using CT, the area of induced tissue necrosis appears as an area of ill-defined hypodensity on the immediate postablation images and becomes better defined only on delayed follow-up CT scans (Fig. 5).

Other than its ability to define the treatment end point during ablation procedures, MR guidance is also advantageous in certain situations, such as when a tumor is not adequately visualized on US or CT; when the complex anatomic location of a tumor renders multiplanar image guidance a safer approach, such as in liver dome lesions (Fig. 6); and when a tumor demonstrates transient arterial enhancement with early washout, such as in hepatocellular carcinoma and hypervascular metastases, thereby precluding image guidance for RFA. In the latter case, the high soft tissue contrast offered by MR imaging can be used to assign tissue landmarks that indicate the location of a transiently enhancing lesion.

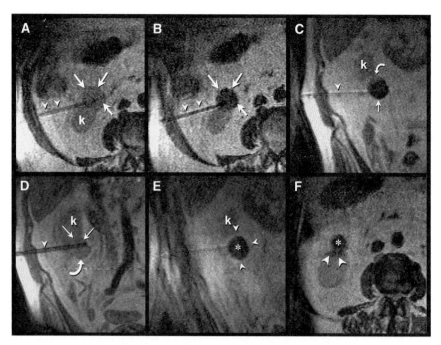

Fig. 3. MR imaging scans obtained intermittently during RF-interstitial thermal ablation of an exophytic anterior lower pole right-sided clear-cell carcinoma in a 75-year-old male patient. (*A*) Transverse fast spin echo (FSE) T2-weighted image (repetition time [TR]/echo time [TE]: 3465/105 milliseconds, number of signal averages [NSA] = 4, echo train length [ETL] = 17) after MR-guided insertion of electrode (*arrowheads*) but before ablation demonstrates intermediate-signal anterior exophytic tumor (*arrows*) involving the lower pole of the right kidney (k). (*B*) Transverse FSE T2-weighted imaging scan (TR/TE: 3465/105 milliseconds, NSA = 4, ETL = 17) after two ablation cycles lasting 15 and 6 minutes at the same electrode location demonstrates complete thermal damage of the tumor at this transverse level as indicated by the development of uniformly low signal (*arrows*) around the needle electrode (*arrowheads*). (*C*) When evaluated on coronal FSE T2-weighted imaging (TR/TE: 1856/105 milliseconds, NSA = 4, ETL = 17) acquired immediately after the transverse images shown in (*B*), most of the tumor is treated as indicated by the development of hypointensity (*straight arrow*) around the needle electrode (*arrowhead*), but a residual untreated portion of the tumor is detected by the intermediate signal crescent (*curved arrow*) seen capping the ablation zone near the junction of the tumor with the kidney (k). Transverse images also documented an untreated zone in a superoposterior location. (*D*) Coronal fast imaging with steady-state precession (FISP) image (TR/TE: 17.8/8.1 milliseconds, NSA = 3, flip angle of 90°) demonstrates the RF electrode position (*arrowhead*) after interactive repositioning superoposteriorly into residual tumor tissue (*straight arrows*). Guidance into residual tumor was based on localization from T2-weighted images (*C*) and was confirmed with additional FSE T2-weighted images before the next ablation cycle, because the treated tumor (*curved arrow*) does not appear hypointense on FISP images. When mirrored fast imaging with steady-state precession images are used for guidance, as was routinely done later in the trial, the ablation zone could be defined on guidance images in addition to the confirmatory FSE T2-weighted study. A third ablation cycle was performed at this location for 12 additional minutes. (*E*) Coronal FSE T2-weighted image (TR/TE: 1898/105 milliseconds, NSA = 4, ETL = 17) after the third RF application reveals complete replacement of the tumor by hypointense thermally damaged tissue (*) surrounded by a faint hyperintense rim of reactive tissue changes (*arrowheads*). (*F*) Transverse FSE T2-weighted image (TR/TE: 1898/105 milliseconds, NSA = 4, ETL = 17) after the third RF application shows a hypointense ablation zone completely replacing the superior portion of the tumor (*) and documents adequate treatment of a margin of normal kidney (*arrowheads*). (*From* Lewin JS, Nour SG, Connell CF, et al. Phase II clinical trial of interactive MR-guided interstitial radiofrequency thermal ablation of primary kidney tumors: initial experience. Radiology 2004;232(3):839; with permission.)

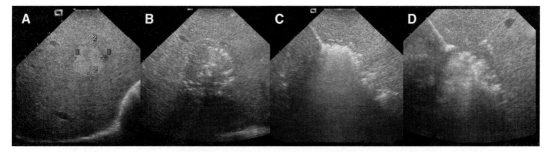

Fig. 4. (*A*) Serial US images obtained during an US-guided radiofrequency ablation of a metastatic lesion within the right lobe of the liver. (*B–D*) Echogenic gas microbubbles form and progressively accumulate in the tissue being treated over the course of the ablation procedure, creating acoustic shadowing that interferes with the visualization of tumor margins, thereby generating uncertainty regarding the exact boundaries of the area of necrosis.

Setup and equipment for MR-guided radiofrequency ablation

Performing RFA procedures under MR imaging guidance involves the same basic requirements for an interventional MR imaging suite as described elsewhere in this issue, including the ability to access the patient through an open-magnet design, the ability to operate the scanner and review images at the patient's bedside, and the ability to implement rapid imaging paradigms to achieve near–real-time interactive guidance (see Fig. 1).

During MR-guided ablation procedures, an RF generator should be kept well outside the 200-G line to prevent magnetic attraction of the metallic components within the generator but can still be conveniently located close to the magnet in the low-field environment. Under higher magnetic field strengths, the RF generator needs to be moved further from the scanner, where special extension cables for the RF electrodes and for the grounding pads should be provided by the RFA system vendor.

MR imaging–compatible RF electrodes have recently been made available, such as the titanium electrodes from Valleylab (Boulder, Colorado; formerly Radionics) and the nitinol electrodes manufactured by RITA Medical Systems (Mountain View, California). The former manufacturer provides electrodes that can be continuously cooled with circulating iced water inside the electrode shaft to reduce charring at the electrode-tissue interface, thereby maximizing the ablation size. The latter manufacturer provides electrodes with multiple active tines that can be deployed in the tissue to produce larger ablation

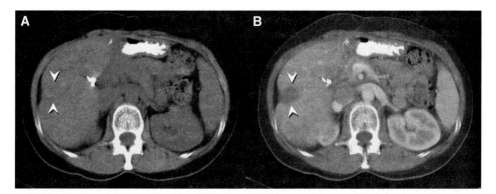

Fig. 5. Follow-up CT scan of a radiofrequency ablation zone within segment 5 of the right lobe of the liver. The zone of coagulation necrosis is seen as a well-defined hypodense area (*arrowheads, A*) that does not enhance on postcontrast scans (*arrowheads, B*). Only chronic ablation zones demonstrate this well-circumscribed appearance on contrast-enhanced CT scans, whereas acute zones of ablation appear less defined. Note the capsular depression overlying the ablation zone, denoting tissue retraction associated with chronicity of the lesion.

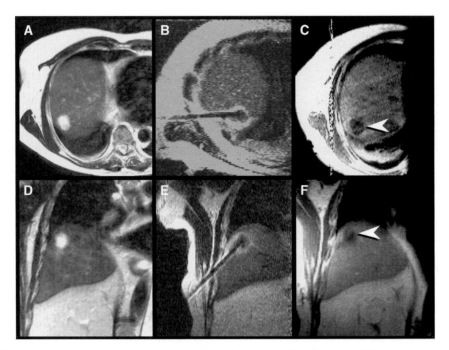

Fig. 6. Hepatic dome metastasis. Turbo spin echo T2-weighted axial (*A*) and coronal (*D*) images of the abdomen demonstrate hyperintense metastasis in the posterior dome of the right lobe of the liver. Turbo spin echo T2-weighted oblique axial-sagittal (*B*) and coronal (*E*) images with similar parameters along the course of the MR imaging–compatible RF electrode confirm the electrode position within the tumor. The effects of RF-interstitial thermal ablation (RF-ITA) are noted as marked hypointensity developed around the active distal 3 cm of the electrode, surrounded by a rim of hyperintensity reflecting edema and (*arrowheads*) hyperemia. After RF-ITA, contrast-enhanced T1-weighted axial (*C*) and coronal (*F*) images demonstrate hypointensity corresponding to an avascular area of tumor necrosis. This approximates the volume of the originally identified tumor, along with a small margin of surrounding normal parenchyma. (*From* Lewin JS, Connell CF, Duerk JL, et al. Interactive MR-guided radiofrequency interstitial thermal ablation of abdominal tumors: clinical trial for evaluation of safety and feasibility. J Magn Reson Imaging 1998;8(1):46; with permission.)

zones. The shaft of the "Semiflex" RF electrode provided by RITA Medical Systems can also be bent to improve the capability for electrode navigation in the rather tight space usually available during interventional MR imaging procedures (Fig. 7).

Susceptibility artifacts from the grounding pads are usually of no concern during intraprocedural imaging because they are typically placed outside the field of interest (eg, on the thighs) during intra-abdominal ablation procedures. Additionally, the interference between the RF generator and the MR imager can be eliminated via the use of a switching circuit that allows simultaneous imaging during RFA [28] or by simply acquiring interrupted intraprocedural imaging in alternation with the ablation cycles. In the latter case, disconnecting the RF generator power plug during imaging is recommended to avoid RF artifacts.

Intraprocedural MR imaging guidance and monitoring

An MR-guided RFA procedure typically has three phases: the guidance, confirmation, and ablation phases.

Guidance phase

The process of guiding an MR imaging–compatible RF electrode into a targeted tumor under MR fluoroscopy is similar in principle to performing an MR-guided biopsy or aspiration procedure and requires attention to the same user-defined imaging parameters and electrode trajectory decisions as described elsewhere in this issue because they can significantly affect electrode visibility and thereby the accuracy and safety of the procedure. RF electrode guidance is typically performed using the freehand technique, although other modes of MR imaging guidance are technically applicable.

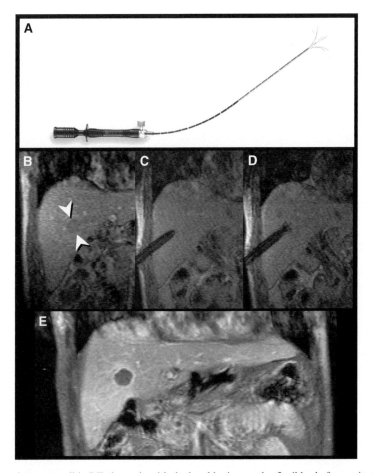

Fig. 7. (*A*) MR imaging–compatible RF electrode with deployable tines and a flexible shaft permits liberal navigation within the usually tight space available during interventional MR imaging procedures (Starbust Semiflex; RITA Medical Systems, Mountain View, California). (*B*) Coronal fast low-angle shot images demonstrates a faintly hypointense colorectal metastasis (*arrowheads*) at the junction of the right and left lobes of the liver. The RF electrode is being inserted into the liver with the tines retracted (*C*), followed by partial deployment of the tines (*D*). (*E*) Coronal postablation gadolinium-enhanced spin echo T1-weighted image demonstrates the hypointense area of induced necrosis with an enhancing marginal rim. (*A*, Courtesy of RITA Medical Systems, Fremont, CA; with permission.)

With the patient under conscious sedation, an RF electrode of the appropriate exposed tip(s) length is percutaneously placed within the tissue or organ of interest and advanced into the targeted tumor under MR "fluoroscopic" guidance, usually using short repetition time (TR)/ short echo time (TE) gradient echo sequences, such as fast imaging with steady-state precession (FISP) (see Fig. 3), true-FISP, mirrored fast imaging with steady-state precession (PSIF), or fast low-angle shot (FLASH). The choice of these sequences is based on the best tumor conspicuity as evaluated on a case-by-case basis. This guidance phase consists of continuous imaging with automated sequential acquisition, reconstruction, and in-room display of multiple sets of contiguous parallel thin-section slices in two orthogonal scan planes oriented along the shaft of the electrode. We typically use sets of three contiguous 5-mm thin slices centered on the electrode shaft to detect and correct slight trajectory deviations during RF electrode navigation.

Confirmation phase

Once the RF electrode is delivered into the targeted tumor, we confirm the electrode tip position in at least two planes using the higher

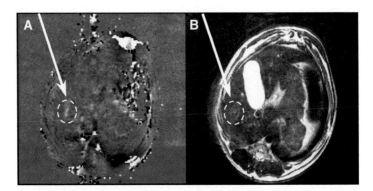

Fig. 8. Phase maps and turbo spin echo magnitude image during thermal ablation. MR imaging parameters, including T1, T2, diffusion, and the resonant frequency of the protons, vary with temperature. (*A*) In these images, the water proton resonant frequency method is used to generate images that can be used quantitatively to measure temperature. Here, the image gray scale is proportional to the temperature in the canine liver undergoing thermal ablation (*arrow*). (*B*) Although the conventional MR imaging scan shows edema and coagulative necrosis at the site of the ablation (*arrow*), no direct assessment of temperature is possible. (*From* Chung YC, Duerk JL, Shankaranarayanan A, et al. Temperature measurement using echo-shifted FLASH at low field for interventional MRI. J Magn Reson Imaging 1999;9(1):138–45; with permission.)

spatial resolution yet relatively lengthy turbo spin echo (TSE) scans before commencing the actual ablation phase (see Fig. 3).

Ablation phase

When the electrode tip is confirmed to be adequately placed within the targeted tumor, the deployment of RF energy can be confidently instituted. Using a standard nonperfused electrode, interstitial RFA is performed at an electrode tip temperature of $90°C \pm 2°C$. Ablation zone length is dependent on the exposed tip length, whereas the ablation zone diameter is limited to approximately 2 cm [29]. This limited ability to achieve a larger ablation zone diameter is thought to be attributable to charring at the electrode-tissue interface, which, in turn, impairs energy transfer. Using the water-cooled electrode system (Cool-tip; Valleylab), a pump is used to circulate chilled water inside the electrode shaft to cool the tip temperature to 10°C to 20°C, thereby preventing charring at the interface and allowing energy to be transmitted further from the source electrode. Ablation zones can be created with this electrode design that would have required multiple ablations with intervening electrode repositioning using a standard RF electrode. To maximize the area of the resulting necrosis, we usually combine the use of the Cool-tip electrode with pulsed application of RF energy, where brief periods of current interruption are automatically triggered when

tissue impedance rises beyond a preset threshold. Again, the intention is to prevent the tissue charring and cavitation that lead to the cessation of RF current deposition. At the conclusion of ablation sessions using Cool-tip electrodes, a second application of RF energy at the same electrode position may be necessary without cooling once the desired margins are achieved so as to destroy the area adjacent to the cooled electrode. A practical method to test the necessity for such additional RF application is to continue measuring the RF electrode tip temperature for 2 minutes after the RF power and water-cooled circulation have been turned off. We reablate "the center of the doughnut" if its temperature falls below 60°C before 2 minutes have elapsed.

Other methods to create a large ablation zone by electrode insertion include the use of a cluster of three straight electrodes (Valleylab) or the use of an electrode with multiple expandable tines, where the tines can be deployed to form a virtual sphere of a small diameter (eg, 2 cm) as indicated on the shaft of the electrode. RF energy is then deployed until the targeted temperature is achieved; at that time, the electrode tines are pushed further to the next larger sphere position (eg, 3 cm) and energy is deployed again. MR imaging–compatible versions of this electrode (Starburst MRI and Starbust Semiflex; RITA Medical Systems) that allow the creation of up to 5-cm ablation zones are available (see Fig. 7). The deployment of the active tines within the targeted tumor is, however, a more

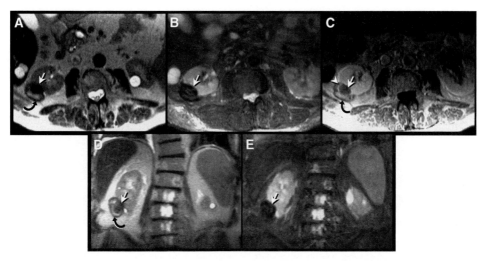

Fig. 9. Follow-up images at 20.6 months after RFA of renal cell carcinoma. Transverse (*A*) and coronal (*D*) half-Fourier acquisition single-shot turbo spin echo images (TR/TE: 4.4/90 milliseconds, number of signal averages [NSA] = 1). Transverse (*B*) and coronal (*E*) fast spin echo STIR images (TR/TE: 7172/60 milliseconds, NSA = 5). (*C*) Transverse contrast-enhanced spin echo T1-weighted images (TR/TE: 770/17 milliseconds, NSA = 3). Images demonstrate the typical long-term MR imaging follow-up appearance of ablation zones. Adequately treated tumors appear dark on all pulse sequences (*straight arrows, A–E*) and may display smooth marginal rim enhancement (benign periablational enhancement) (*arrowhead, C*) on postcontrast studies. The appearance of an ovoid hypointensity surrounded by hyperintensity and peripherally marginated by a thin hypointense rim as seen in (*A*), (*C*), and (*D*) results from perinephric fat included within the ablation zone that tends to regain its normal signal intensity, being surrounded by a fibrous capsule (*curved arrows, A, C, D*) that delineates the original extent of thermal injury. The fat suppression resulting from the STIR technique explains the lack of such appearance in (*B*) and (*E*). (*From* Lewin JS, Nour SG, Connell CF, et al. Phase II clinical trial of interactive MR-guided interstitial radiofrequency thermal ablation of primary kidney tumors: initial experience. Radiology 2004;232(3):842; with permission.)

complicated process compared with the insertion of a straight electrode, and careful review of the confirmation images should thus be performed before ablation to avoid situations like the tumor being pushed away rather than penetrated by the deployed tines; the tines being clustered together or unevenly deployed; or one of the tines extending into an undesirable location, such as close to the colon or gallbladder.

The ablation time usually ranges from 6 to 20 minutes at each electrode location before repositioning for larger tumors. The exact duration of an individual session is based on the MR imaging monitoring during that session, however, so as to achieve the maximal area of tissue necrosis expected for the RF electrode in use.

Electrode repositioning into persistent foci of a high-signal tumor, as detected on intraprocedural T2-weighted and short tau inversion recovery (STIR) images, is performed in the scanner under continuous MR imaging guidance in an interactive manner similar to that used for initial electrode placement (see Fig. 3). The "guide-confirm-ablate" sequence is repeated until the induced thermal ablation zone is noted to encompass the entire tumor and a small cuff of normal adjacent tissue or when the developing thermal ablation zone approaches adjacent vital structures. The RF electrode is then withdrawn, and repeat images are obtained with the addition of gadopentetate dimeglumine–enhanced T1-weighted images to confirm the final extent of devitalized tissue and exclude complications (see Fig. 6).

After the ablation and postprocedure scanning, the patient is usually observed overnight before being discharged the following morning at our institution, as part of our clinical trial protocol. For many patients with uncomplicated procedures, discharge after 5 or 6 hours of observation should suffice.

MR imaging of tissue necrosis

The ability to visualize the effects of thermal damage around the electrode tip directly, to detect

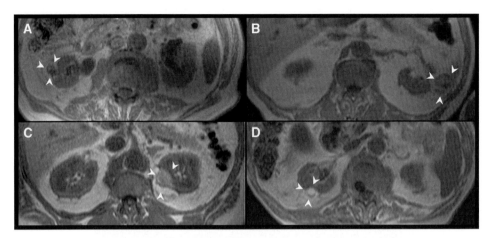

Fig. 10. T1-weighted in-phase gradient echo images of four different ablated renal cell carcinomas (*arrowheads, A–D*) demonstrate the spectrum of possible MR imaging signal characteristics on high-field (1.5 T) scans. Thermal ablation zones may appear hypointense (*A*), isointense (*B*), or hyperintense (*C*) on high-field gradient echo in-phase imaging. (*From* Merkle EM, Nour SG, Lewin JS. MR imaging follow-up after percutaneous radiofrequency ablation of renal cell carcinoma: findings in eighteen patients during first 6 months. Radiology 2005;235(3):1068; with permission.)

inadequately treated foci of the tumor, and to reposition the RF electrode into these areas during therapy interactively are central features for using MR imaging to guide and monitor RFA procedures because they enable treatment of the entire tumor on a single-visit basis while minimizing the risk of complications from unduly aggressive therapy. This manner of controlled ablation is different from the reported US- or CT-guided ablations [30,31], where the duration of the RF application at a given electrode location is based on the manufacturer's recommendations and the number of RF electrode insertions required to treat a given tumor is based on a subjective estimate reflecting the interventionalist's experience with the size and shape of an individual tumor. As such, residual tumors seen on follow-up imaging and necessitating further ablation with up to a total of four visits are not infrequent after US- and CT-guided RFA [30].

The relation of MR imaging signal intensity change to tissue temperature is a complex phenomenon, and although precise MR imaging measurement of temperature is difficult, temperature-sensitive MR imaging sequences have been developed to enable accurate on-line monitoring of heat deposition (Fig. 8) [32–34]. Conversely, MR imaging can directly monitor the lethal effect of hyperthermia on viable tissues rather than measuring the temperature change itself, through detecting the changes in the tissue relaxation parameters that accompany the phase transition

from the viable to the necrotic state [35,36]. The accuracy of MR imaging findings in defining the extent of thermally induced tissue necrosis using several different energy sources has been repeatedly demonstrated and validated in reference to histopathologic analysis [37–41].

The development of tissue necrosis associated with RFA entails, among a wider spectrum of tissue damage processes [42,43], denaturation, shrinkage, aggregation of cytoplasmic proteins, and increased hydrophobic interactions resulting in the extrusion of water. The latter effect, along with binding between the denatured proteins and any residual free water, most likely represents the underlying cause for the shortening of the T2 relaxation time after thermal ablation, which ultimately leads to the uniform hypointense appearance of ablation zones seen on the T2-weighted and STIR images (see Fig. 3) acquired intermittently during the procedure. This feature allows direct observation of the size and configuration of the developing thermal ablation zone and permits the identification of any foci of residual viable tumor, which appear as relatively hyperintense areas (see Fig. 3) compared with the hypointense effectively ablated zones.

The cellular changes associated with the heating process, although permanent in fibroglandular and muscular tissues, may seem reversible in adipose tissues with predominant triglyceride content [42]. This explains the previously reported resumption of normal T2-weighted signal intensity within the

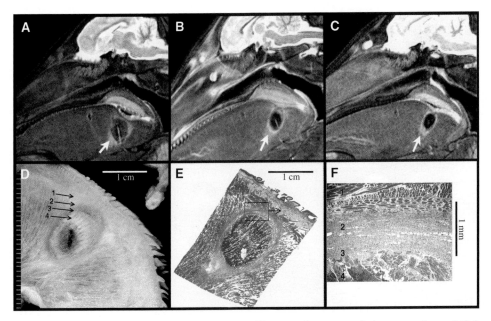

Fig. 11. Example of the temporal involution of an RFA zone illustrates the process of edge maturation on MR imaging with histopathologic correlation from sequential follow-up studies of tongue base RFA in a porcine model. Sagittal turbo spin echo short tau inversion recovery images (repetition time/echo time: 5300/35 milliseconds, echo train length = 7, number of signal averages = 1) acquired on a high-field MR imaging scanner (1.5 T) show a 2.8-mL volume thermal lesion on the immediate postablation scan (*A*) that has shrunken to 1.7 mL on the 2-week scan (*B*) and continued to shrink to reach 0.8 mL on the 1-month scan (*C*) (*arrows, A–C*). Note the gradual resolution and the progressive definition of the marginal reactive tissue changes (*A–C*). Corresponding gross pathologic (*D*) and low-power (*E*) and high-power (*F*) trichrome-stained histologic specimens obtained immediately after the 1-month scan, demonstrating tissue changes associated with the early healing process as represented by the circumferential encasement of the area of coagulation necrosis by fibrous tissue giving rise to four distinct layers of pathologic and histologic findings (*D, F*) as follows: (1) normal muscle tissue of the base of the tongue, (2) mature fibrous tissue, (3) active granulation tissue, and (4) coagulated (mummified) muscle tissue. (*From* Nour SG, Lewin JS, Gutman M, et al. Percutaneous MR-guided radiofrequency interstitial thermal ablation of tongue base in porcine models: implications for obstructive sleep apnea syndrome. Radiology 2004;230(2):367; with permission.)

perinephric fat after ablation procedures [8], although it does not explain the persistence of a thin, presumably fibrotic, hypointense rim marking the original extent of ablation on these images (Fig. 9).

The appearance of thermal ablation zones on precontrast T1-weighted MR imaging scans is, conversely, variable (Fig. 10), where an ablation zone may appear hypointense, isointense, or slightly or markedly hyperintense [42]. Reduction of the T1 relaxation time during thermal ablation is most likely related to the amount of inevitable hemorrhage that occurs within the tissues during the ablation process and seems to correlate with the degree of target organ vascularity [43]. Additionally, blood itself exhibits an abrupt decrease in T1 and T2 relaxation times at temperatures greater than 60°C, resulting in a hyperintense appearance on T1-weighted imaging [43].

Several investigators have demonstrated the development of an acute inflammatory reaction associated with edema, hyperemia, and the foci of hemorrhage surrounding the zones of thermal ablation on histopathologic analysis [41,44–46]. This inflammatory response can be instantly appreciated on MR imaging monitoring of thermal ablation zones as a bright rim marginating the area of necrosis on T2-weighted and STIR images that demonstrates significant enhancement on the postgadolinium T1-weighted scans. The inner margin of this rim is typically sharp, whereas its outer margin usually fades gradually into the adjacent intact tissues [8]. Although we have demonstrated that the extent of actual cell death does eventually extend to the outer margin of the inflammatory rim [41], we always use the sharp inner margin as a reliable indicator of the definite extent of tissue necrosis on our intraprocedural

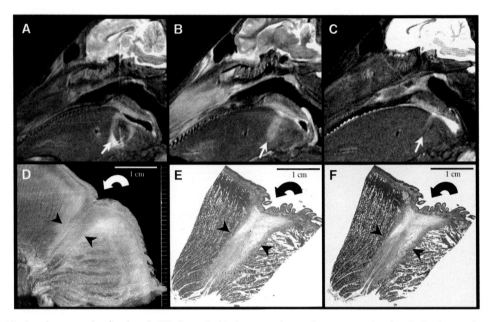

Fig. 12. Another example of a chronic RF-thermal ablation zone that underwent complete involution into a shrunken fibrous scar. Sagittal turbo spin echo short tau inversion recovery images (repetition time/echo time: 5300/35 milliseconds, echo train length = 7, number of signal averages = 1) acquired on a high-field MR imaging scanner (1.5 T) immediately (*A*), 2 weeks (*B*), and 1 month (*C*) after percutaneous RFA of the tongue base. Note the rapid rate of thermal lesion shrinkage from 3.7 mL on the immediate postablation scan (*A*) to 1 mL at 2 weeks (*B*) and ending up as a thin band of enhancing scar tissue on the 1-month scan (*arrows, A–C*). Corresponding gross pathologic (*D*) and hematoxylin-eosin–stained (*E*) and trichrome-stained (*F*) histologic specimens demonstrating the total replacement of the area of necrosis by a grayish dense fibrous tissue (*arrowheads, D*) that lacks inflammatory cells, denoting a healed scar (*arrowheads, E*) and stains blue on the trichrome stain (*arrowheads, F*). Note the inward traction of the still intact surface mucosa by the contracting scar tissue (*curved arrows, D–F*). (*From* Nour SG, Lewin JS, Gutman M, et al. Percutaneous MR-guided radiofrequency interstitial thermal ablation of tongue base in porcine models: implications for obstructive sleep apnea syndrome. Radiology 2004;230(2):366; with permission.)

T2-weighted and STIR images as well as on the confirmatory postablation imaging that includes the gadolinium-enhanced T1-weighted series to ensure the complete treatment of the targeted tumor. Careful observation of the extent of this inflammatory signal change is critical when ablation is performed close to a vital structure, such as the colon or gallbladder, however.

Later, the reactive tissue inflammation surrounding the area of acute thermal injury subsides and starts to be gradually invaded by granulation tissue laid concentrically around the devitalized core. This ring of granulation tissue then undergoes active organization resulting in progressive maturation into fibrous tissue, a process that proceeds from the periphery of the ablation zone inward (Fig. 11) [46]. These tissue changes are reflected on the follow-up MR imaging scans as a gradual resolution of the hyperintense rim seen on T2-weighted and STIR images until it becomes

barely detectable after approximately 3 months in most cases [8]. On postgadolinium scans, uniform marginal enhancement within the granulation tissue and, subsequently, within the fibrous scar should be expected to last for longer periods. Ultimately, the chronic thermal ablation zone involutes into an area of featureless "mummified" coagulated tissue encased by a variable amount of fibrous tissue. The latter may further progress to replace the entire ablation zone, thus rendering it into a small contracted scar (Fig. 12) [46].

Postablation follow-up MR imaging scans should be carefully scrutinized for evidence of early tumor recurrence, which should be generally sought at the margins rather than at the center of the thermal ablation zone. Any marginal irregularity should be interpreted with suspicion, particularly if associated with focal loss of the uniform hypointense signal expected on T2-weighted and STIR images (Fig. 13).

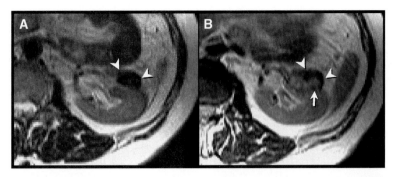

Fig. 13. Careful evaluation of the margins of thermal ablation zones on follow-up MR imaging scans is essential to detect any new edge irregularity. Only hypointense signals on T2-weighted or short tau inversion recovery images are equivalent to coagulation necrosis. (*A*) Axial T2-weighted image obtained 15 months after radiofrequency ablation of renal cell carcinoma. The regularly ovoid and diffusely hypointense area (*arrowheads*) seen along the anterior margin of the interpolar segment of the left kidney is consistent with a completely necrotic ablation zone. (*B*) Another T2-weighted image obtained 1 year later demonstrates the previously seen hypointense necrotic zone (*arrowheads*) with interval development of an isointense nodule (*arrow*) along the posterior margin of the ablation zone. This appearance is typical for local tumor recurrence. The length of tumor-free period in this patient (27 months) should stress the value of carefully scrutinizing the margins of ablation zones on each follow-up scan. Comparison with prior scans, especially the first postablation (baseline) scan, is indispensable.

Additionally, on postgadolinium scans, only uniform marginal enhancement is a normal finding, whereas any focal enhancement along the margin of the ablation zone should be interpreted as residual tumor or recurrence (Fig. 14). MR imaging is a well-suited modality to evaluate for early tumor recurrence because it allows assessment of the margins in multiple planes and with different tissue contrast weightings in addition to the information provided on the gadolinium-enhanced scans.

There are, however, factors that may render the evaluation for tumor recurrence a quite complicated task. Ablation zones may demonstrate irregular outlines rather than the expected perfectly spherical or ovoid appearance. This occurs when the energy distribution is modified during the ablation procedure by the presence of an adjacent sizable blood vessel exerting a focal "heat sink" effect at one side of the ablation zone. Irregular areas of necrosis are also encountered when large-volume ablations are attempted by performing multiple overlapped ablations or through the use of techniques like saline perfusion, which increases the ionic concentration in the tissues to enhance RF current flow. The development of postoperative infection, hematomas, or a seroma adjacent to the site of ablation is another factor that can complicate the interpretation of follow-up MR imaging scans. Review of prior scans, particularly the first postablation

baseline scans, should therefore be a routine practice that can help to monitor interval development of new iso- or hyperintense areas within the premises of the hypointense ablation zone on T2-weighted and STIR images or the development of a new focal enhancement along a uniformly thick regular or irregular margin.

Patient safety during MR-guided radiofrequency ablation

Safe clinical application of MR-guided RFA requires careful consideration of a number of measures related to the interventional use of MR imaging and the medical application of RF energy.

Safety issues for the interventional use of MR imaging

General safety measures for interventional MR imaging suites

Although interventional radiologists performing MR-guided RFA essentially use the basic skills they developed during their earlier experience with the more conventional US- and CT-guided interventions, they should always be aware of the major basic difference (ie, the magnetic field). Although risks are less prominent on the low- and medium-field strength (0.2–0.5 T) magnets typically used for MR-guided RFA, hazardous consequences can result when ferromagnetic

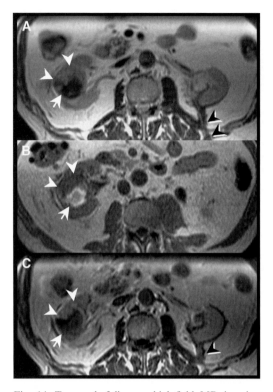

Fig. 14. Two-week follow-up high-field MR imaging scans of the first of two debulking thermal ablation procedures performed to palliate this patient with a large centrally located renal cell carcinoma of the right kidney and global impairment of renal function. The ablated zone (*arrows, A–C*) demonstrates hypointense signal on fast spin echo (FSE) T2-weighted image (*A*), hyperintense blood signal on a T1-weighted gradient echo in-phase image (*B*), and no enhancement on a postgadolinium scan (*C*). The area of residual tumor tissue (*white arrowheads, A–C*) can be readily identified on all three pulse sequences as hyperintense tissue capping the anterior aspect of the ablated zone on FSE T2-weighted images (*A*) and as an isointense area on the in-phase image (*B*) that enhances on the postgadolinium scan (*C*). Note the left-sided nephrostomy tube (*black arrowheads, A, C*). (*From* Merkle EM, Nour SG, Lewin JS. MR imaging follow-up after percutaneous radiofrequency ablation of renal cell carcinoma: findings in eighteen patients during first 6 months. Radiology 2005; 235(3):1070; with permission.)

instruments become accelerated in the fringe field of the scanner, because they can cause serious or even fatal injuries. As a rule, no ferromagnetic materials should be brought within the 5-G line of any scanner. Scalpels, needles, RF electrodes, and anesthesia equipment should be made of MR imaging–compatible materials. Physiologic

monitors should be nonferromagnetic or be kept outside the fringe field of the magnet.

Electric burns can result from direct electromagnetic induction in a conductive loop, induction in a resonant conducting loop, or electric field resonant coupling with a wire (the antenna effect) [47–49]. The last mechanism is more relevant when performing interventions with catheters and guide wires rather than with rigid needles and electrodes. Generally, the risk of electric burns may be minimized by limiting conductive loops, wire-patient contact, and cable lengths.

Finally, acoustic noise during interventions on open low– and medium–field strength scanners does not normally reach the occupational exposure limit (15 min/d at 115 dB), and ear protection is therefore generally not needed during routine MR-guided RFA in contrast to other high-field interventions. Acoustic noise is increased with decreased slice thickness, field of view (FOV), TR, and TE.

Specific safety measures for percutaneous MR-guided radiofrequency electrode navigation

In addition to the general measures discussed previously, knowledge of a number of operator-dependent factors and the effects of their modification during procedure planning and execution is central to the conduction of safe and efficient tumor ablation using MR imaging guidance. These factors are best addressed under the two broad categories of those pertinent to tumor visualization and those pertinent to visualization of the RF electrode.

Adequate visualization of the target pathologic findings and surrounding anatomy. Because speed is important in pulse sequences designed primarily for the guidance phase of RF electrode placement, the resultant images do not have the explicit quality expected from a purely diagnostic sequence. They should provide sufficient anatomy and/or pathology contrast along with good vascular conspicuity to provide safe device navigation toward the target tumor, however. Different near–real-time pulse sequences are available that allow multiple tissue contrasts to be obtained depending on the implemented pulse sequence parameters [50–52]. As indicated previously, the most commonly used sequences to guide electrode navigation during MR-guided RFA procedures are FISP, true FISP, PSIF, and FLASH. Adequate visualization of anatomy and pathologic findings varies in different applications and

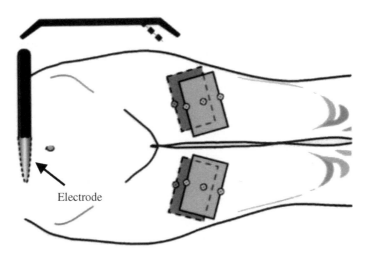

Fig. 15. Proper placement of grounding pads for RFA. The schematic drawing depicts the placement of the grounding pads (*gray rectangles*) in relation to the RF electrode. To minimize grounding pad burn, multiple pads should be placed horizontally with their long axis facing the electrode. This facilitates a more even distribution of heat dissipation, minimizing untoward heating along the grounding pad surface. (*From* Goldberg SN. Radiofrequency tumor ablation: principles and techniques. Eur J Ultrasound 2001;13(2):141; with permission.)

requires selection of the appropriate pulse sequence and tissue contrast mechanism. We typically dedicate a separate "planning session" before the actual "ablation session" for selection of the optimal sequence to depict the anatomy and/or pathology contrast and the ideal RF electrode trajectory and treatment position for each patient.

Adequate visualization of the radiofrequency electrode. Safe manipulation of the RF electrode under MR imaging guidance requires attention to several parameters that may markedly alter the visibility of the electrode and hamper accurate localization of the active tip or interfere with the precise appreciation of the extent and configuration of the deployed tines. These parameters, many of which are controllable, relate to the magnetic field strength, RF electrode composition, and orientation at a given time relative to the main magnetic field (B_0), pulse sequence design, sampling bandwidth, and frequency-encoding direction. The reader is referred to the article on biopsy and aspiration in the current issue for a detailed discussion on the effect of each of these parameters on the visualization of needles and electrodes.

Safety issues for the use of radiofrequency energy

Adequate system grounding

The deposition of high currents during RFA procedures can result in serious burns at the grounding pad site [53]. This is attributable to the fact that when RF current passes through its complete electric circuit, an equal amount of current is deposited at the return electrodes (grounding pads) as at the source electrode. Therefore, the amount of heat deposited at the grounding pads is actually equivalent to that used for "cooking the tumor" at the source electrode. Heating is maximal at the edges of the pads, particularly at the leading edges facing the RF electrode [54]. To avoid serious burns at the grounding pad site, multiple foil pads with a large surface area should be placed on well-prepared skin and oriented with the longest surface edge facing the RF electrode (Fig. 15) [53].

Adequate radiofrequency current deposition

The optimal outcome of an RFA session is to be able to create a thermal lesion that covers the whole targeted tumor plus a rim of safety margin comparable to the 0.5- to 1-cm rim generally targeted during surgery. Although undertreatment is obviously an unacceptable outcome, over-ablation is also not free from risks. Injury of vital structures adjacent to the target tumor can complicate the treatment, and organs like the gallbladder and biliary radicles as well as bowel loops are particularly sensitive to thermal injury [54]. Careful planning and image guidance, particularly with MR imaging in which the induced thermal lesion can be observed as it forms in near real-time, are important to avoid such complications. In addition to the concern regarding collateral damage, it is important when planning extensive ablations to consider whether sufficient organ function can be preserved and to be aware that large-volume tissue necrosis is associated with a higher incidence of infection and postablation syndrome. Keltner et al [55] reported a case of prolonged RFA of the liver for a metastatic carcinoid tumor complicated by hemolysis, rhabdomyolysis, and transient acute renal failure.

University Hospitals of Cleveland/Case Western Reserve University experience

Experience with RFA performed under the exclusive guidance and monitoring of MR imaging began soon after the inception of the interventional MR imaging program at the University Hospitals of Cleveland/Case Western Reserve University approximately a decade ago. The primary focus at our institution has been the advancement of minimally invasive interstitial RF thermotherapy of tumors of the liver and retroperitoneum with electrode placement performed under direct MR imaging guidance within the MR imager. The concept of the interventional MR imaging suite was introduced to test the ability to scan the patient, plan the optimum RF electrode trajectory, interactively guide the electrode into the tumor, obtain on-line intraprocedural feedback on the result of treatment, and modify the RF electrode position to treat residual tumor, all being performed during one session without having the patient or the interventionalist leave the MR imager at any point. Results of a phase I clinical trial were published in 1998 [7] and demonstrated the feasibility and safety of RFA performed completely within an MR imaging suite (see Fig. 6). A phase 2 clinical trial was then instituted to evaluate the efficacy of these procedures, with the primary focus being the evaluation of MR-guided RFA of renal tumors in patients with contraindications to or who had refused surgery. The initial results of the phase II trial have recently been published (see Figs. 3 and 9) [8]. Patients experienced only minimal intraprocedural discomfort that was totally controlled by intravenous sedation and local anesthesia. Few patients required oral acetaminophen for analgesia on the evening after treatment. No patients required pain medication on discharge the following morning. According to the thermal ablation protocol at our institution, we bring the patients

back for follow-up clinical examination and MR imaging scanning at 2 weeks and then again at 3 months after ablation, quarterly during the first year, and semiannually thereafter. Long-term follow-up of the first 10 patients showed no evidence of tumor recurrence for follow-up durations up to 41.7 months. In our experience, RFA is best suited for the treatment of circumscribed tumors less than 4 cm in greatest dimension. It should be noted, however, that even tumors within this size limit may fail therapy because of location adjacent to sources of heat sink, such as flowing blood or the renal collecting system, or because of contact with structures like the colon or gallbladder, thereby compromising the feasibility of adequate margin treatment.

Current research and future directions

The developed clinical expertise in image-guided RFA of tumors and the acknowledgment of the obvious advantages that MR imaging offers in this setting (Box 1) have sparked researchers' interest in further investigating the full potential of this technique of RFA.

The feasibility and safety of performing RFA in various body organs under the sole guidance of MR imaging have been investigated in animal models. Several reports have shown that the applicability of this technique extends beyond the results already achieved in the current clinically recognized applications. Encouraging results

---

Box 1. Advantages of MR imaging during the guidance and monitoring of radiofrequency interstitial thermal ablation

During the guidance of radiofrequency electrode into the target tumor
High soft tissue contrast
High spatial resolution
Multiplanar capabilities
High vascular conspicuity
Lack of ionizing radiation

During the monitoring of thermal tissue destruction
Ability to define treatment end point by providing immediate feedback about the extent of necrosis during ablation
Feasibility of temperature mapping

from pancreatic [56], long bone [57], vertebral [58] (Fig. 16), and other organ ablations promise an expanding future of cancer treatment, exploiting the advantage of the minimally invasive nature of RFA along with the superb value of MR imaging for guiding and monitoring therapy.

Developing the RF technology needed to create larger thermal ablation zones with the least number of RF electrode insertions is another research topic that attempts to address an important existing limitation to the more widespread use of RF energy for tumor ablation. Overcoming this limitation is essential to reduce risks, such as tumor seeding, bleeding, and infection, that may potentially complicate multiple RF electrode repositionings to create overlapping ablation zones. The ability to create larger ablation zones is also important to reduce the procedure time and thus improve patient compliance and reduce morbidity when managing large tumors.

Techniques already investigated include the use of multiple probe RF electrode arrays [59], electrodes with multiple expandable tines, or internally cooled (Cool-tip) RF electrodes that prevent charring at the electrode-tissue interface, thereby allowing higher maximum energy to be deposited into the tissue [60,61]. These electrodes are already commercially available and are widely used in current clinical practice. Other investigators have proposed the creation of larger thermal ablation zones through the reduction of the blood supply to an organ so as to reduce perfusion-mediated tissue cooling (ie, heat sink) [62] or through direct intraparenchymal injection of normal saline or hypertonic sodium chlorine (NaCl) solution as a bolus before or a continuous infusion during ablation to create a high local ion concentration in the tissue being treated [63–65]. Several designs of perfusion electrodes that permit continuous intraprocedural irrigation of ablated

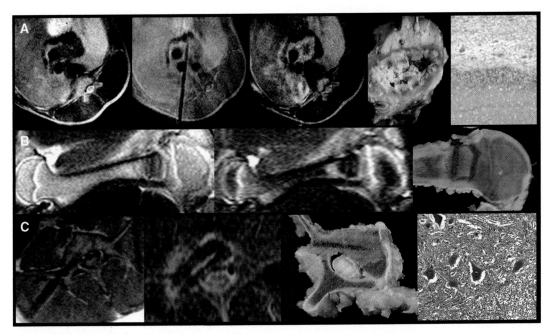

Fig. 16. Experimental work has demonstrated the feasibility and safety of performing RFA of a wide array of body organs under the sole guidance and monitoring of MR imaging. Scans are from MR-guided pancreatic (*A*), long bone (*B*), and vertebral (*C*) RFA procedures with pathologic correlation. The MR imaging appearance of thermal ablation zones is generally similar regardless of the target organ or tissue and consists of a hypointense zone on all pulse sequences (although a varying degree of hyperintensity can be seen on precontrast T1-weighted images as shown in Fig. 6), surrounded by a T2-weighted bright rim that enhances on postgadolinium scans. (*A, From* Merkle EM, Haaga JR, Duerk JL, et al. MR-guided radio-frequency thermal ablation in the pancreas in a porcine model with a modified clinical C-arm system. Radiology 1999;213(2):463–4; with permission. *B, From* Aschoff AJ, Merkle EM, Emancipator SN, et al. Femur: MR-guided radio-frequency ablation in a porcine model-feasibility study. Radiology 2002;225(2):474; with permission. *C, From* Nour SG, Aschoff AJ, Mitchell IC, et al. MR-guided radio-frequency thermal ablation of the lumbar vertebrae in porcine models. Radiology 2002;224(2):456; with permission.)

tissues with saline through multiple holes located on the electrode shaft or on expandable tines are also commercially available. Histopathologic analysis has demonstrated the reliability of NaCl-enhanced ablation techniques to produce complete uniform tissue necrosis in the larger ablation zones thus created [66]. Nevertheless, a significant present limitation to the clinical application of these techniques is the irregular and irreproducible shape of the resultant ablation zones. Current research is ongoing to address this issue.

Parallel to these investigations, there has been continuing research to justify the future utility of MR imaging in light of the developing technology of RF thermal treatment. MR imaging has been reported to guide and monitor the effect of reduced tissue perfusion on the induced thermal ablation zone size accurately in parenchymal organs of animal models [67,68]. Previous work in our laboratory has also already demonstrated the feasibility of interactive MR imaging monitoring of intraparenchymally injected hypertonic saline in ex vivo tissues [69] and has proven the capability of MR imaging to monitor a thermal ablation zone as it develops in vivo within the altered local tissue biology after the injection of hypertonic NaCl solution [70].

A fourth interesting subject related to the validity of MR imaging as an excellent real-time predictor of tumor necrosis, is the three-dimensional registration of thermal ablation zones as they appear on MR imaging scans compared with the actual cellular damage seen histologically. Results from analysis of acute (nonsurvival) thermal ablation zones created in animal models have shown that the central hypointense region seen on T2-weighted and STIR images reliably corresponds to the area of actual cell death [40]. Further survival animal experiments have also demonstrated that cellular elements within the bright enhancing rim marginating the thermal ablation zone also eventually progress to complete necrosis [41].

Finally, the practice of RFA under MR imaging guidance is backed by extensive complementary MR imaging physics research focused primarily on MR imaging pulse sequence development [50–52] and device tracking optimization. Interactive MR imaging scan plane definition during freehand navigation of rigid interventional devices, such as RF electrodes and biopsy needles, without the need for stereotactic cameras, is now possible using a software interface that serves to link the measurement unit of the imager with prototype wireless fiducial markers tuned to the resonance frequency of the scanner and mounted to the interventional device [71].

Summary

Performing RFA procedures under MR imaging involves two distinct processes: interactive guidance of the RF electrode into the targeted tumor and monitoring the effect of therapy. The justification for using MR imaging for electrode guidance is quite similar to its use to guide biopsy and aspiration procedures, where MR imaging offers advantages related to superior soft tissue contrast, multiplanar capabilities, and high vascular conspicuity that facilitate safe and accurate guidance in selected lesions. The major contribution of MR imaging to thermal ablation procedures is its ability to monitor tissue changes associated with the heating process instantaneously, an attribute that is not paralleled by any other currently available imaging modality. Such ability facilitates a controlled approach to ablation by helping to detect inadequately treated tumor foci for subsequent interactive repositioning of the RF electrode during therapy. As such, MR imaging guidance and monitoring enable treatment of the entire tumor on a single-visit basis while avoiding undue overtreatment and preserving often critically needed organ function.

Although knowledge of interventional MR imaging concepts and familiarity with its technology and with the related safety issues are indispensable for interventional radiologists attempting thermal ablation procedures in the MR imaging environment, understanding the tissue basis of necrosis imaging is becoming an essential part of the knowledge base for the larger sector of general radiologists who are required to interpret the follow-up MR imaging scans of the increasing number of thermal ablation patients.

Acknowledgments

The authors acknowledge the members of the Interventional MR Imaging Research Program at the University Hospitals of Cleveland/Case Western Reserve University for their ongoing commitment to the development of interventional MR imaging techniques. The authors also thank Bonnie Hami for her invaluable editorial assistance.

References

[1] Allport JR, Weissleder R. In vivo imaging of gene and cell therapies. Exp Hematol 2001;29(11): 1237–46.

[2] Yang X, Atalar E, Li D, et al. Magnetic resonance imaging permits in vivo monitoring of catheter-based vascular gene delivery. Circulation 2001; 104(14):1588–90.

[3] Floeth FW, Aulich A, Langen KJ, et al. MR imaging and single-photon emission CT findings after gene therapy for human glioblastoma. AJNR Am J Neuroradiol 2001;22(8):1517–27.

[4] Guerquin-Kern JL, Volk A, Chenu E, et al. Direct in vivo observation of 5-fluorouracil release from a prodrug in human tumors heterotransplanted in nude mice: a magnetic resonance study. NMR Biomed 2000;13(5):306–10.

[5] Calvo BF, Semelka RC. Beyond anatomy: MR imaging as a molecular diagnostic tool. Surg Oncol Clin N Am 1999;8(1):171–83.

[6] Fuss M, Wenz F, Essig M, et al. Tumor angiogenesis of low-grade astrocytomas measured by dynamic susceptibility contrast-enhanced MRI (DSC-MRI) is predictive of local tumor control after radiation therapy. Int J Radiat Oncol Biol Phys 2001;51(2): 478–82.

[7] Lewin JS, Connell CF, Duerk JL, et al. Interactive MRI-guided radiofrequency interstitial thermal ablation of abdominal tumors: clinical trial for evaluation of safety and feasibility. J Magn Reson Imaging 1998;8(1):40–7.

[8] Lewin JS, Nour SG, Connell CF, et al. Phase II clinical trial of interactive MR imaging-guided interstitial radiofrequency thermal ablation of primary kidney tumors: initial experience. Radiology 2004; 232(3):835–45.

[9] Eichler K, Mack MG, Straub R, et al. Oligonodular hepatocellular carcinoma (HCC): MR-controlled laser-induced thermotherapy. Radiologe 2001;41(10): 915–22.

[10] Huber PE, Jenne JW, Rastert R, et al. A new noninvasive approach in breast cancer therapy using magnetic resonance imaging-guided focused ultrasound surgery. Cancer Res 2001;61(23):8441–7.

[11] Chen JC, Moriarty JA, Derbyshire JA, et al. Prostate cancer: MR imaging and thermometry during microwave thermal ablation-initial experience-Radiology 2000;214(1):290–7.

[12] Mala T, Edwin B, Samset E, et al. Magnetic-resonance-guided percutaneous cryoablation of hepatic tumours. Eur J Surg 2001;167(8):610–7.

[13] Curley SA. Radiofrequency ablation of malignant liver tumors. Oncologist 2001;6(1):14–23.

[14] Bischof J, Christov K, Rubinsky B. A morphological study of cooling rate response in normal and neoplastic human liver tissue: cryosurgical implications. Cryobiology 1993;30(5):482–92.

[15] Steeves RA. Hyperthermia in cancer therapy: where are we today and where are we going? Bull NY Acad Med 1992;68(2):341–50.

[16] Zervas NT, Kuwayama A. Pathological characteristics of experimental thermal lesions. Comparison of induction heating and radiofrequency electrocoagulation. J Neurosurg 1972;37(4):418–22.

[17] Farahani K, Mischel PS, Black KL, et al. Hyperacute thermal ablation zones: MR imaging evaluation of development in the brain. Radiology 1995; 196(2):517–20.

[18] Aronow S. The use of radio-frequency power in making ablation zones in the brain. J Neurosurg 1960;17:431–8.

[19] Zervas NT. Eccentric radio-frequency ablation zones. Confin Neurol 1965;26(3):143–5.

[20] Chung YC, Duerk JL, Lewin JS. Generation and observation of radio frequency thermal ablation zone ablation for interventional magnetic resonance imaging. Invest Radiol 1997;32(8):466–74.

[21] Nicoli N, Casaril A, Marchiori L, et al. Treatment of recurrent hepatocellular carcinoma by radiofrequency thermal ablation. J Hepatobiliary Pancreat Surg 2001;8(5):417–21.

[22] Elias D, Debaere T, Muttillo I, et al. Intraoperative use of radiofrequency treatment allows an increase in the rate of curative liver resection. J Surg Oncol 1998;67(3):190–1.

[23] Yohannes P, Pinto P, Rotariu P, et al. Retroperitoneoscopic radiofrequency ablation of a solid renal mass. J Endourol 2001;15(8):845–9.

[24] Schenck JF, Jolesz FA, Roemer PB, et al. Superconducting open-configuration MR imaging system for image-guided therapy. Radiology 1995;195(3): 805–14.

[25] Cline HE, Schenck JF, Watkins RD, et al. Magnetic resonance-guided thermal surgery. Magn Reson Med 1993;30(1):98–106.

[26] Cline HE, Hynynen K, Watkins RD, et al. Focused US system for MR imaging-guided tumor ablation. Radiology 1995;194(3):731–7.

[27] Rossi S, Di Stasi M, Buscarini E, et al. Percutaneous RF interstitial thermal ablation in the treatment of hepatic cancer. AJR Am J Roentgenol 1996;167(3): 759–68.

[28] Zhang Q, Chung YC, Lewin JS, et al. A method for simultaneous RF ablation and MRI. J Magn Reson Imaging 1998;8(1):110–4.

[29] McGahan JP, Schneider P, Brock JM, et al. Treatment of liver tumors by percutaneous radiofrequency electrocautery. Semin Interv Radiol 1993; 10:143–9.

[30] Gervais DA, McGovern FJ, Wood BJ, et al. Radiofrequency ablation of renal cell carcinoma: early clinical experience. Radiology 2000;217(3):665–72.

[31] Pavlovich CP, Walther MM, Choyke PL, et al. Percutaneous radio frequency ablation of small renal tumors: initial results. J Urol 2002;167(1):10–5.

[32] Vogl TJ, Muller PK, Hammerstingl R, et al. Malignant liver tumors treated with MR imaging-guided laser-induced thermotherapy: technique and prospective results. Radiology 1995;196(1):257–65.

[33] Chung YC, Duerk JL, Shankaranarayanan A, et al. Temperature measurement using echo-shifted FLASH at low field for interventional MRI. J Magn Reson Imaging 1999;9(1):138–45.

[34] Botnar RM, Steiner P, Dubno B, et al. Temperature quantification using the proton frequency shift technique: in vitro and in vivo validation in an open 0.5 Tesla interventional MR scanner during RF ablation. J Magn Reson Imaging 2001;13(3):437–44.

[35] Matsumoto R, Oshio K, Jolesz FA. Monitoring of laser and freezing-induced ablation in the liver with T1-weighted MR imaging. J Magn Reson Imaging 1992;2(5):555–62.

[36] Bleier AR, Jolesz FA, Cohen MS, et al. Real-time magnetic resonance imaging of laser heat deposition in tissue. Magn Reson Med 1991;21(1):132–7.

[37] Anzai Y, Lufkin RB, Hirschowitz S, et al. MR imaging-histopathologic correlation of thermal injuries induced with interstitial Nd:YAG laser irradiation in the chronic model. J Magn Reson Imaging 1992; 2(6):671–8.

[38] Matsumoto R, Selig AM, Colucci VM, et al. MR monitoring during cryotherapy in the liver: predictability of histologic outcome. J Magn Reson Imaging 1993;3(5):770–6.

[39] Tracz RA, Wyman DR, Little PB, et al. Comparison of magnetic resonance images and the histopathological findings of ablation zones induced by interstitial laser photocoagulation in the brain. Lasers Surg Med 1993;13(1):45–54.

[40] Breen MS, Lancaster TL, Lazebnik RS, et al. Three-dimensional method for comparing in vivo interventional MR images of thermally ablated tissue with tissue response. J Magn Reson Imaging 2003;18(1):90–102.

[41] Breen MS, Lazebnik RS, Fitzmaurice M, et al. Radiofrequency thermal ablation: correlation of hyperacute MR ablation zone images with tissue response. J Magn Reson Imaging 2004;20(3): 475–86.

[42] Merkle EM, Nour SG, Lewin JS. MR imaging follow-up after percutaneous radiofrequency ablation of renal cell carcinoma: findings in eighteen patients during first 6 months. Radiology 2005;235(3): 1065–71.

[43] Graham SJ, Stanisz GJ, Kecojevic A, et al. Analysis of changes in MR properties of tissues after heat treatment. Magn Reson Med 1999;42(6):1061–71.

[44] Boaz TL, Lewin JS, Chung YC, et al. MR monitoring of MR-guided radiofrequency thermal ablation of normal liver in an animal model. J Magn Reson Imaging 1998;8(1):64–9.

[45] Merkle EM, Shonk JR, Duerk JL, et al. MR-guided RF thermal ablation of the kidney in a porcine model. AJR Am J Roentgenol 1999;173(3):645–51.

[46] Nour SG, Lewin JS, Gutman M, et al. Percutaneous MR imaging-guided radiofrequency interstitial thermal ablation of tongue base in porcine models: implications for obstructive sleep apnea syndrome. Radiology 2004;230(2):359–68.

[47] Dempsey MF, Condon B, Hadley DM. Investigation of the factors responsible for burns during MRI. J Magn Reson Imaging 2001;13(4):627–31.

[48] Dempsey MF, Condon B. Thermal injuries associated with MRI. Clin Radiol 2001;56(6):457–65.

[49] Nitz WR, Oppelt A, Renz W, et al. On the heating of linear conductive structures as guide wires and catheters in interventional MRI. J Magn Reson Imaging 2001;13(1):105–14.

[50] Duerk JL, Lewin JS, Wendt M, et al. Remember true FISP? A high SNR, near 1-second imaging method for T2-like contrast in interventional MRI at .2 T. J Magn Reson Imaging 1998;8(1):203–8.

[51] Chung YC, Merkle EM, Lewin JS, et al. Fast T (2)-weighted imaging by PSIF at 0.2 T for interventional MRI. Magn Reson Med 1999;42(2): 335–44.

[52] Duerk JL, Butts K, Hwang KP, et al. Pulse sequences for interventional magnetic resonance imaging. Top Magn Reson Imaging 2000;11(3):147–62.

[53] Goldberg SN, Solbiati L, Halpern EF, et al. Variables affecting proper system grounding for radiofrequency ablation in an animal model. J Vasc Interv Radiol 2000;11(8):1069–75.

[54] Goldberg SN. Radiofrequency tumor ablation: principles and techniques. Eur J Ultrasound 2001;13(2): 129–47.

[55] Keltner JR, Donegan E, Hynson JM, et al. Acute renal failure after radiofrequency liver ablation of metastatic carcinoid tumor. Anesth Analg 2001; 93(3):587–9.

[56] Merkle EM, Haaga JR, Duerk JL, et al. MR imaging-guided radio-frequency thermal ablation in the pancreas in a porcine model with a modified clinical C-arm system. Radiology 1999;213(2):461–7.

[57] Aschoff AJ, Merkle EM, Emancipator SN, et al. Femur: MR imaging-guided radio-frequency ablation in a porcine model-feasibility study. Radiology 2002;225(2):471–8.

[58] Nour SG, Aschoff AJ, Mitchell IC, et al. MR imaging-guided radio-frequency thermal ablation of the lumbar vertebrae in porcine models. Radiology 2002;224(2):452–62.

[59] Goldberg SN, Gazelle GS, Dawson SL, et al. Tissue ablation with radiofrequency using multiprobe arrays. Acad Radiol 1995;2(8):670–4.

[60] Goldberg SN, Gazelle GS, Solbiati L, et al. Radiofrequency tissue ablation: increased ablation zone diameter with a perfusion electrode. Acad Radiol 1996;3(8):636–44.

[61] Lorentzen T. A cooled needle electrode for radiofrequency tissue ablation: thermodynamic aspects of improved performance compared with conventional needle design. Acad Radiol 1996;3(7):556–63.

[62] Goldberg SN, Hahn PF, Tanabe KK, et al. Percutaneous radiofrequency tissue ablation: does perfusion-mediated tissue cooling limit coagulation necrosis? J Vasc Interv Radiol 1998;9(1 Part 1):101–11.

[63] Livraghi T, Goldberg SN, Monti F, et al. Saline-enhanced radio-frequency tissue ablation in the treatment of liver metastases. Radiology 1997; 202(1):205–10.

[64] Goldberg SN, Ahmed M, Gazelle GS, et al. Radiofrequency thermal ablation with NaCl solution injection: effect of electrical conductivity on tissue heating and coagulation-phantom and porcine liver study. Radiology 2001;219(1):157–65.

[65] Miao Y, Ni Y, Mulier S, et al. Ex vivo experiment on radiofrequency liver ablation with saline infusion through a screw-tip cannulated electrode. J Surg Res 1997;71(1):19–24.

[66] Rafie S, Nour SG, Rodgers M, et al. Reliability of NaCl-enhanced radiofrequency thermal ablation to achieve homogeneous tissue necrosis. In: Proceedings of the Radiological Society of North America (RSNA) 90th Scientific Meeting. Chicago: Radiological Society of North America; 2004. p. 208.

[67] Aschoff AJ, Merkle EM, Wong V, et al. How does alteration of hepatic blood flow affect liver perfusion and radiofrequency-induced thermal ablation zone size in rabbit liver? J Magn Reson Imaging 2001; 13(1):57–63.

[68] Aschoff AJ, Sulman A, Martinez M, et al. Perfusion-modulated MR imaging-guided radiofrequency ablation of the kidney in a porcine model. AJR Am J Roentgenol 2001;177(1):151–8.

[69] Nour SG, Lewin JS, Duerk JL. Saline injection in ex-vivo liver: monitoring with fast gradient echo sequences at 0.2 T. In: Proceedings of the International Society for Magnetic Resonance in Medicine (ISMRM) Ninth Scientific Meeting. Berkeley (CA): International Society for Magnetic Resonance in Medicine; 2001. p. 2186.

[70] Nour SG, Goldberg SN, Mitchell IC, et al. MR guidance and monitoring of saline-augmented radiofrequency interstitial thermal ablation. In: Proceedings of the Radiological Society of North America (RSNA) 88th Scientific Meeting. Oak Brook (IL): Radiological Society of North America; 2002. p. 218.

[71] Flask C, Elgort D, Wong E, et al. A method for fast 3D tracking using tuned fiducial markers and a limited projection reconstruction FISP (LPR-FISP) sequence. J Magn Reson Imaging 2001;14(5):617–27.

ELSEVIER
SAUNDERS

Magn Reson Imaging Clin N Am
13 (2005) 583–594

MAGNETIC
RESONANCE
IMAGING CLINICS
of North America

MR-Guided Laser Ablation

Martin G. Mack, MD, PhD*, Thomas Lehnert, MD,
Katrin Eichler, MD, Thomas J. Vogl, MD, PhD

*Department of Diagnostic and Interventional Radiology, Universitätsklinikum Frankfurt/Main,
Theodor-Stern-Kai 7, 60590 Frankfurt, Germany*

Percutaneous MR-guided laser-induced interstitial thermotherapy (LITT) has received increasing attention as a promising technique for the treatment of a variety of primary and secondary malignant liver tumors. In many cases, LITT can be used instead of more invasive and expensive surgical techniques.

The liver is the most common site of metastatic disease from colorectal carcinoma, and it is rare that metastases are present at other sites if the liver and lung are free of tumor [1]. In 1994 in the United States, colorectal carcinoma developed in approximately 149,000 people; approximately 56,000 patients died of this neoplasm. Weiss and colleagues [1] estimated that at least 20% of patients who have this disease die with metastases exclusively in the liver.

In many patients, the degree of hepatic involvement is the main determinant of survival [2–4]. The median survival for patients who have liver metastases from colorectal carcinoma is 4 to 12 months from the time of diagnosis of metastatic disease. Among those patients who have a solitary metastasis, 45% are alive at 2 years, whereas only 12% are alive at 3 years.

Breast cancer has a significant tendency to spread to the lungs, bones, and liver, and breast cancer liver metastases usually indicate the presence of disseminated cancer with a poor prognosis, even if it appears to be limited to a single organ. It

has been reported, however, that in 5% to 12% of patients, metastases can be confined to the liver [5,6].

Surgical resection of liver metastases from breast cancer is still a subject of discussion, but several studies have shown that surgical treatment of hepatic metastases from breast cancer may prolong survival in certain subgroups of patients to a greater extent than standard or nonsurgical therapies [7–11]. The number and the size of hepatic metastases, the interval between treatment of the primary lesion and hepatectomy, and the existence of extrahepatic metastasis were not adverse prognostic factors [12].

In patients who are not candidates for hepatectomy, the palliative management of hepatic metastases remains unsatisfactory. There is a need for an efficient, minimally invasive technique that succeeds in retarding, if not halting, growth of metastases.

LITT is a minimally invasive technique suitable for local tumor destruction within solid organs that uses optical fibers to deliver high-energy laser radiation to the target lesion [13,14]. Due to light absorption, temperatures of up to 150°C are reached within the tumor, leading to substantial thermocoagulation. MR imaging is used for placement of the laser applicator in the tumor and for monitoring progress of thermocoagulation. The thermosensitivity of certain MR sequences is the key to real-time monitoring, allowing accurate estimation of the actual extent of thermal damage [15–18].

This article presents the results of local lesion control with MR-guided minimally invasive LITT and associated survival data.

---

* Corresponding author.

E-mail address: M.Mack@em.uni-frankfurt.de (M.G. Mack).

Material and methods

Laser system and application set

An irrigated power laser system (SOMATEX, Teltow, Germany) was used for MR-guided minimally invasive percutaneous LITT of soft tissue tumors. It consists of an MR-compatible cannulation needle (length, 20 cm; diameter, 1.3 mm) with a tetragonally beveled tip and stylet; a guidewire (length, 100 cm); a 9-French sheath with stylet; and a 7-French double-tube thermostable (up to 400°C) protective catheter (length, 40 cm), also with a stylet, which enables internal cooling with saline solution (Fig. 1A). Cooling of the surface of the laser applicator modifies the radial temperature distribution so that the maximum temperature shifts into deeper tissue layers (see Fig. 1B). This was evaluated by computer simulations that calculated the temperature distribution of different

types of applicators in pig liver by defining the input power required to achieve a maximum tissue temperature of 100°C. The temperature distribution at the cooled applicator is a combined effect of deep optical penetration of Nd:YAG laser and cooling of the applicator surface. Hence, the cooled applicator can be used at higher laser powers than noncooled systems without exceeding critical temperatures. The protective catheter is flexible, transparent to near-infrared radiation, and made of Teflon. Marks on the sheath and the protective catheter allow exact positioning of the sheath and the protective catheter in the patient. The protective catheter has a sharpened tip that, in combination with an adapted mandarin, allows repositioning of the system.

Furthermore, a flexible laser applicator (SOMATEX) with a tip diameter of 1.0 mm and an active zone length between 10 and 40 mm was

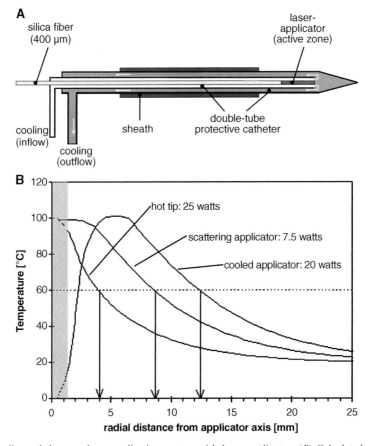

Fig. 1. (A) Internally cooled power laser application system with laser applicator. (B) Calculated radial temperature profile of different applicators in porcine liver (simulation for Nd:YAG laser).

specially designed to keep the entire device as small as possible. The laser applicator was placed at least 3 mm before the distal end of the protective catheter to enable sufficient cooling of the distal tip.

Laser coagulation was performed using an Nd-YAG laser (MediLas 5060, MediLas 5100, Dornier, Germering, Germany) with a wavelength of 1064 nm.

Patients and lesions

LITT was performed between June 1993 and October 2004 in 1568 patients who had a total of 4169 liver metastases that were treated in 3602 treatment sessions. The lesions were ablated with 9508 laser applicators and 17,094 laser applications. There were 821 male patients and 747 female patients whose mean age was 59 years (range, 6–89). The largest patient group had colorectal liver metastases (n = 805). The mean age in this group was 61.2 years (range, 34–84 years). This group had 2397 colorectal liver metastases ablated in 2068 treatment sessions with 5869 laser applicators and 10,696 laser applications. The size of the lesions was 2 cm or less in 33% of the cases, between 2 and 3 cm in 33%, between 3 and 4 cm in 18%, and larger than 4 cm in diameter in 16%. Inclusion criteria for the 805 patients who had colorectal liver metastases were the five major indications for LITT: patients who had recurrent liver metastases after partial liver resection (n = 271), metastases in both liver lobes (n = 288), locally nonresectable lesions (n = 104), general contraindications for surgery (n = 30), or patients who refused surgical resection (n = 111).

The second largest patient group included patients who had breast cancer liver metastases. There were 308 patients treated in this group (mean age, 54.8 years; range, 27–79 years) who had a total of 721 liver metastases; 1594 laser application systems were inserted.

The remaining patients had a variety of different primary tumors including hepatocellular carcinoma, melanoma, gastric cancer, pancreatic cancer, and so forth.

The authors' institutional review board approved this study. Informed consent was obtained from all patients to use combined MR- and CT-guided LITT.

MR imaging

Unenhanced and contrast-enhanced (0.1 mmol/kg body weight gadolinium diethylenetriamine pentaacetic acid) MR imaging was performed in all cases before the interventions to evaluate the size, localization, and number of lesions and after the intervention to verify the obtained necrosis. The imaging protocol included a T2-weighted breath-hold turbo-spin echo (TSE) sequence (repetition time/time to echo [TR/TE], 3000 ms/92 ms; matrix, 154 mm × 256 mm; flip angle, 150°) in transverse slice orientation; a half-Fourier acquisition single-shot turbo spin echo sequence (TR/TE, 1000 ms/60 ms; matrix, 178 mm × 256 mm; flip angle, 147°); and a T1-weighted unenhanced and contrast-enhanced gradient echo sequence (fast low-angle shot [FLASH] 2D; TR/TE, 110 ms/5 ms; matrix, 178 mm × 256 mm; flip angle, 90°) in transverse and sagittal slice orientation. The first follow-up MR imaging study was performed on the day after the LITT treatment. Further follow-up studies were performed every 3 months after the intervention. All follow-up studies were performed with a 1.5 T scanner (Symphony Quantum, Siemens Medical Solutions, Erlangen, Germany).

Treatment protocol and setup

The placement of the laser application systems was done under CT-guidance in most patients (Somatom Volume Zoom, Siemens Medical Solutions). In some patients, ultrasound guidance or MR-guidance was used.

The LITT treatment itself was performed under MR guidance using a 0.5-T scanner (Privilig, Escint, Israel) by T1-weighted gradient echo sequences (TR/TE, 140 ms/12 ms; flip angle, 80°; matrix, 128 mm × 256 mm; number of slices, 5; slice thickness, 8 mm; interslice gap, 30%; acquisition time, 15 seconds) in axial slice orientation and parallel to the laser applicators. These two sequences were repeated at least every minute.

In all patients, the ablation procedure was performed by using T1-weighted thermal imaging to monitor the LITT procedures and the procedure was modified concerning the duration of ablation [19]. Moreover, the pull-back procedure was calculated on the basis of the thermal imaging. The pull-back procedure was used to enlarge the coagulation necrosis in the longitudinal axis by pulling back the laser fiber between 1 and 3 cm (depending on the size of the lesion, the relationship to surrounding structures, and the thermal imaging) within the protective catheter. In no case was the ablation procedure performed on a time or energy basis.

The entire LITT treatment was performed using local anesthesia and intravenously injected analgesics (meperidine, 10–80 mg; or piritramid, 5–15 mg) and sedation (midazolam, 2–10 mg). Local anesthesia was achieved with 1% mepivacaine (20–30 mL).

After switching off the laser, T1-weighted and contrast-enhanced gradient echo images were obtained for determining the degree of induced necrosis. After the procedure, the needle track was closed with fibrin glue (Tissucol Duo S Immuno, Baxter AG, Wien, Austria).

Follow-up examinations using nonenhanced and contrast-enhanced sequences were performed typically on the next day and then every 3 months after the LITT procedure. Quantitative and qualitative parameters, including size, morphology, signal behavior, and contrast enhancement, were evaluated for deciding whether further treatments were necessary or whether treatment could be terminated.

Medications

> Intravenous antibiotics: cefotiam (2 g). The effectiveness of perioperative antibiotic prophylaxis is proven; recent recommendations for abdominal surgery are first-generation cephalosporines such as cefotiam
> Intravenous pain medication: piritramid, meperidine
> Local anesthesia: mepivacaine
> Intravenous conscious sedation: diazepam, midazolam
> Intravenous antiemetic medication: metoclopramide
> Oral pain medication (over-the-counter): metamizol, tramadol
> Fibrin glue: Tissucol Duo S Immuno (2 mL) (Baxter AG), a biologic tissue glue consisting of two frozen components (human fibrinogen and thrombin) prepared in practical sets

Complications

Complications and side effects were identified on routine clinical follow-up examinations, chart evaluation, and on follow-up imaging studies performed routinely after the laser ablation. The evaluation was done by one of the authors independently. Complications that required further treatment (eg, tube drainge for pleural effusion or liver abscess) were defined as clinically relevant.

Small nonsymptomatic subcapsular hematomas were not classified as clinically relevant.

Statistical analysis

Tumor volume and volume of coagulation necrosis were calculated based on measurements in three dimensions. The three greatest dimensions (referred to as x, y, and z) were then used to calculate the volume of an ellipsoid [20]:

$$\text{Ellipsoid volume} = (4\pi/3)(x/2)(y/2)(z/2)$$

Local tumor control was determined using unenhanced and contrast-enhanced MR images obtained 3, 6, and 12 months after LITT treatment.

Survival rates were calculated for all patients who had colorectal liver metastases and breast cancer liver metastases using the Kaplan-Meier method [21]. Subset analysis was based on the following indications for performing the study: primary lymph node stage, development of metachronous metastases, number of initial metastases, and the different patient groups. The Breslow test, the Tarone Ware test, and the log rank test were used to calculate the statistical significance for the differences between the groups. $P < .05$ was considered to be statistically significant.

The estimated mean survival times are biased due to the number of censored cases. In these cases, the event in question had not yet been noted in the patient by the end of the period of observation. For the purposes of the mean survival time, these cases are treated as if the event occurred at that time. The median time could not be estimated in a number of groups due to the small number of occurrences of the event in the group or to the censoring of the longest times observed. The authors present both mean and median survival, when possible, to allow the reader some idea (although biased) of the trend when some of the medians are not estimated.

Results

Colorectal liver metastases

The mean survival rate for all treated patients—starting the calculation at the date of diagnosis of the metastases treated with LITT—was 3.8 years (95% confidence interval [CI]: 3.5–4.1 years; 1-year survival, 93%; 2-year survival, 72%; 3-year survival, 47%; 5-year survival, 24%) (Fig. 2). The mean survival after the first LITT

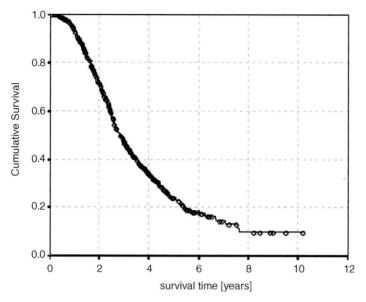

Fig. 2. Graph shows 5-year cumulative survival curves for 805 patients who had 2397 colorectal liver metastases. Curves were calculated with the Kaplan-Meier method, starting the calculation at the date of diagnosis of the metastases treated with LITT.

treatment was 3.3 years (95% CI: 3.0–3.6 years; 1-year survival, 82%; 2-year survival, 54%; 3-year survival, 37%; 5-year survival 19%) (Fig. 3).

There was statistically significant better survival seen in patients who had one or two initial metastases (n = 449; mean survival, 4.3 years; 95% CI: 3.9–4.7 years) than in patients who had three or four initial metastases (n = 228; mean survival, 3.3 years, 95% CI: 2.9–3.7 years) or patients who had five initial metastases (n = 129; mean survival, 2.8 years; 95% CI: 2.5–3.1 years) (Fig. 4).

There also was statistically significant better survival in patients who refused surgery (n = 111;

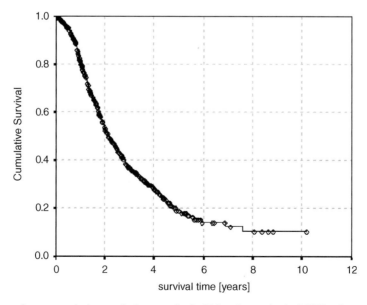

Fig. 3. Graph shows 5-year cumulative survival curves for in 805 patients who had 2397 colorectal liver metastases. Curves were calculated with the Kaplan-Meier method, starting the calculation at the date of the first LITT treatment.

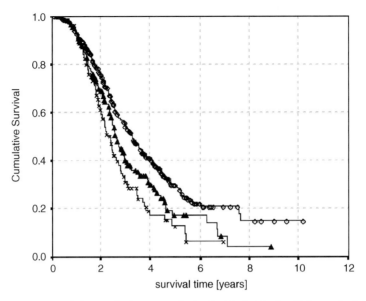

Fig. 4. Graph shows 5-year cumulative survival curves, calculated with the Kaplan-Meier method, in accordance with the number of initially treated metastases in 805 patients who had 2397 colorectal liver metastases. The difference was statistically significant ($P < .05$). ◇, one or two metastases, censored cases; ▲, three or four metastases, censored cases; ×, five metastases, censored cases.

mean survival, 5.5 years) than in patients who were not candidates for surgery due to difficult localization of the metastases for surgery (mean survival, 3.4 years), bilobar metastases (mean survival, 3.2 years), or recurrent liver metastases after partial liver resection (mean survival, 3.6 years) or in patients who had general contraindications for surgery (mean survival, 2.6 years) (Fig. 5).

In evaluating the effect of the primary lymph node stage, it can be shown that patients with N0 or N1 primary lymph node stages (65.5%) had statistically significant better survival compared with patients with N2 and N3 stages (34.5%). The mean survival in patients with N0 and N1 lymph node stage was 3.9 years (95% CI: 3.6–4.3 years). The mean survival in patients with N2 and N3 lymph node stage was 3.6 years (95% CI: 3.1–4.0 years).

Patients who had metachronous metastases (metastases developed more than 6 months after detection of primary tumor; n = 346) showed statistically significant better survival rates compared with patients who had synchronous metastases (n = 459). The mean survival in patients who had metachronous metastases was 4.1 years (95% CI: 3.6–4.0 years). The mean survival in patients who had synchronous metastases was 3.5 years (95% CI: 3.2–4.8 years; log rank test, $P = .0049$; Tarone Ware test, $P = .0030$; Breslow test, $P = .0062$).

There were no statistically significant differences based on patient sex or size of treated metastases ($P > .05$).

Breast cancer liver metastases

The mean survival rate for all 308 treated patients—starting the calculation at the date of diagnosis of the metastases treated with LITT—was 4.9 years (95% CI: 4.3–5.4 years; 1-year survival, 95%; 2-year survival, 78%; 3-year survival, 60%; 5-year survival, 39%) (Fig. 6). The median survival was 4.3 years (95% CI: 3.4–5.3 years). The mean survival after the first LITT treatment was 4.3 years (95% CI: 3.7–4.8 years; 1-year survival, 85%; 2-year survival, 66%; 3-year survival, 50%; 5-year survival, 28%) (Fig. 7).

There were no statistically significant differences in survival rate for patients who had one or two initial metastases (n = 182) versus patients who had three or four initial metastases (n = 82) or patients who had five initial metastases (n = 45; log rank test, $P = .5145$; Tarone Ware test, $P = .3304$; Breslow test, $P = .2218$) (Fig. 8).

Patients who had metachronous metastases (metastases developed more than 6 months after detection of primary tumor; 80.8%) showed no statistically significant improved survival

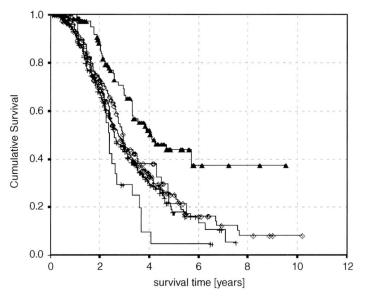

Fig. 5. Graph shows 5-year cumulative survival curves, calculated with the Kaplan-Meier method, in accordance with the indication for LITT in 805 patients who had 2397 colorectal liver metastases. The difference was statistically significant (log rank test, Breslow test, Tarone Ware test: $P < .001$). ◇, recurrence after partial liver resection, censored cases; +, metastases in both liver lobes, censored cases; ×, general contraindications for surgery, censored cases; ▲, patient refused resection of liver metastases, censored cases; ○, difficult localization for surgery but limited disease, censored cases.

compared with patients who had synchronous metastases (19.2%; $P > .05$).

There were no statistically significant differences based on the size of treated metastases ($P > .05$).

For patients who had no evidence of bone metastases at time of inclusion (n = 230), the mean survival was 4.8 years (95% CI: 4.1–5.2 years). For patients who had controlled bone metastases (n = 78), the mean survival was 4.3 years (95%

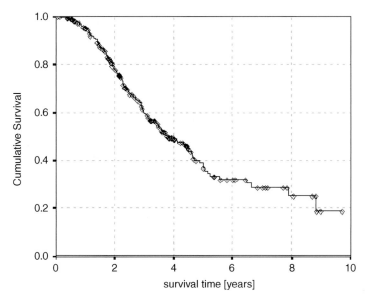

Fig. 6. Graph shows 5-year cumulative survival curves for 308 patients who had 721 breast cancer liver metastases. Curves were calculated with the Kaplan-Meier method, starting the calculation at the date of diagnosis of the metastases treated with LITT. ◇, censored cases.

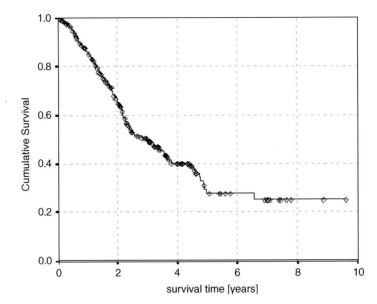

Fig. 7. Graph shows 5-year cumulative survival curves for 308 patients who had 721 breast cancer liver metastases. Curves were calculated with the Kaplan-Meier method, starting the calculation at the date of the first LITT treatment. $\diamond$, censored cases.

CI: 3.4–5.1 years). The difference, however, was not statistically significant when assessed with the log rank, Tarone Ware, and Breslow tests for equality of survival distribution (log rank test, $P = .36$; Tarone Ware test, $P = .33$; Breslow test, $P = .34$).

Discussion

For many years, surgical resection of liver metastases has been the "gold standard" for radical treatment of malignant liver tumors; however, only 20% of patients are suitable for

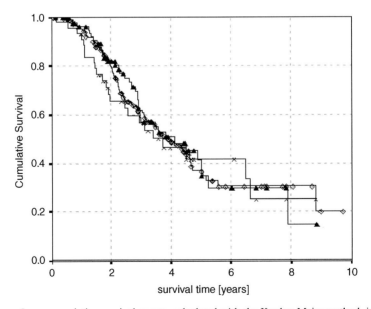

Fig. 8. Graph shows 5-year cumulative survival curves, calculated with the Kaplan-Meier method, in accordance with the number of initially treated metastases in 308 patients who had 721 breast cancer liver metastases. The difference was not statistically significant ($P > .05$). $\diamond$, one or two metastases, censored cases; $\blacktriangle$, three or four metastases, censored cases; $\times$, five metastases, censored cases.

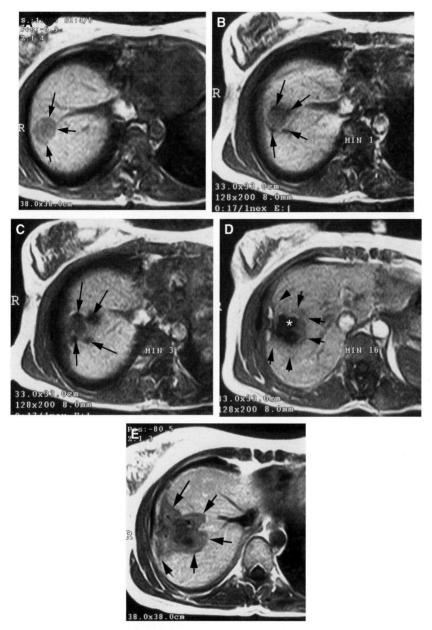

Fig. 9. (*A*) Transverse noncontrast gradient echo image (TR/TE, 140 ms/12 ms; flip angle, 80°) before LITT shows the liver metastases of a colorectal cancer (*arrows*) in liver segment 8. (*B*) Transverse noncontrast T1-weighted gradient echo image (TR/TE, 140 ms/12 ms; flip angle, 80°) obtained 1 minute after starting the laser treatment demonstrates an already-decreased signal intensity in the lesion (*arrows*) and surrounding tissue. (*C*) Transverse noncontrast T1-weighted gradient echo image (TR/TE, 140 ms/12 ms; flip angle, 80°) obtained 3 minutes after starting the laser treatment demonstrates obvious signal intensity decrease in the lesion (*arrows*) and surrounding tissue. (*D*) Transverse noncontrast T1-weighted gradient echo image (TR/TE, 140 ms/12 ms; flip angle, 80°) obtained 3 minutes after starting the laser treatment demonstrates obvious signal intensity decrease in the lesion and surrounding tissue (*arrows*) due to the increase in tissue temperature. The temperature of the lesion is approximately 110°C in the center (*) and 60°C to 70°C in the peripheral zone. (*E*) Transverse contrast-enhanced T1-weighted gradient echo image 24 hours after LITT demonstrates the induced coagulation area (*arrows*). A reliable safety margin was coagulated around the lesion.

surgical resection. Clinical conditions such as the presence of lesions in both hepatic lobes or the reduced clinical condition of a patient exclude surgical treatment. In addition, liver surgery is a method that has an associated mortality rate of approximately 5%. These facts have led to therapeutic alternatives in the treatment of liver metastases that are divided into oncologic strategies (eg, systemic or locoregional chemotherapy) and interventional techniques (eg, percutaneous alcohol injection, chemoembolization, or percutaneous laser treatment).

The clinical success of the MR-guided LITT depends on three factors: the optimal localization of the applicator in the center of the lesion controlled in all dimensions, an optimal on-line monitoring of the temperature elevation in the tumor and surrounding tissue, and exact documentation of the local tumor control rate. The on-line thermometry allows an exact guidance of the interventional procedure. The MR image provides unparalleled topographic accuracy due to its excellent soft tissue contrast and high spatial resolution. Therefore, early detection of local complications (eg, bleeding and hemorrhage) and treatment effects (eg, coagulative necrosis) is possible (Fig. 9).

The main benefits of this kind of treatment include the minimally invasive character of MR-guided LITT, the missing short- or long-term side effects related to the treatment, and short hospital stay.

Several factors may influence the size and morphology of the areas of induced necrosis, including tumor geometry and adjacent structures such as arteries, portal and hepatic veins, and the biliary tree. The relationship of the tumor to the liver capsule is an essential factor in planning treatment of the lesion.

Although the intention of LITT was originally palliative, its favorable survival rates compared with those obtained with surgical resection of liver metastases based on analyses of large surgical series [22–29] with lower complication rates are most encouraging. These data suggest that the indication for LITT in favor of surgery can be extended also to potentially curative patients who have colorectal liver metastases, including surgical candidates, if not more than five metastases with a maximum diameter of 5 cm are present.

An analysis of the true incidence of complications of interventional treatment for malignant liver tumors is essential for establishing the safety and utility of interventional radiologic techniques that are classified as minimally invasive. Improved application techniques have yielded enlargements of the volume of induced coagulation necrosis up to 8 cm in laser therapy and radiofrequency ablation but they are accompanied by an increased rate of complications. Many of these complications are imaging findings or minor complications such as subcutaneous hematomas, bilioma, and local infections at the puncture site. Pleural effusions were the most frequently observed major complication after LITT, and large effusions of more than 1000 mL causing clinical symptoms were indications for thoracocentesis or chest tube placement. Considering the large number of puncture procedures, vascular complications were rare. These results are consistent with most of the complication reports of other interventional study groups [30–32]. In the authors' experience, tumors in the upper liver segments 8, 7, 4a, and 2 are predisposed for such reactions, especially in those lesions having contact with the diaphragm. Careful preinterventional planning, preparation of the interventional access route, and avoiding penetration or thermal damage to pleural spaces may reduce the severity of this side effect. Regarding the deep inferior position of the costodiaphragmal pleural spaces in maximal inspiration (ie, the usual breath-hold situation of diagnostic CT examination), the authors prefer to use the "expiration" breath-hold for CT-guided catheter positioning. CT-guidance is very helpful for the puncture of liver lesions, especially in segment 8, using a deep caudocranial approach without touching the pleural spaces. Therapy for affected patients included intensive breathing exercises and daily control of body temperature. The rate of pleural effusion was reduced slightly by early mobilization and outpatient management.

Large surgical series were associated with morbidity and mortality of approximately 16% and 5%, respectively, in a wide range and depending on the center. Subphrenic and liver abscesses, hematoma, and bile duct injuries were major specific complications; pulmonary embolism, deep vein thrombosis, renal failure, and acute cardiac failure were general health complications [27,28,33,34].

Summary

MR-guided LITT is a safe and effective treatment modality that improves survival in well-selected patients who have liver metastases. A major advantage of MR-guided LITT is that it can be easily performed under local anesthesia in an outpatient setting with a low complication rate.

References

[1] Weiss L, Grundmann E, Torhorst J, et al. Haematogenous metastatic patterns in colonic carcinoma: an analysis of 1541 necropsies. J Pathol 1986;150: 195–203.

[2] Goslin R, Steele G Jr, Zamcheck N, et al. Factors influencing survival in patients with hepatic metastases from adenocarcinoma of the colon or rectum. Dis Colon Rectum 1982;25:749–54.

[3] Jaffe BM, Donegan WL, Watson F, et al. Factors influencing survival in patients with untreated hepatic metastases. Surg Gynecol Obstet 1968;127:1–11.

[4] Steele G Jr, Ravikumar TS. Resection of hepatic metastases from colorectal cancer. Biologic perspective. Ann Surg 1989;210:127–38.

[5] Hoe AL, Royle GT, Taylor I. Breast liver metastases: incidence, diagnosis and outcome. J R Soc Med 1991;84:714–6.

[6] Zinser JW, Hortobagyi GN, Buzdar AU, et al. Clinical course of breast cancer patients with liver metastases. J Clin Oncol 1987;5:773–83.

[7] Bathe OF, Kaklamanos IG, Moffat FL, et al. Metastasectomy as a cytoreductive strategy for treatment of isolated pulmonary and hepatic metastases from breast cancer. Surg Oncol 1999;8:35–42.

[8] Carlini M, Lonardo MT, Carboni F, et al. Liver metastases from breast cancer. Results of surgical resection. Hepatogastroenterology 2002;49: 1597–601.

[9] Kondo S, Katoh H, Omi M, et al. Hepatectomy for metastases from breast cancer offers the survival benefit similar to that in hepatic metastases from colorectal cancer. Hepatogastroenterology 2000;47: 1501–3.

[10] Maksan SM, Lehnert T, Bastert G, et al. Curative liver resection for metastatic breast cancer. Eur J Surg Oncol 2000;26:209–12.

[11] Pocard M, Pouillart P, Asselain B, et al. Hepatic resection in metastatic breast cancer: results and prognostic factors. Eur J Surg Oncol 2000;26: 155–9.

[12] Yoshimoto M, Tada T, Saito M, et al. Surgical treatment of hepatic metastases from breast cancer. Breast Cancer Res Treat 2000;59:177–84.

[13] Mack MG, Straub R, Eichler K, et al. Breast cancer metastases in liver: laser-induced interstitial thermotherapy—local tumor control rate and survival data. Radiology 2004;233(2):400–9.

[14] Puls R, Stroszczynski C, Gaffke G, et al. Laser-induced thermotherapy (LITT) of liver metastases:

MR-guided percutaneous insertion of an MRI-compatible irrigated microcatheter system using a closed high-field unit. J Magn Reson Imaging 2003;17:663–70.

[15] Castren Persons M, Lipasti J, Puolakkainen P, et al. Laser-induced hyperthermia: comparison of two different methods. Lasers Surg Med 1992;12: 665–8.

[16] Jolesz FA, Bleier AR, Jakab P, et al. MR imaging of laser-tissue interactions. Radiology 1988;168: 249–53.

[17] Le Bihan D, Delannoy J, Levin RL. Temperature mapping with MR imaging of molecular diffusion: application to hyperthermia. Radiology 1989;171: 853–7.

[18] Vogl TJ, Mack MG, Hirsch HH, et al. In-vitro evaluation of MR-thermometry for laser-induced thermotherapy. Fortschr Röntgenstr 1997;167:638–44.

[19] Vogl TJ, Mack MG, Hirsch HH, et al. In vitro evaluation of MR thermometry in the implementation of laser-induced thermotherapy. Fortschr Rontgenstr 1997;167:638–44.

[20] Dachman AH, MacEneaney PM, Adedipe A, et al. Tumor size on computed tomography scans: is one measurement enough? Cancer 2001;91:555–60.

[21] Kaplan EL, Meier P. Nonparametric estimation from incomplete observation. J Am Stat Assoc 1958;53:457–81.

[22] Butler J, Attiyeh FF, Daly JM. Hepatic resection for metastases of the colon and rectum. Surg Gynecol Obstet 1986;162:109–13.

[23] Adson MA. Resection of liver metastases—when is it worthwhile? World J Surg 1987;11:511–20.

[24] Adson MA, Heerden van J, Adson MH, et al. Resection of hepatic metastases from colorectal cancer. Arch Surg 1984;119:647–51.

[25] Doci R, Gennari L, Bignami P, et al. One hundred patients with hepatic metastases from colorectal cancer treated by resection: analysis of prognostics determinants. Br J Surg 1991;78:797–801.

[26] Hohenberger P, Schlag P, Schwarz V, et al. [Leberresektion bei Patienten mit Metastasen colorektaler Carcinome. Ergebnisse und prognostische Faktoren]. Chirurg 1988;59:410–7.

[27] Nordlinger B, Guiguet M, Vaillant JC, et al. Surgical resection of colorectal carcinoma metastases to the liver. A prognostic scoring system to improve case selection, based on 1568 patients. Association Francaise de Chirurgie. Cancer 1996;77:1254–62.

[28] Scheele J, Altendorf-Hofmann A, Stangl R, et al. Surgical resection of colorectal liver metastases: gold standard for solitary and completely resectable lesions. Swiss Surg Suppl 1996;4:4–17.

[29] Stangl R, Altendorf Hofmann A, Charnley RM, et al. Factors influencing the natural history of colorectal liver metastases. Lancet 1994;343: 1405–10.

[30] Livraghi T, Giorgio A, Marin G, et al. Hepatocellular carcinoma and cirrhosis in 746 patients:

long-term results of percutaneous ethanol injection. Radiology 1995;197:101–8.

[31] Oshowo A, Gillams A, Lees W, et al. Radiofrequency ablation extends the scope of surgery in colorectal liver metastases. Eur J Surg Oncol 2003;29: 244–7.

[32] Barry BD, Kell MR, Redmond HP. Tumor lysis syndrome following endoscopic radiofrequency interstitial thermal ablation of colorectal liver metastases. Surg Endosc 2002;16:1109.

[33] Sarantou T, Bilchik A, Ramming KP. Complications of hepatic cryosurgery. Semin Surg Oncol 1998;14:156–62.

[34] Scheele J, Stangl R, Altendorf-Hofmann A. Surgical interventions in liver metastases. Langenbecks Arch Chir Verh Dtsch Ges Chir 1990;Suppl II:217–25.

ELSEVIER
SAUNDERS

Magn Reson Imaging Clin N Am
13 (2005) 595–600

MAGNETIC
RESONANCE
IMAGING CLINICS
of North America

MR-Guided Percutaneous Sclerotherapy of Low-Flow Vascular Malformations in the Head and Neck

Daniel T. Boll, MD[a], Elmar M. Merkle, MD[b], Jonathan S. Lewin, MD[c],*

[a]Department of Radiology, University Hospitals of Ulm, Steinhövelstrasse 9, 89075 Ulm, Germany
[b]Department of Radiology, Duke University, Trent Drive, Durham, NC 27710, USA
[c]The Russell H. Morgan Department of Radiology and Radiological Science, The Johns Hopkins University Hospital, 600 North Wolfe Street, Baltimore, MD 21287, USA

Vascular sclerotherapy, performed through the injection of sclerosant agents into abnormally dilated vessels, causes thrombosis, fibrosis, stenosis, and ultimately scarring of the treated vessels by irritating and damaging the endothelial lining. Sclerotherapeutic treatment is usually performed under fluoroscopic guidance, with cross-sectional imaging reserved for preinterventional planning and postinterventional control [1]. More recently, however, the use of MR imaging for needle guidance and monitoring of sclerosant injection has been advocated and evaluated [2–4]. In this manuscript, the underlying pathophysiology of low-flow malformations is reviewed, followed by a summary of the MR imaging guidance and monitoring technique. Finally, the outcome data from the authors' experience at Case Western Reserve University and University Hospitals of Cleveland is summarized.

Low-flow malformations

Soft-tissue vascular anomalies are part of a spectrum of commonly found congenital malformations in the head and neck that can be found in children and adults [1]. From a diagnostic and therapeutic perspective, an unambiguous classification scheme is crucial to differentiate between and to identify vascular tumors and vascular malformations [5]. Vascular tumors such as hemangiomas histologically show endothelial hyperplasia and undergo an initial proliferative phase during early childhood and later involute with age, making any invasive treatment unnecessary [5–7]. This anomaly is in contrast to vascular malformations, which histologically present with chromosomal-induced errors in endothelial development but demonstrate normal endothelial turnover and thin-walled, dilated channels with sparse smooth muscle cells and adventitial fibrosis [1,8]. Such vascular malformations in the head and neck remain stable or slowly grow proportionally over time and require therapy when pain, functional impairment, bleeding, airway obstruction, dental distortion, or cosmetic disfigurement occur [1,9]. Furthermore, facial or cervical vascular malformations show differing hemodynamic patterns that are of paramount importance in the choice of appropriate treatment. High-flow vascular anomalies such as arteriovenous fistulae and arteriovenous malformations are adequately addressed by transarterial embolization, whereas low-flow malformations found to be solitary or combined in capillary, venous, or lymphatic vessels are more effectively treated with percutaneous sclerotherapy [10–12].

Imaging evaluation

MR imaging has proved useful for defining the extent and spatial relationships of soft-tissue vascular anomalies [13]. Furthermore, over the last several years, there has been a substantial increase in interest in interventional MR imaging as a minimally invasive treatment modality due to its excellent soft-tissue contrast, good spatial and

---

* Corresponding author.
E-mail address: jlewin2@jhmi.edu (J.S. Lewin).

temporal resolution, and multiplanar slice selection for guidance of needle insertion and monitoring of drug injection [14,15]. Pilot studies have proved the technical feasibility and safety of using MR imaging for facial and cervical malformation characterization, target localization, guidance and monitoring of percutaneous sclerotherapy, and postinterventional control [2–4].

The role of imaging in the sclerotherapy procedure must include the detection of extravasation of the sclerosing agent into the regional soft tissues or draining veins. If undetected, this extravasation may result in complications such as skin necrosis, neuropathy, muscle atrophy and contracture, deep vein thrombosis, pulmonary embolus, disseminated intravascular coagulation, and cardiopulmonary collapse [16,17].

The MR-guided sclerotherapy procedure

MR-guided sclerotherapy can be performed on a number of imaging systems. The key requirement is accessibility to the anatomic area of interest to allow the placement of a needle and direct visualization during the injection of sclerosant. In the following description of the authors' technique, all imaging for the purpose of lesion characterization, target localization, guidance and monitoring of the sclerotherapy, and postprocedural follow-up was performed on a 0.2-T, C-arm imaging system (Magnetom Open, Siemens Medical Solutions, Erlangen, Germany) equipped with an in-room MR-compatible, high-resolution monitor. The room was also equipped with patient monitoring including pulse oximetry and noninvasive blood pressure monitoring capabilities.

For initial lesion characterization, turbo spin-echo (TSE) imaging with T2 weighting (repetition time (TR)/echo time (TE), 4914 ms/102 ms; slices/slice thickness, 19/5 mm; matrix/field of view (FoV), 252 mm × 256 mm/200 mm × 200 mm; number of signal averages (NSA), 2; acquisition time (AT), 6 minutes, 0 seconds) and T1 weighting (TR/TE, 532 ms/15 ms; slices/slice thickness, 19/5 mm; matrix/FoV, 256 mm × 256 mm/200 mm × 200 mm; NSA, 2; AT, 4 minutes, 36 seconds) were employed. The low-flow patterns of the vascular malformations were diagnosed by noting the absence of flow-void artifacts on T2-weighted TSE imaging (Fig. 1A) [2,3].

Target localization was performed by moving a water-filled syringe over the skin surface above the vascular malformation while rapidly and continuously imaging the tip of the syringe until the desired needle pass was identified, employing a fast imaging with steady precession (FISP) gradient-echo sequence (TR/TE/flip angle, 17.8 ms/8.1 ms/90°; slices/slice thickness, 3/5 mm; matrix/FoV, 128 mm × 256 mm/250 mm × 250 mm; NSA, 1; AT, 9 seconds) oriented along the needle shaft (see Fig. 1B) [2,4].

The same gradient-echo sequence was used for guidance of MR-compatible needle advancement (22-gauge, E-Z-EM, Westbury, New York) after subcutaneous infiltration of 1% lidocaine for local anesthesia. After final needle placement within the low-flow vascular malformation, the position was confirmed using a T1-weighted spin echo (SE) sequence (TR/TE, 500 ms/24 ms; slices/slice thickness, 3/4 mm; matrix/FoV, 250 mm × 256 mm/250 mm × 250 mm; NSA, 3; AT, 1 minute, 19 seconds) [2,4].

To allow monitoring of the sclerotherapy by means of MR imaging, the sclerosing agent, ethanolamine oleate (50 mg/mL; Questcor Pharmaceuticals, Union City, California), was mixed with 2 µmol of the contrast agent, gadopentetate dimeglumine (0.5 mol/L; Berlex Laboratories, Wayne, New Jersey), per milliliter of sclerosing agent, a concentration typically used for MR arthrography [18]. Percutaneous sclerotherapy was performed under rapid and continuous imaging using the FISP sequence while slowly injecting 2 to 6 mL of the tagged sclerosing agent until various-sized targeted portions of the malformation were completely filled (see Fig. 1C) [4].

For postinterventional imaging, the T1-weighted SE sequence of the malformation characterization protocol was used (see Fig. 1D).

Clinical results—the Case Western Reserve University experience

The following is a summary of the results from 64 MR-guided sclerotherapy procedures in patients referred to the radiologic department for MR imaging evaluation and subsequent MR-guided treatment of low-flow vascular malformations in the head and neck outside the central nervous system. The facial and cervical low-flow vascular malformations that were examined and treated were localized in the masticator space, the parapharyngeal space, the parotid space, the carotid space, and the face [4]. Clinical symptoms included cosmetic disfigurement (n = 15), distorted

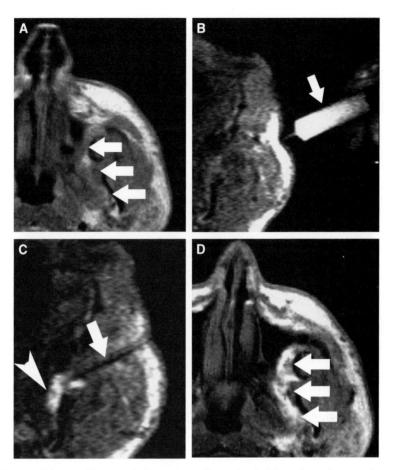

Fig. 1. Thirty-five-year-old man with congenital vascular malformation in bilateral masticator and parotid spaces. (*A*) Vascular malformation within right masticator space (*arrows*) as visualized on preinterventional transverse T1-weighted SE imaging (TR/TE, 532 ms/15 ms; slices/slice thickness, 19/5 mm; matrix/FoV, 256 mm × 256 mm/200 mm × 200 mm; NSA, 2; AT, 4 minutes, 36 seconds). (*B*) Localization of target malformation with water-filled syringe (*arrow*). (*C*) Subsequent MR-guided needle (*arrow*) placement employing FISP gradient-echo interventional imaging sequences (TR/TE/flip angle, 17.8 ms/8.1 ms/90°; slices/slice thickness, 3/5 mm; matrix/FoV, 128 mm × 256 mm/250 mm × 250 mm; NSA, 1; AT, 9 seconds) oriented along the needle shaft. MR-monitored injection of contrast-tagged sclerosing agent (*arrowhead*) by way of MR-compatible needle. (*D*) Transverse T1-weighted SE imaging (TR/TE, 532 ms/15 ms; slices/slice thickness, 19/5 mm; matrix/FoV, 256 mm × 256 mm/200 mm × 200 mm; NSA, 2; AT, 4 minutes, 36 seconds) visualized the vascular malformation (*arrows*) in the right masticator space filled with contrast-tagged sclerosing agent. (*From* Boll DT, Merkle EM, Lewin JS. Low-flow vascular malformations: MR-guided percutaneous sclerotherapy in qualitative and quantitative assessment of therapy and outcome. Radiology 2004;233(2):379; with permission.)

dentition/dental problems (n = 2), impaired chewing (n = 2), speech problems (n = 2), cheek numbness (n = 1), intermittent hemorrhage (n = 12), and pain (n = 15) [4].

The patients were followed with clinical examinations and MR imaging 12 ± 2.4 weeks after treatment employing the malformation characterization protocol and, owing to the size of the vascular malformations, further treatments were performed until all initial clinical symptoms were successfully addressed [4].

After the initial MR-guided sclerotherapy session, individual patient interviews and clinical examinations addressed the therapeutic progress before every subsequent treatment. Attention was focused on improving the presenting symptoms, such as decrease of hemorrhaging and pain and improvement of function (Fig. 2) [4]. All results were documented and decisions on further sclerotherapeutic stages were based on an improvement of the most relevant and disturbing symptoms. Transient increases in pain after sclerotherapy in

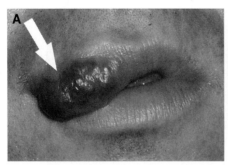
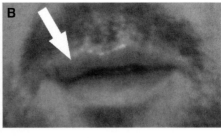

Fig. 2. Thirty-four-year-old man with congenital vascular malformation in the right upper lip. (*A*) Initial preinterventional photograph showing extension of initial skin discoloration (*arrow*) and cosmetic disfigurement. (*B*) Photograph taken after three MR-guided sclerotherapy treatment sessions shows a decrease in size of the low-flow vascular malformation (*arrow*) and partial regaining of physiologic lip vermilion. (*From* Boll DT, Merkle EM, Lewin JS. Low-flow vascular malformations: MR-guided percutaneous sclerotherapy in qualitative and quantitative assessment of therapy and outcome. Radiology 2004;233(2):381; with permission.)

addition to marked acute swelling of the treated portion of the low-flow vascular malformation were not considered complications [19].

MR-guided sclerotherapy–induced intravascular perfusion changes including thrombosis, fibrosis, and scarring were assessed through calculation of the contrast-to-noise ratios on T2-weighted image datasets [4,20]. The signal intensities were compared with preprocedural perfused regions and postprocedural sclerosed portions of the vascular malformation (Fig. 3) [4].

The volume of the malformation was determined on T1-weighted preinterventional image datasets. Segmentation and volume assumption

were performed before treatment and on consecutive follow-up examinations (see Fig. 3) [4].

Outcome of the sclerotherapy procedures

Bleeding into the oral cavity and cosmetic disfigurement were the most disturbing symptoms noted by the patients with low-flow vascular malformations in the head and neck. Oral bleeding was successfully addressed in all cases by MR-guided sclerotherapy; in addition, all patients noted an improvement in cosmetic appearance, especially a decrease in facial swelling and

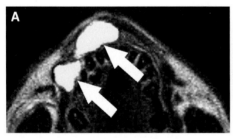
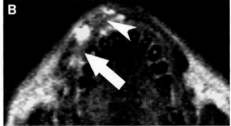

Fig. 3. Same patient as in Fig. 2. (*A*) Preinterventional transverse T2-weighted MR-TSE imaging (TR/TE, 4914 ms/102 ms; slices/slice thickness, 19/5 mm; matrix/FoV, 252 mm × 256 mm/200 mm × 200 mm; NSA, 2; AT, 6 minutes, 0 seconds) visualized the cavernous anterior portion and the lateral portion (*arrows*) of the vascular malformation with high signal intensities without apparent flow voids. (*B*) Follow-up transverse T2-weighted MR-TSE imaging after initial sclerotherapy treatment session (TR/TE, 4914 ms/102 ms; slices/slice thickness, 19/5 mm; matrix/FoV, 252 mm × 256 mm/200 mm × 200 mm; NSA, 2; AT, 6 minutes, 0 seconds) visualized intravascular thrombus (*arrowhead*) within the larger portion of the vascular malformation and complete thrombosis of the smaller portion (*arrow*), with significant overall shrinkage. (*From* Boll DT, Merkle EM, Lewin JS. Low-flow vascular malformations: MR-guided percutaneous sclerotherapy in qualitative and quantitative assessment of therapy and outcome. Radiology 2004;233(2):381; with permission.)

skin discoloration. In two patients, vascular malformations surrounding teeth in need of dental therapy were successfully treated, making subsequent dental care possible [4].

Chewing dysfunction and speech problems in one patient with buccal swelling from an underlying vascular malformation were successfully treated using MR-guided therapy by decreasing the size of the abnormal vessels. This shrinkage led to a subjectively recognized improvement in speech clarity and mastication [4].

MR-guided sclerotherapy itself produced only minimal individual discomfort as assessed through patient interviews immediately after the procedure; however, all patients experienced pain and marked acute soft-tissue swelling immediately following MR-guided sclerotherapy, which was treated locally with application of an ice-pack in addition to oral analgesics. No severe complications were observed. Increased sensitivity in the area of the treated portion of the vascular malformation subsided during the subsequent 1 to 2 weeks [4].

The evaluation of alterations in flow patterns within the treated portions of low-flow vascular malformations proved the ability of MR imaging to successfully depict induced thrombosis and subsequent fibrosis. In addition, the perfused volume of the treated portions of the low-flow vascular malformations decreased in all patients [4].

MR-guided percutaneous sclerotherapy of low-flow vascular malformations in the head and neck

Congenital vascular malformations present with a characteristic serpentine pattern of endothelium-lined vascular channels with internal striations and fibrofatty septations; they may also potentially contain intravascular thrombosis, hemosiderin deposits, and phleboliths [21]. Vascular malformations show a subcutaneous fatty prominence; however, a propensity for discontinuous multifocal involvement, with a tendency to follow neurovascular distributions, suggests a more diffuse congenital dysplasia rather than an isolated dysplasia to the malformed vascular spaces [22]. In particular, low-flow vascular malformations are characterized by the absence of dilated feeding arteries and draining veins.

The abnormal mural muscular anatomy of congenital vascular malformations (consisting of sparse smooth-muscle clumps) is most likely responsible for the gradual vascular expansion [8]. An escalated, malformed vascular growth might be induced by hemodynamic alterations caused by various previously performed treatment attempts [1]; however, any form of vascular malformation expansion directly affects the surrounding tissue. Adjacent musculature has shown strains of fatty infiltration and subsequent atrophy, fascial involvement, and infiltration into associated tendons, whereas adjacent bones may present with intramedullary vascular components [22].

Therefore, complex anatomy and its spatial relationships with adjacent structure, various intravascular perfusion patterns, and functionally induced changes of morphology over time emphasize that successful planning and guiding of minimally invasive sclerotherapy rely on an imaging modality that fulfills the requirements of providing sufficient spatial and temporal resolution, lesion characterization, and a high degree of reproducibility [4].

Evaluation of data from the authors' experience shows that MR imaging succeeded in vascular malformation characterization, target localization for the sclerotherapy, and sclerotherapeutic guidance and monitoring. The process of vascular malformation characterization was crucial in identifying the causative portion of the extended network of interconnected dilated veins responsible for the predominant clinical symptoms [4]. Identifying subcutaneous vascular targets that were not too superficial or too profoundly hidden within the complex anatomic environment prevented the development of skin necrosis or the rapid systemic drainage of the sclerosing agent.

Summary

MR-guided sclerotherapy is an excellent approach for the treatment of the predominant symptoms of congenital low-flow vascular malformations in the head and neck. In the authors' experience, this mode of treatment appears to be safe and efficient and allows the quantitative verification of therapeutic success during follow-up examinations.

References

[1] Dubois J, Soulez G, Oliva VL, et al. Soft-tissue venous malformations in adult patients: imaging and therapeutic issues. Radiographics 2001;21(6): 1519–31.

[2] Lewin JS, Merkle EM, Duerk JL, et al. Low-flow vascular malformations in the head and neck: safety and feasibility of MR imaging-guided percutaneous sclerotherapy—preliminary experience with 14 procedures in three patients. Radiology 1999;211(2): 566–70.

[3] Hayashi N, Masumoto T, Okubo T, et al. Hemangiomas in the face and extremities: MR-guided sclerotherapy—optimization with monitoring of signal intensity changes in vivo. Radiology 2003;226(2): 567–72.

[4] Boll DT, Merkle EM, Lewin JS. Low-flow vascular malformations: MR-guided percutaneous sclerotherapy in qualitative and quantitative assessment of therapy and outcome. Radiology 2004;233(2): 376–84.

[5] Mulliken JB, Zetter BR, Folkman J. In vitro characteristics of endothelium from hemangiomas and vascular malformations. Surgery 1982;92(2):348–53.

[6] Mulliken JB, Glowacki J. Classification of pediatric vascular lesions. Plast Reconstr Surg 1982;70(1): 120–1.

[7] Kaplan PA, Williams SM. Mucocutaneous and peripheral soft-tissue hemangiomas: MR imaging. Radiology 1987;163(1):163–6.

[8] Mulliken JB, Fishman SJ, Burrows PE. Vascular anomalies. Curr Probl Surg 2000;37(8):517–84.

[9] Enjolras O. Classification and management of the various superficial vascular anomalies: hemangiomas and vascular malformations. J Dermatol 1997; 24(11):701–10.

[10] Dubois JM, Sebag GH, De Prost Y, et al. Soft-tissue venous malformations in children: percutaneous sclerotherapy with Ethibloc. Radiology 1991; 180(1):195–8.

[11] Berenguer B, Burrows PE, Zurakowski D, et al. Sclerotherapy of craniofacial venous malformations: complications and results. Plast Reconstr Surg 1999;104(1):1–11.

[12] O'Donovan JC, Donaldson JS, Morello FP, et al. Symptomatic hemangiomas and venous malformations in infants, children, and young adults: treatment with percutaneous injection of sodium tetradecyl sulfate. AJR Am J Roentgenol 1997; 169(3):723–9.

[13] Meyer JS, Hoffer FA, Barnes PD, et al. Biological classification of soft-tissue vascular anomalies: MR correlation. AJR Am J Roentgenol 1991;157(3): 559–64.

[14] Chung YC, Merkle EM, Lewin JS, et al. Fast T(2)-weighted imaging by PSIF at 0.2 T for interventional MRI. Magn Reson Med 1999;42(2):335–44.

[15] Lewin JS, Petersilge CA, Hatem SF, et al. Interactive MR imaging-guided biopsy and aspiration with a modified clinical C-arm system. AJR Am J Roentgenol 1998;170(6):1593–601.

[16] Yakes WF, Haas DK, Parker SH, et al. Symptomatic vascular malformations: ethanol embolotherapy. Radiology 1989;170(3 Pt 2):1059–66.

[17] Takayasu K, Mizuguchi Y, Muramatsu Y, et al. Late complication of a large simple cyst of the liver mimicking cystadenocarcinoma after sclerotherapy. AJR Am J Roentgenol 2003;181(2):464–6.

[18] Helgason JW, Chandnani VP, Yu JS. MR arthrography: a review of current technique and applications. AJR Am J Roentgenol 1997;168(6): 1473–80.

[19] Donnelly LF, Bisset GS III, Adams DM. Marked acute tissue swelling following percutaneous sclerosis of low-flow vascular malformations: a predictor of both prolonged recovery and therapeutic effect. Pediatr Radiol 2000;30(6):415–9.

[20] Corti R, Osende JI, Fayad ZA, et al. In vivo non-invasive detection and age definition of arterial thrombus by MRI. J Am Coll Cardiol 2002; 39(8):1366–73.

[21] Cohen EK, Kressel HY, Perosio T, et al. MR imaging of soft-tissue hemangiomas: correlation with pathologic findings. AJR Am J Roentgenol 1988; 150(5):1079–81.

[22] Rak KM, Yakes WF, Ray RL, et al. MR imaging of symptomatic peripheral vascular malformations. AJR Am J Roentgenol 1992;159(1):107–12.

ELSEVIER
SAUNDERS

Magn Reson Imaging Clin N Am
13 (2005) 601–604

**MAGNETIC
RESONANCE
IMAGING CLINICS
of North America**

Index

Note: Page numbers of article titles are in **boldface** type.

Changing Your Address?

Make sure your subscription changes too! When you notify us of your new address, you can help make our job easier by including an exact copy of your Clinics label number with your old address (see illustration below.) This number identifies you to our computer system and will speed the processing of your address change. Please be sure this label number accompanies your old address and your corrected address—you can send an old Clinics label with your number on it or just copy it exactly and send it to the address listed below.

We appreciate your help in our attempt to give you continuous coverage. Thank you.

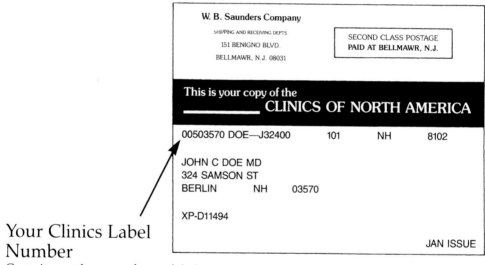

Your Clinics Label Number

Copy it exactly or send your label
along with your address to:
W.B. Saunders Company, Customer Service
Orlando, FL 32887-4800
Call Toll Free 1-800-654-2452

Please allow four to six weeks for delivery of new subscriptions and for processing address changes.

Practice, Current, Hardbound:
SATISFACTION GUARANTEED

YES! Please start my subscription to the **CLINICS** checked below with the ❏ first issue of the calendar year or ❏ current issues. If not completely satisfied with my first issue, I may write "cancel" on the invoice and return it within 30 days at no further obligation.

Please Print:

Name _____

Address_____

City_____ State _____ ZIP _____

Method of Payment

❏ Check (payable to **Elsevier**; add the applicable sales tax for your area)

❏ VISA   ❏ MasterCard   ❏ AmEx   ❏ Bill me

Card number _____ Exp. date _____

Signature _____

Staple this to your purchase order to expedite delivery

❏ **Adolescent Medicine Clinics**
  ❏ Individual $95
  ❏ Institutions $133
  ❏ *In-training $48

❏ **Anesthesiology**
  ❏ Individual $175
  ❏ Institutions $270
  ❏ *In-training $88

❏ **Cardiology**
  ❏ Individual $170
  ❏ Institutions $266
  ❏ *In-training $85

❏ **Chest Medicine**
  ❏ Individual $185
  ❏ Institutions $285

❏ **Child and Adolescent Psychiatry**
  ❏ Individual $175
  ❏ Institutions $265
  ❏ *In-training $88

❏ **Critical Care**
  ❏ Individual $165
  ❏ Institutions $266
  ❏ *In-training $83

❏ **Dental**
  ❏ Individual $150
  ❏ Institutions $242

❏ **Emergency Medicine**
  ❏ Individual $170
  ❏ Institutions $263
  ❏ *In-training $85
    ❏ Send CME info

❏ **Facial Plastic Surgery**
  ❏ Individual $199
  ❏ Institutions $300

❏ **Foot and Ankle**
  Individual $160
  Institutions $232

❏ **Gastroenterology**
  ❏ Individual $190
  ❏ Institutions $276

❏ **Gastrointestinal Endoscopy**
  ❏ Individual $190
  ❏ Institutions $276

❏ **Hand**
  ❏ Individual $205
  ❏ Institutions $319

❏ **Heart Failure (NEW in 2005!)**
  ❏ Individual $99
  ❏ Institutions $149
  ❏ *In-training $49

❏ **Hematology/ Oncology**
  ❏ Individual $210
  ❏ Institutions $315

❏ **Immunology & Allergy**
  ❏ Individual $165
  ❏ Institutions $266

❏ **Infectious Disease**
  ❏ Individual $165
  ❏ Institutions $272

❏ **Clinics in Liver Disease**
  ❏ Individual $165
  ❏ Institutions $234

❏ **Medical**
  ❏ Individual $140
  ❏ Institutions $244
  ❏ *In-training $70
    ❏ Send CME info

❏ **MRI**
  ❏ Individual $190
  ❏ Institutions $290
  ❏ *In-training $95
    ❏ Send CME info

❏ **Neuroimaging**
  ❏ Individual $190
  ❏ Institutions $290
  ❏ *In-training $95
    ❏ Send CME inf0

❏ **Neurologic**
  ❏ Individual $175
  ❏ Institutions $275

❏ **Obstetrics & Gynecology**
  ❏ Individual $175
  ❏ Institutions $288

❏ **Occupational and Environmental Medicine**
  ❏ Individual $120
  ❏ Institutions $166
  ❏ *In-training $60

❏ **Ophthalmology**
  ❏ Individual $190
  ❏ Institutions $325

❏ **Oral & Maxillofacial Surgery**
  ❏ Individual $180
  ❏ Institutions $280
  ❏ *In-training $90

❏ **Orthopedic**
  ❏ Individual $180
  ❏ Institutions $295
  ❏ *In-training $90

❏ **Otolaryngologic**
  ❏ Individual $199
  ❏ Institutions $350

❏ **Pediatric**
  ❏ Individual $135
  ❏ Institutions $246
  ❏ *In-training $68
    ❏ Send CME info

❏ **Perinatology**
  ❏ Individual $155
  ❏ Institutions $237
  ❏ *In-training $78
    ❏ Send CME inf0

❏ **Plastic Surgery**
  ❏ Individual $245
  ❏ Institutions $370

❏ **Podiatric Medicine & Surgery**
  ❏ Individual $170
  ❏ Institutions $266

❏ **Primary Care**
  ❏ Individual $135
  ❏ Institutions $223

❏ **Psychiatric**
  ❏ Individual $170
  ❏ Institutions $288

❏ **Radiologic**
  ❏ Individual $220
  ❏ Institutions $331
  ❏ *In-training $110
    ❏ Send CME info

❏ **Sports Medicine**
  ❏ Individual $180
  ❏ Institutions $277

❏ **Surgical**
  ❏ Individual $190
  ❏ Institutions $299
  ❏ *In-training $95

❏ **Thoracic Surgery (formerly Chest Surgery)**
  ❏ Individual $175
  ❏ Institutions $255
  ❏ *In-training $88

❏ **Urologic**
  ❏ Individual $195
  ❏ Institutions $307
  ❏ *In-training $98
    ❏ Send CME info

BUSINESS REPLY MAIL

FIRST-CLASS MAIL   PERMIT NO 7135   ORLANDO FL

POSTAGE WILL BE PAID BY ADDRESSEE

PERIODICALS ORDER FULFILLMENT DEPT
ELSEVIER
6277 SEA HARBOR DR
ORLANDO FL 32821-9816